'Joan Duveen masterfully explains the complexities and subtleties of this ancient system that lies at the heart of Chinese medicine. He smartly unfolds the workings of the heavenly stems and earthly branches, allowing practitioners to utilize this effective information in their personal cultivation and clinical practice. I highly recommend this book to people looking for understanding of the universal *qi* flow.'
– *CT Holman, author of* Treating Emotional Trauma with Chinese Medicine *and* Shamanism in Chinese Medicine

'The theory and practice of stems and branches belongs to the oldest, most complex foundations of acupuncture and Chinese medicine. Few acupuncturists know and master this ancient theory of "the rhythm of the laws of *qi*" as well as Joan Duveen. In this book, he has succeeded in explaining this difficult subject in a clear, structured and pleasantly readable way, so that it can also be applied in daily practice. It is a book that should be a standard part of every acupuncture course, in order to understand what Chinese medicine is all about.'
– *Yan Schroën, practitioner, lecturer and researcher of Chinese medicine*

'"Mind-blowing" was my first impression of Joan's teachings, almost 30 years ago... "Mind-blowing" is my impression again, upon laying down this fascinating book. With love, compassion and humility, Joan shares with us his knowledge – gained through decades of diligent study, clinical experience and personal development. This is a book about constitutional acupuncture and healing; but even more so, it is a book of humanity and humaneness, written by a master acupuncturist and a truly inspiring teacher. I believe it will be a cornerstone for deeper understanding and an inspiration for generations of acupuncturists to come.'
– *Rani Ayal, constitutional acupuncturist and teacher*

'Chinese medicine, as defined by the *Yellow Emperor's Classic of Medicine*, embodies a holistic system of scientific knowledge that regards the human body as a microcosm in the context of an all-encompassing cosmic environment. It represents one of the world's most time-honoured alchemical traditions, examining the phenomenon of human existence in the process of its continuous fusion with heaven and earth. At a time when the limits of the monodimensional approach of materialist science and its repercussions in the field of modern medicine have become more apparent than ever, Joan Duveen's excellent introduction to the intricate macrocosmic background sciences of Chinese medicine is cause for celebration. His monograph on the stems and branches system of cyclical energy calculation not only honours the lineage of J.D. van Buren, one of the first European master teachers of this wisdom tradition, but also makes this once hermetic information approachable by enriching it with a lifetime of clinical insights from a senior practitioner of acupuncture. I highly recommend this book for every student and practitioner of Chinese medicine!'
– *Heiner Fruehauf, PhD, Lac, founding professor, College of Classical Chinese Medicine, National University of Natural Medicine, Portland, Oregon*

'I have read this book with pleasure and at times could not put it down, which is rare for a study book. Joan is able to grip the reader and explain the different aspects of the stems and branches theory in a concise and understandable way, which will help many who read this book.

Furthermore, he forces the reader to look at their personal development, which to my mind is irrevocably linked to this theory. You cannot work with this material without looking at yourself. Then it will grow and you can make it your own. I believe that has always been the aim of Dr van Buren. It is wonderful to see little aspects of "the great master" mirrored in Joan's words and attitude.

Joan also makes it very clear that you have to read the pulses correctly and to the best of your ability to be able to apply stems and branches. That was something Dr van Buren was a master at. He would always listen to the pulses above all else and adapt his treatment accordingly. He always said "stems and branches mean nothing if it does not fit the pulses".'

– Pauline van Buren, wife of Dr J.D. van Buren (deceased) and former principal of the
International College of Oriental Medicine (ICOM)

'In a subject where written works are few and the original texts in the *Neijing Suwen* give little guidance on their application to clinical practice, Joan Duveen's mature and thoughtful book is a welcome addition to the literature, backed as it is by years of clinical and teaching experience. If you have been curious about stems and branches acupuncture but don't know where to begin, this book provides an excellent entry point into that world.'

– Peter Firebrace FBAcC, acupuncturist, writer, lecturer, director of Guan Academy, past
principal of the International College of Oriental Medicine (UK)

'The heavenly stems and earthly branches *(GanZhi),* a rich and multi-layered system with roots soundly embedded in the ancient Chinese cosmological sciences, has been used for thousands of years to codify the patterns of life. The *GanZhi* are the building blocks that allow us to dive ever deeper into the arts of Chinese astrology, Chinese cosmology, classical Chinese medicine and more. In this work, Joan Duveen shares decades' worth of study and clinical experience to guide practitioners in learning how to use the *GanZhi* to both gain insight into the constitutional patterns that shape a person's health and wellbeing throughout their life stages, and to guide effective treatment. Demonstrated through valuable case studies, this book is an important manual for Chinese medicine students and practitioners and all those who are interested in the practical application of the time-honoured *GanZhi* arts.'

– Master Zhongxian Wu, lifelong Daoist practitioner and author of
15 books on Chinese wisdom traditions

'Joan Duveen is a leading practitioner and scholar of Chinese medicine. His new text, *Applying Stems and Branches Acupuncture in Clinical Practice,* takes us on a deep dive into an important, and often neglected, dimension of clinical practice. Joan presents Chinese medicine in an ecological context, embracing a deeply compassionate and integral view of the self. This work should improve our grasp of the subtleties of physiology and the relationship between constitutional endowment and life experience in the evolution of the self. I have waited 20 years for Joan to complete this work and am delighted with its depth and humanity.'

– Lonny Jarrett, practitioner, scholar and author of Nourishing Destiny, Clinical
Practice, and Deepening Perspectives on Chinese Medicine

Applying Stems and Branches
Acupuncture in Clinical Practice

of related interest

The Way of the Five Seasons
Living with the Five Elements for Physical, Emotional, and Spiritual Harmony
John Kirkwood
ISBN 978 1 84819 301 7
eISBN 978 0 85701 252 4

Shamanism in Chinese Medicine
Applying Ancient Wisdom to Health and Healing
CT Holman M.S., L.Ac.
Foreword by Master Zhongxian Wu
ISBN 978 1 78775 137 8
eISBN 978 1 78775 138 5

Treating Emotional Trauma with Chinese Medicine
Integrated Diagnostic and Treatment Strategies
CT Holman M.S., L.Ac.
ISBN 978 1 84819 318 5
eISBN 978 0 85701 271 5

APPLYING STEMS and BRANCHES ACUPUNCTURE in CLINICAL PRACTICE

Dynamic Dualities in Classical Chinese Medicine

JOAN DUVEEN

Foreword by Tae Hunn Lee

SINGING DRAGON

LONDON AND PHILADELPHIA

First published in Great Britain in 2022 by Singing Dragon
An imprint of Jessica Kingsley Publishers
An imprint of Hodder & Stoughton Ltd
An Hachette Company

I

Front cover image source: Maurice Rijnen. The cover image is for
illustrative purposes only, and any person featuring is a model.

A CIP catalogue record for this title is available from the
British Library and the Library of Congress

ISBN 978 1 78775 370 9
eISBN 978 1 78775 371 6

Printed and bound in Great Britain by CPI Group

Jessica Kingsley Publishers' policy is to use papers that are natural, renewable and recyclable
products and made from wood grown in sustainable forests. The logging and manufacturing
processes are expected to conform to the environmental regulations of the country of origin.

Jessica Kingsley Publishers
Carmelite House
50 Victoria Embankment
London EC4Y 0DZ

www.singingdragon.com

This book is dedicated to

Dr Johannes Diedericus (Dick) van Buren,
a pioneering acupuncturist

27 November 1921 – 12 May 2003

Contents

PART I: THE TEN GREAT MOVEMENTS AND TEN HEAVENLY STEMS

Foreword

After proofreading the manuscript for this book, Joan kindly asked me if I was willing to write a foreword from the perspective of a reader and student. It felt like a tall order to give a comment on a subject and teacher that are so close to my heart, but I agreed and felt that it might help fellow students, colleagues and readers to navigate through the content.

My journey into constitutional acupuncture started with an interest and questions about life and human nature and what constitutes health, disease, joy and suffering. I guess it was a search for meaning. I started to read philosophical texts and books and my first exposure to Chinese medicine was through Traditional Chinese Medicine (TCM). I then decided to enrol in the International College of Oriental Medicine in England. At that time, Dr van Buren and his wife Pauline were still overseeing the organization and running of the college, and the ethos that Chinese medicine and acupuncture are applied philosophy was strongly felt and seen. Looking back though, these concepts were merely words to me, but with time and work they have become more alive within me and I am sure that this will continue to be the case. More and more I start to appreciate and understand the depth and value of what was given to us.

Dr van Buren passed away in 2003, the year I graduated, and a few years after that I started teaching at the college with the encouragement of Pauline, for which I am very grateful. It has provided invaluable learning experiences for me through the exchange with students and colleagues.

I have been a student of Joan Duveen's for the last twenty years, and during this time I had the honour and pleasure not only to attend his lectures, seminars and retreats, but also to spend time over walks, talks and meals and to experience Joan with his family and as a friend. It became very obvious to me that the teaching and material presented in this book is not only for treating patients in clinic, but also and maybe even more importantly for self-understanding and self-cultivation. The book is rooted in a truly alive tradition and a philosophy that can reach and enrich every aspect of our being and life. It may lead to freedom, not in the sense of being able to do what we desire, but freedom to be who we really are and from there engage with fellow human beings and life with joy, love and respect and use this understanding to treat patients who seek us out for help and support. I was able to observe and experience the application of the teachings and philosophy not only with patients in clinic, but also in Joan himself and in the way he engaged with students, colleagues, family and friends.

As such, what is being presented in this book is a true labour of love, a sharing of experience and an invitation to a dialogue and exchange. The text is not a mere presentation of facts, but Joan's own experience gained from the many years of deep study, observation and practical application of the philosophy. It is not a book to be taken at face value, to be read and memorized and blindly accepted as truth, but it is an invitation to work and engage with it so we can reach an inner understanding of the underlying philosophy.

The fact that we pick up this book, for whatever reason, means that there is already an interest and calling to engage in this subject. If we are open and let go of preconceived ideas and knowledge we might already have, we truly allow the words to enter our hearts and vibrate within ourselves. This may arouse a curiosity to explore what these words mean to us.

We are taken on a journey to look at the principles of this philosophy from different angles and perspectives, helped by practical examples which bring it alive and show us how it can be applied to treat patients. This then starts a process of reflection. Feelings, emotions and thoughts might arise, which means that we are starting to embody, feel and experience the meaning of the words, which is different from pure intellectual knowledge. The process of digestion, assimilation and integration has started. From here, we begin to see it from our own being and perspective with discrimination and discernment, and in this way a real dialogue can take place, from author to reader, a self-dialogue within the reader and, with new perspective and understanding, we can then answer back to the author and to life itself.

I believe this is the meaning of a living tradition and, if we are open to the process, it can also happen through written words. This is my experience of reading and engaging with this book. We have to remind ourselves that this book represents a snapshot in time, part of an ongoing process and is by no means a finished product, and by making space in our heart we can all contribute to its further development.

I did not find it easy to read the manuscript and it took me a long time to go through each chapter. I often got stuck on a sentence or paragraph, trying to figure out what was really meant by the words, knowing that there has been a lot of careful consideration and thought by Joan in choosing words and expressions. It helped me to research and familiarize myself with general concepts and terms used in philosophy and psychology. I also keep going back to the basic principles of yin and yang, Heaven–Earth–Man, Four Emanations and Five Elements to help me to put things into context and not get lost in the complexity. Deep understanding of these basic fundamental principles is the fertile soil from which the more complex concepts can grow and flower which in turn enriches the soil again.

There are so many levels of understanding, so many different associations and perspectives, that it would often mess with my head and I literally couldn't get my head around it. I realized that what stopped me from grasping the meaning was my own knowledge and ideas through which I looked at the words; I wasn't open and receptive but wanted to confirm and apply my own knowledge and ideas. It helps to forget myself for a while and try to 'walk a mile in Joan's shoes'. Other times, I just needed to give it some time and space, to let it settle and rest within me, go for a walk and disengage from the material. Help in understanding can come in many different ways: a conversation we have, experiences we remember, music we listen to, looking at plants, trees or the sunset, in other words through the beauty of life and nature itself. Intellect is a great tool but can also be a hindrance in assimilating and understanding from within.

Reading each chapter from beginning to end in order to get an overview first before getting into the details was also helpful. Often the meaning of certain passages revealed itself later on. I don't claim to have assimilated and understood everything that has been written, but I trust that it will come with time and work. Learning and understanding does not happen in a linear fashion, and there is certainly no end to it. Understanding of one aspect will affect everything else, and when the penny dropped, I found myself going back to other chapters or paragraphs with new depth and vision. Just like life, knowledge and depth of understanding are cyclical in nature.

The process doesn't stop here, as we have to apply and work with what we have gained, not only with patients, but within ourselves and our lives. This is probably the most important part of the process, through which, as Dr van Buren often said, 'the philosophy will start to work within us' and we will be able to make our own experiences and manage to apply it in our own individual ways.

Despite all the complexity, we mustn't forget that this philosophy comes out of life, describes life and thus can be discovered through curiosity, awareness and observation of life and self. I already value this book as a companion and friend, and I know that I can and will always pick it up again to engage in a renewed dialogue to look for inspiration and understanding and I hope that it can do the same for you too.

Tae Hunn Lee

Acknowledgements

Looking out over the meadows, the sun having just risen, I sit at my computer. At the beginning of 2019, in this very spot in the holiday home Elzenhof on the Dutch Island of Ameland, I started to write the first words of this book. This time I am accompanied by my love, my wife Marjolein. She's been by my side through all my ups and downs during my writing process. I want to thank her for her patience and for accepting my almost daily confinement in my office. But, even more, I want to thank her for the long dialogues at the kitchen table and during long walks we took together. Our conversations about topics that emerge in the book, such as self-knowledge, shame, guilt, hope, loneliness and fear, have made an indelible impression on me. Without her insights, wisdom, reflections we shared and her relentless support, this book wouldn't be here.

In January 2019 I was here alone. I had to get used to the idea of writing a book that I repeatedly said would never come. After all, constitutional acupuncture is an oral tradition, in which the student learns directly from a teacher. Development of knowledge and self-knowledge then takes place simultaneously under the inspiring leadership of the teacher. And although I had been teaching for years in line with my promise to J.D. van Buren to pass on his body of thought, I still had doubts. What do I have to add to the books that already exist on this topic? Is it at all possible to convey the essential value of self-knowledge through a book? How can I make it clear that knowing and understanding one's own constitutional challenges and pitfalls are indispensable when working with patients through constitutional acupuncture?

At the British Acupuncture Council Congress in 2018 I met CT Holman. During a conversation about our work and passions over a joint breakfast, he said, as others have also increasingly been urging me, that I should write down my knowledge and experiences of the practical use of heavenly stems and earthly branches. I resisted, using the arguments of oral teaching and tradition. But CT persisted. 'You know, why don't you talk to Claire Wilson from Singing

Dragon?' CT's book *Treating Emotional Trauma with Chinese Medicine* had just been published with Singing Dragon and I had seen the announcement of a presentation at the congress. 'She's here too, and she's probably interested.' It was remarkable that he mentioned this publishing house, because I had once said to a friend: 'If I ever wanted to write a book, I'd like to publish it through Singing Dragon.'

I thank CT who gave me the last incentive to really sit down and develop the routine of writing. I want to thank Claire and the staff at Singing Dragon for their faith in this book. When I spoke to Claire, I told her it wasn't going to be a book with just factual knowledge. 'I would like to do my best to engage with the reader, not only to transfer knowledge, but to challenge the reader to reflect. It won't be an easy-to-read book.' Her answer was short and friendly. 'Of course, whatever you think is right.' Her open confidence and evident experience gave me the courage to get started. I want to thank her for that. Since that day I have been thinking about the content of this book, having many conversations with colleagues and other professionals, conducting research and writing in my office almost every day.

I would like to thank Tae Hunn Lee for his tremendous support, proof-reading, corrections, advice and assistance in editing the text, creating all the diagrams and tables and for accepting my request to write a foreword from the reader's perspective. And Anna McAnndra for proofreading, editing, providing suggestions and correcting the text. Both were inspiring sparring partners. I am grateful to them for their unwavering dedication, commitment and support to this project. They have immensely contributed to making this complex topic more accessible.

Maurice Rijnen, thank you for your help in designing the cover. After a 20-minute conversation, you understood the essence of the book and the next day the first draft was in my email. Your design does justice to Dr J.D. van Buren, who once said about this upside-down tree: 'This is what it's all about, nothing more and nothing less.'

I thank my family, Marjolein, Judith, Rozemarijn, Deva, Sem and the grand-children Olli, Noam, Eddi and Benjamin. You are the ever-present inspiration of my heart, you are the happiness of my existence.

I stand on the shoulders of everyone who has been my teacher: My main teachers J.D. van Buren and his wife Pauline, Leon Hammer, Julian Scott, my *qigong* and *tai chi* teachers, books, videos and movies about Chinese medicine, psychology and philosophy, friends and loved ones, but even more so the students and patients who trusted me. Without being aware of it, they were my very important teachers. I am grateful for what I have been able to observe, experience and learn from you through conversations, observations, treatments and above all your openness. This book is a tribute to all of you.

My writing is a testimony to years of study, encounters, observations and treatments, to the respect for the material and the way it was and is applied. I am deeply grateful for all the times I have been able to observe the impressive way Dick van Buren treated. His lessons are unforgettable, just like the joint dinners and the delicious chocolate cakes and long conversations that I have had the pleasure of experiencing with Dick and Pauline van Buren. I am grateful for the opportunities I have been given to work with them. It called on my inner mission to keep J.D. van Buren's legacy flourishing continuously.

And although in this book I deviate from the tradition of learning to observe and acquire knowledge through oral teaching, I do my best to connect with you, the reader, in such a way that the spirit of tradition may vibrate in our hearts. I want to thank you for your willingness to engage in and walk this path together.

Preface

There is only one path.

Professional football player. My future was set. Playing football was my passion. For hours I practised alone in a field next to our house. After school, we played matches with friends where the goalposts were made from jerseys and a small dead tree. Never was I tired, I imitated Pelé, felt like Pelé and mastered his tricks, which I had seen on one of the then rare televisions at a friend's house. My parents weren't that much into football and they didn't think we needed a TV. Every Wednesday I went to watch children's programmes on television with my childhood friend Arij, and if my parents agreed we could watch a football match together in the evening.

We lived in Laren in the Netherlands in a beautiful bungalow with a thatched roof which was built in 1950 with the inherited money of my mother's parents who were killed in World War II. I lived close to nature, felt free as a bird and enjoyed the warmth of a cup of tea when I came home from school. This cup of tea and a chat with my mother is one of my fond memories of a safe and cosy childhood.

It must have been difficult for my parents to provide a safe childhood for us without expressing the fear, grief and anger they carried inside. It wasn't until much later in my life that I understood that avoiding those emotions about the loss of their parents and other horrors of the war also affected us, my sister, my brother and me. But when I was a kid I had no idea. We had a pleasant, perfectly normal upbringing. No questions or doubts about that. Home and family were the foundations we stood on and gave us a sense of playfulness and, for me, that was mostly playing football.

I was football, breathed football, thought football, felt football; every free moment I played with a football and even the trainers at the club were convinced that I would become a professional football player.

When other clubs showed interest, my plan seemed to work, until suddenly I was forced to quit. I was 13 years old at the time. Due to a nasty knee injury my plans for the future collapsed and I felt lost. It was not only because I couldn't play football anymore. It was me, my identity. My whole being was injured. Football wasn't just something I practised, it was something I lived.

Years later I was very happy that this knee injury had forced my destiny in a different direction. Although, was it a different direction? It taught me to follow my passion. That young boy's passion for training, playing and learning is similar to the life of the man who learned to practise as a constitutional acupuncturist. It started with learning techniques, reading books, training pulse diagnosis, finding good teachers, discussions with peers, learning that there is success and failure and yet to continue to learn. Just because I like it so much.

It began with a certain monomaniac way of studying, in a way that the *shen* and the self were infused with the philosophical approach that was called working with 'stems and branches'.

At first, constitutional acupuncture seemed very mathematical because it requires a calculation that leads to a 'birth chart' describing the pattern of *qi* at the time of birth. But the basis of this method is a philosophical-spiritual model that is applied in practice. Constitutional acupuncture is based on knowledge and calculation, but even more on spiritual anthropogenesis and thus love, a gift from humanity to itself. Applying constitutional acupuncture in clinic is a human contribution to the development of becoming more human and a great method of treating the wholeness of people. Besides healing people, it offers opportunities to get closer to yourself.

There was a reason that the founder of this method in our Western world, J.D. van Buren, never wrote a book about it. He believed that this knowledge was and should be transferred through oral teaching, watching a teacher, experiencing the teacher's way of making diagnosis and treatment, his way of communicating, his way of talking or being silent.

It is not through copying his ways and methods I had observed that I walk this path of practising acupuncture. Only through understanding myself in this process of learning was I able to make it my own. It was not because I had to, but because I felt the drive from within.

After completing my physiotherapy studies, I started studying Chinese medicine and philosophy in 1975. One of my first acupuncture teachers in 1978 was a very knowledgeable person. He liked to transfer knowledge to his students and used many words and examples. I felt overwhelmed by his knowledge and his success in treating his patients. I wanted to copy his knowledge, I wanted to be able to 'look into his brain and gain his understanding'.

Meeting and listening to J.D. van Buren the first time in 1982 was a different experience. Here he stood, a tall, charismatic but shy and calm man. He gave an introduction to Chinese medicine and started with the beginning of Life. He talked about life that comes from fragmentation of the Universal Spark of Life and how it feeds people. But above all, he talked about the responsibility of humans in the mutual relationship with the Universal Spark. This was the very first time of many times that he started a lecture with the Universal Spark.

I felt overwhelmed again. Not because of his knowledge, quite the opposite. My heart was reopened. I didn't understand what he was talking about at all, but every fibre in my body and soul resonated with his words. On a subtle level, I knew I had the chance to fulfil an unknown destiny by becoming his student, not knowing that this relationship would last for 21 years and only physically end on the day he died in 2003. Even now, when writing these words and reading my notes, or remembering conversations with him, or when I feel pulses or treat patients, I feel his presence as a resonance in my heart from the past in the present.

As a young football player, I had to practise and practise, till I was finally able to master the tricks of Pelé. It repeated as a student of Dr van Buren. Working with my abilities and qualities over and over again, getting to know my shortcomings, understanding the magnitude of my emotions, mental, physical and spiritual qualities and limitations, likes and dislikes as landmarks on my path. And I knew that if I ever thought I had mastered the method and stopped learning, I'd lose the essence of it. It really is so and remains a constant learning path. Being a pupil of Pelé or van Buren is not what it is about. It's about being a student of life, being open to the challenges of life, living and breathing this life of opportunities to make the world a little bit better by doing my utmost to be who I am.

And here we are, you and me.

How do I transfer the *jing* and *shen*, the essence and spirit of the method of 'Heavenly Stems and Earthly Branches' to you? What are the tools, method and content to show you both the material and spiritual aspects of it? This depends not only on the choices I make here, but also on the perception of you, reader, as a possible fellow student of life. Knowledge and theories are expected to describe reality, but quantum mechanics, space travel and Eastern medicine have made it clear that individual perception influences mutual experience. Knowledge, reality and perception are inextricably linked and influence each other.

Technical details and knowledge give people enough tools to work with stems and branches. And I am very grateful for the many translations of the *Yellow Emperor's Classics of Internal Medicine* that allow acupuncturists around the world to study and apply this ancient knowledge. For the writing of this book I mainly used the translations of Dr Henry Lu (1990) and of Bing Wang, Nelson Liansheng Wu and Andrew Qi Wu (1997). Both books are treasuries of information and knowledge about the five phases, heavenly stems and earthly branches. I recommend them wholeheartedly, but the theoretical knowledge is only part of the information. At the end, the theory might turn out to be a burden, a load of knowledge weighing on the shoulders. And despite our desire to heal people, the theory alone won't give us enough tools to treat with stems and branches satisfactorily.

Insight, intellect, intuition, intelligence, interaction, integrity and introspection, along with a transparent and stable 'I', are guidelines on the path to wholeness and they grow mainly through self-knowledge. The eight 'I's are indispensable for greater efficiency and fulfilment, and they do not grow by theory. I invite you to make the given information alive by using it to explore yourself, to get to know better the possibilities and limitations of your own perception and observation and to look at yourself more clearly.

This book is intended as an inspiration to freely navigate the material of stems and branches, but I hope that it also inspires you, in the spirit of my teacher's lessons, to inner growth, in which the interconnectedness of theory, knowledge and personal perceptions and feelings all turn out to be part of the indwelling self.

The word self-knowledge gives the impression that something is investigating the self, but that something is also the self. The path of self-knowledge is the path of finding unity and togetherness in the internal and external world of diversity and oppositions. Through self-knowledge, the theory of the stems and branches comes to life and constitutional acupuncture treatments become your very own method. That may seem strange, but we all bring with us our own energy and our own birth chart with its unique and meaningful consequences for relationships and the way we make choices.

The practitioner's personal insights and observations of the interaction of birth energies are at the same time subjective as they are objective. Chinese medicine gives very accurate descriptions of observations, but the implementation and treatments always depend on the mutual exchange between practitioner and patient.

The theory of stems and branches describes both the reality of the patient and the condition of the practitioner. In addition to a theoretical basis, practical and individual observations are based on wisdom, love and inner development. They colour all perceptions and conditions that create a living unity as a starting point for a treatment.

This book will regularly discuss topics as self-understanding, self-perception, self-knowledge and self-cultivation, togetherness and love because the natural expression of the self and reciprocity of relationships are expressions of the oneness of all selves that transcends knowledge and theories. Learning to work with stems and branches is an endless personal and collective path, the *Dao*, that enriches all. Through open communication and constantly finding new pathways in the vastness of the material, we can experience the ultimate art of healing ourselves and others.

Dr J.D. van Buren was already an osteopath, naturopath and a homeopath before he started studying acupuncture in 1952. He travelled to many different countries to gain as much knowledge as possible which resulted in him receiving a Doctorate of Acupuncture in Taiwan in 1969. In 1974 he travelled to Korea to visit the Oriental Medical School of Kyung Hee University in Seoul. He received a book written by Professor Chang Bin Lee, director of the medical school, which introduced him to the traditional teachings of heavenly stems and earthly branches. The origin of 'Stems and Branches acupuncture' that is nowadays taught in the world is from the *Huang Di Nei Jing Su Wen*[1] and from the book *System of a New Philosophy by the Dualistic Monism* (1982) by Chang Bin Lee. J.D. van Buren's life's work was to develop the practical and clinical applications of the many theoretical texts and pictures in Chang Bin Lee's book.

This paradigm of thinking and treating was and is still not common among most Chinese medicine practitioners, even today. Philosophy was banned in China during the Cultural Revolution, but due to J.D. van Buren's efforts we are able to apply this philosophy in clinic today. For most of his practical life, besides treating patients, he was committed to making this ancient system available to acupuncture practitioners again. He shared with me, not long before he passed away, that 'Many students learn about Chinese philosophy but lack the tools to apply it' and 'Treatments should be philosophy-based only'. These are some of his spoken legacies.

The core idea of this system, known in the Western world as 'Stems and Branches acupuncture', is discussed in classics such as *Wu Yun Liu Qi*, 'five movements and six *qi*'. I prefer to call it constitutional acupuncture, because people then almost immediately understand that this form of acupuncture diagnoses and treats through respect for the natural innate condition of the patient. The significance of this philosophy is hidden mainly within Chapters

---

1   'The Yellow Emperor's classic (*jing*) of internal (*nei*) medicine.'

66–74 of *Huang Di Nei Jing Su Wen*, without really giving proper tools for how it can be practised in the acupuncture clinic.

The practical implications of this philosophy were originally only given orally during a teacher's observation. I had the privilege of being in regular contact with J.D. van Buren and was able to study, ask questions and observe his work for many years. It was common in the teacher-student tradition for the student not to ask questions during the early years of the apprenticeship. This wasn't from a hierarchical point of view or out of respect for the teacher (which, by the way, I did have enormously), but out of respect for the possibilities and power of self-knowledge.

By not asking questions, a conversation started in myself and I became aware of my doubts and uncertainties that normally would have led to questions being asked. Through being silent and gaining the courage to learn from my insecurities, there was room for self-insight and, with that, for more essential questions that became increasingly clear over the years. Of course, I was allowed to ask questions while observing him, but during the early years I mostly observed and studied, besides my notes and books, his clinical work in silence. What I essentially learned from him during these early years was that wonderment, in addition to hard work and doing your very best, is essential to empower those entrusted to you with the courage to increase self-knowledge which then is at service of healing. During my first years of study at the International College of Oriental Medicine, I hardly dared to go to Dr van Buren. I first wanted to focus more on the basics of pulse diagnosis with his partner Pauline and his other assistant Ruud Moester, before I had the guts to observe his work. And I hoped that in this way I could learn more from his skills later.

J.D. van Buren never lost the mindset of being a student of life. He was a charismatic person with a lot of knowledge and intuition. In addition, he learned from every patient, even though he had known that patient for over thirty years. Each consultation was like a first meeting that he approached with renewed curiosity. The more we got to know each other, the more he shared and, after a while, I felt more free to ask him questions. I suspect that those questions also led him to study, because sometimes I only received answers after a few days or weeks.

What will be discussed in this book is not intended to establish the only truth or way of working. It is intended to invite you to compare it with your already acquired knowledge and experience and above all to put into practice the power of wonder, questions and self-knowledge. When questions arise, I invite you to first take a closer look at your own intuition, comprehension and awareness.

After van Buren's death in 2003, I have continued to study and further develop the material. Always remembering that he repeatedly emphasized that it is not only about theories and knowledge, but rather about applying stems and branches *philosophy* in clinical practice and that patients reveal the qualities of the practitioner. For me, that means that I treat, teach and write with his motto in mind: 'Treat the ill person, not the illness.'

The TEN GREAT MOVEMENTS and TEN HEAVENLY STEMS

Life flows from the upside-down tree out of Heaven
and meets the tree on Earth, the symbol for all forms.
The unity of life and form are
the core of a living togetherness.

CHAPTER 1

THE FIELD OF STEMS AND BRANCHES

THE DYNAMICS BETWEEN SEASONS AND HUMANS[1]

The year in the Chinese calendar has different subdivisions in seasons: the four seasons of winter, spring, summer and autumn; the five seasons of winter, spring, summer, late summer and autumn; and the six seasons of *tai yang*, *jué yin*, *shao yin*, *shao yang*, *tai yin* and *yang ming*. The 24 solar terms also divide up the year, lasting 14 days each, and start in January with Great Cold, followed by Beginning of Spring, Rain Water, Awakening of Beings, Spring-Equinox and so on. The great movement, heavenly stem and earthly branch that govern the whole year influence the character of each season. This implies that some seasonal variations can be considered normal for that year, even when they seem exceptional.

For example, a year dominated by the active great movement metal should be more dry. Compared to 'normal' seasons some seasons might be more dry and hot. It is expected that there will be less rain and humidity. In addition, throughout the year the dominant metal subdues wood; growth and regeneration will be less exuberant, especially in the spring.

Signs and symptoms can occur when metal dominance increases, especially when the dominance is accompanied by weakness and fragility of wood in a birth chart.[2] Pains occur below the flanks along with lower abdominal pain as well as diseases in the eyes and ears. The wood is even more subdued and nature withers when the influence of metal on the year becomes extremely dominant. Complaints spread and become stronger, such as more intense pains, coughing with *qi* that moves counter-current or stagnates, and the organs become tense.

---

1   This topic is discussed in detail in Chapters 66–74 of the *Huang Di Nei Jing Su Wen*.
2   The birth chart is a snapshot of the movement of time and space at the moment of birth. See Chapter 2.

The practitioner working with stems and branches can determine whether deviations are foreseeable. For this, the calendar with all its influences needs to be well understood. Excess or insufficiency in a particular season can be considered normal or pathological for that year. And if the birth chart is interpreted correctly and people's constitutional weaknesses and strengths become apparent, the practitioner can then understand the impact of the seasons on patients, explain symptoms and illnesses and, in fact, prevent disease from occurring in the future.

THE DYNAMICS OF THE BIRTH CHART

The Chinese calendar is a metaphysical system created by humans based on the observation and perception of heaven and earth. Stars, orbits of planets, sun, phases of the moon, nature, cycles of seasons and so forth are the basic parameters of the calendar. Each year, season, month, day, hour is determined and characterized by the properties of a heavenly stem and earthly branch,[3] giving each time period its unique character. In China, the calendar was more than just a divider of time. It was seen as an entity, an intermediary between heaven and humanity. The emperor was the only one allowed to adjust the calendar, of course in consultation with his astronomers and advisers. Important emperors became more important when they provided adjustments, because it was a testament to their greatness.

For centuries, people only knew the energetic description of their date of birth, instead of the exact day, month and year. When asked for the birthday you got the answer, for example, born in year *Jia/Wu*, in month *Ren/Shen* on the day *Wu/Yin*.[4] The nature of those time periods marks the character and abilities of the person in question, which was considered more important than knowing the particular date.

In the past, creating a birth chart took a lot more time than it does today. On

---

3   The Chinese calendar as we know it today has been developed and constantly adapted over the centuries. For example, the first month of the calendar was attributed to the time of the lung and springtime in the Han Dynasty, the gallbladder in the Shang Dynasty, and the *san jiao* in the Chin Dynasty. During the reign of Emperor Wei Ti in 104 BCE the second new moon after the winter solstice was determined as the new year, along with the *qi* of the lungs. Between the seventh and fifth centuries BCE there was only a calendar based on the 24 'seasons', the 24 solar terms. It wasn't until around 800 BCE that the Chinese zodiac animals were added. There has been a 10-day week until the first attempts to build a 7-day week were made around 1000 CE during the Sung Dynasty. Observations of the stars, planets and nature have been the common factor of Chinese calendars over centuries.

4   Successively heavenly stem *Jia*, gallbladder and earthly branch *Wu*, heart, the heavenly stem *Ren*, bladder, earthly branch *Shen*, bladder, the heavenly stem *Wu*, stomach and earthly branch *Yin*, lung.

the internet, there are many websites where a birth chart with the four pillars of destiny appears within seconds.[5] You have to pay attention though, because some websites calculate the time back to Beijing time. This makes no sense to me because the calendar is a universal concept and related to the actual place of residence.[6]

In addition it is a bit complicated to create a birth chart for someone born around the turn of the year (late January, early February) because some websites start the year on 5 February,[7] others on 20 January.[8] Others, such as J.D. van Buren, take the Chinese New Year, the second new moon after the winter solstice, as the beginning of the new year. The *Huang Di Nei Jing Su Wen* is unclear about the start of the year. Some components of the calendar start on 20 January and other components some weeks later. In short, it requires the experience and special diagnostic skills of the practitioner to make and interpret birth charts around the end of January and early February.

The constitutional stronger and weaker aspects, which are based on the configuration of *qi* at the date and time of birth, along with the diagnosis of the body, behaviour and pulse, provide insight into the process of health and disease of a patient and provide directions for treatment.

Heavenly and earthly qualities that are present at the time of birth can perform a more active and powerful influence or be less present, more passive and weaker. Especially in light of the fact that the time of birth is considered constitutional, the dynamics between these stronger and weaker aspects pose a challenge to the general health of the individual.

An example of such a challenge: Between 11 a.m. and 1 p.m. and during summer the heart *qi* is more active and the gallbladder *qi* of the opposite time of the day and season is more passive.[9] Due to the time and season of birth, the heart *qi* may naturally be more active. Then the gallbladder *qi* is naturally weaker and it will pose a challenge for those individuals to keep that *qi* healthy.

DYNAMICS OF *JING* AND UPBRINGING

The *jing*, the root of life, the vital, pure *qi*, which assists humans to follow the natural order, guides harmonious development of an individual's nature in

---

5   Heavenly stems and earthly branches of year, month, day and hour.
6   However, when someone is born in the southern hemisphere, it is more complicated because there is a six-month time difference in regards to seasons for someone born in the northern hemisphere.
7   The Beginning of Spring in the 24 solar term seasons.
8   Great Cold in the 24 solar term seasons.
9   The heart *qi* is weaker at night between 11 p.m. and 1 a.m. and during winter.

attunement with the history of humanity. In fact, the history of the family and humanity is carried in the essence of the *jing* in every human being.

The pre-natal *jing qi* supplies the material for the creation of a new life and stores the memory of the true self. In other words, it carries the mandate of heaven in humans. The post-natal *jing qi* nourishes the body, controls growth, reproduction and development throughout life and stores the memory of life experiences, which are being passed on to subsequent generations. The *jing* contains the *qi* from heaven and earth that is realized and expressed as love through the heart.

The third aspect that affects people throughout life is upbringing. The role of upbringing appears to be less important than initially thought, partly because many parents appear to stimulate the predisposition of children. Nevertheless, parental upbringing, but certainly also education by schools and influence by peers, influence personality and behaviour, resulting in a unique expression of *qi* and thus of the body, body characteristics and pulse image.

The effects on the *jing*, upbringing, education and influence of others, without the constitutional blueprint having anything to do with it, can lead to issues such as a weak *jing*, great willpower, nervousness, inferiority and superiority problems, digestive problems, emotional deprivation and so on. In other words, the influence of the *qi* configuration at the time of birth is separate from genetic information and upbringing.

This book focuses on some of the components that determine the balance and challenges of the birth chart. Diagnosis and treatment must of course take into account the elements and effects of heredity, life experiences and upbringing.

THE DYNAMICS OF THE BIRTH AND THE CURRENT CHART

The energetic representation of the time of treatment is called the current chart. When the energetic consequences of the birth chart and the current chart are compared, the practitioner can determine which stronger and/or weaker aspects of the patient's birth chart are intensified by the current chart presenting the seasonal *qi* and climate. This provides more insight into the state of health.

For example, if people have an innate weaker kidney *qi*, due to the balance in their birth chart, they need to pay more attention to their kidney *qi* between 5 and 7 a.m. as well as in years when the kidney *qi* is easily subdued due to the energetic configuration of that year and when in the current chart the kidney *qi* is subdued by, for example, too much earth and damp.

THE DYNAMICS OF THE BIRTH CHART
AND CHARTS OF PAST EVENTS

Comparing the birth chart with charts of the prevailing *qi* of the time of illnesses, trauma or other important moments can provide a lot of insight into the vulnerabilities of people. Impressive events often take place in times when the already vulnerable *qi* of the birth chart are even more vulnerable. This may sound strange when it comes to 'accidental' events, but experience has shown that events leave an overpowering impression when someone is going through a constitutionally difficult period of time.

In the curriculum at the International College of Oriental Medicine (ICOM), UK, I used to give a project to the third-year students. Every student was asked to make and interpret their own birth chart. Each student was also given a particular past date – which was calculated as vulnerable for them – to compare with their individual birth chart. They were asked to share what happened at that time in their lives. In almost all cases the students looked at me questioningly: 'How do you know that?' Not infrequently I was asked if I had talked to their mother. The stories of the students included past illnesses, as well as serious car accidents and sudden deaths in the family. The effects of those events had made a deep impression on the students' *shen*, *qi* and *jing*, partly because of the fragile state of the energetic configuration of the constitution at that vulnerable time.

Comparing the charts of major events with the birth charts makes an important contribution to self-understanding. It is interesting to see which *qi* brings about physical, emotional and mental reactions.

THE DYNAMICS OF THE BIRTH CHART
AND THE CHART OF FUTURE

Originally, working with constitutional acupuncture was mainly intended to be preventive. If the weaknesses and strengths of the birth chart are clear, it is not complicated to know what advice someone needs and what treatment will bring the constitution into the optimal state for the coming months. Simply put, someone with weak kidney *qi* will receive nutritional advice for the winter months to strengthen the kidney *qi* and, if necessary, treatment to nourish the kidney *qi*. Of course the birth chart is more nuanced, but once the interpretation has been made and has been compared with the energetic weaknesses and strengths of the coming months, advice and treatment strategies can be just as clear.

THE DYNAMIC OF THE BIRTH CHART AND THE BALANCE OF ORGANS AND CHANNELS

Disease and imbalance of organs or channels can be explored within different concepts such as five phases, Japanese acupuncture, six divisions, French acupuncture, TCM, eight conditions, and so on. In the philosophy of stems and branches, all organs and channels have a unique relationship with a heavenly stem, an earthly branch and one of the six divisions. Diagnosis and interpretation of the birth chart clarify which treatment makes the most sense for each unique person. It is not about the disease, but about the disturbed balance of the personal forces that could cause an illness. Treatment of the balance of innate forces strengthens the constitution so that imbalances can be counteracted.

This book mainly emphasizes the heavenly stems and earthly branches. A book on the six divisions may be published at a future date.

CHAPTER 2

THE BIRTH CHART

We consider the heavenly stems and earthly branches as elements of heaven and earth that divide time into periods. The total cycle of the combination of both leads to a division of sixty possibilities that can be found in the Chinese calendar, which is further composed of yin and yang, the rhythm of the moon, the sun and the stars, the five planets, the zodiac, the five phases or movements, the six *qi* and the eight trigrams.

For many centuries, each time period – year, month, day and hour – has been defined by one heavenly stem and one earthly branch, meaning that each moment in time can be captured by eight elements. In this way the Chinese calendar provides insight into the *qi* present at the time of birth, the so-called 'constitutional *qi*'. The birth chart is a snapshot of the movement of time and space at the moment of birth. In itself, that snapshot means nothing. Interpretation of the birth chart data is performed by someone who can 'read' the interactions of the eight characters – *bazi* or 'four pillars of destiny'. It provides a map on which the challenges, destiny and fate of a person can be determined.

Constitutional acupuncture uses the birth chart to understand the coherence and interactions between the different birth *qi*, which provides insight into the challenges of personal life, but even more how to deal with those challenges related to disease and health. To better understand the meaning of the content of this book, it is recommended that you make some birth charts of different loved ones, friends, patients, people you think you know really well.

This book focuses on the great movement, heavenly stem and earthly branch of the year, which can be found in Table 2.1 as follows:

- Find the year in the diagram
- At the top of the diagram: the great movement, heavenly stem
- At the bottom of the diagram: the related organ
- On the left side of the diagram: the earthly branch

- On the right side of the diagram: the related channel

Example: 2022 is determined by the great movement wood and the heavenly stem *Ren*. The related organ is the bladder. The earthly branch of 2022 is *Yin*, the related channel is lung.

Chart of 2022: '*Ren*, Bl in wood' and *Yin*, lung

IMPORTANT NOTE

The start of the year is a fairly difficult topic because the Chinese year does not start on 1 January and the date of the Chinese New Year (CNY) is open to multiple interpretations; several dates are mentioned for the CNY. There is the official CNY that starts on the day of the second new moon after the winter solstice, which falls between 21 January and 20 February. There is the so-called farmers' New Year that falls on 5 February, called the Beginning of Spring. In addition, there is the start of the great movement of the year on 20 January, which is the start of a 14-day period called Great Cold, one of the 24 solar term periods of 14 days.

This means that the birth chart is evident when people are born after the official CNY. When people are born between 20 January and CNY, it is unclear which great movement, heavenly stem and earthly branch is involved. Dr van Buren once decided to take the CNY (second new moon after winter solstice) as the beginning of the Chinese year, but the reality is different. People born during that period of uncertainty need an experienced practitioner to determine which energies are dominant.

Table 2.1 Heavenly stem and earthly branch combination of the year[1]

Great Movements	Earth	Water	Fire	Metal	Wood	
HS →	*Jia*	*Bing*	*Wu*	*Geng*	*Ren*	
EB ↓						
Zi	1924/1984	1936/1996	1948/2008	1960/2020	1972/2032	Gb
Yin	1974/2034	1926/1986	1938/1998	1950/2010	1962/2022	Lu
Chen	1964/2024	1976/2036	1928/1988	1940/2000	1952/2012	St
Wu	1954/2014	1966/2026	1978/2038	1930/1990	1942/2002	Ht
Shen	1944/2004	1956/2016	1968/2028	1980/2040	1932/1992	Bl
Xu	1934/1994	1946/2006	1958/2018	1970/2030	1982/2042	Hc
	Gb	S.i.	St	L.i.	Bl	

---

1   The yin and yang aspects of this table are further explained in Chapter 5 of this book.

Great Movements	Metal	Wood	Earth	Water	Fire	
HS →	Yi	Ding	Ji	Xin	Gui	
EB ↓						
Chou	1925/1985	1937/1997	1949/2009	1961/2021	1973/2033	Liv
Mao	1975/2035	1927/1987	1939/1999	1951/2011	1963/2023	L.i.
Si	1965/2025	1977/2037	1929/1989	1941/2001	1953/2013	Sp
Wei	1955/2015	1967/2027	1979/2039	1931/1991	1943/2003	S.i.
You	1945/2005	1957/2017	1969/2029	1981/2041	1933/1993	Ki
Hai	1935/1995	1947/2007	1959/2019	1971/2031	1983/2043	Sj
	Liv	Ht	Sp	Lu	Ki	

CHAPTER 3

YUAN HENG LI ZHEN

He was a wanderer
He went where life took him
Only when he was old and looked back
did he understand[1]

Understanding the system and inner meaning of heavenly stems (*tiangan*) and earthly branches (*dizhi*) requires curiosity to understand the philosophical background of Chinese medicine and an interest in its practical application. The main legacy of J.D. van Buren is the practical use of the heavenly stems and earthly branches in the acupuncture clinic. It has been a privilege to be able to study with him and to fulfil a promise to continue his work.

When practising this method it is advisable to also study subjects like free will, responsibility for health, philosophical subjects like the *wu-shen*,[2] texts of and about Chinese philosophers, because this method encompasses all of life: The journey never ends.

The heavenly stems and earthly branches represent the heavenly or cosmic *qi* and earthly *qi*, that influence all natural cycles such as the cyclical system of channels, cycles of *wei qi*, *ying qi*, time, climate and seasons. The heavenly stems and earthly branches are non-visible, energetic expressions of the principles of Time and Space. They were designed by humans to describe nature in all its phenomenal power and are used as tools to define the energetic configuration of moments in time and space, but above all to find balance in health and nutrition for proper vitality. The system of stems and branches or constitutional acupuncture may open the path of health and healing in tune with the authentic *qi*, which is received at time of conception and revealed at birth.

---

1 My mother Sjoe about my father Fred.
2 The five *shen*: heart-*shen* 神, *yi* 意, *po* 魄, *zhi* 志 and *hun* 魂.

BIRTH

Birth is a creative moment that initiates life in a physical body as an expression of the spirit, or it may be better to say that the physical body is animated into the world of the spirit to express the spirit as a physical-mental-emotional being on its path of destiny.

Breathing in for the first time at birth results in the meeting of cosmic *qi* with the *qi* of the newborn. It creates correct *qi* for the channel (meridian) network. At the time of the first inhalation the kidney *qi* grasps the lung *qi* and roots the combination of cosmic *qi* and personal *qi* into a location between the two kidneys. At that special moment the destiny of personal life is defined. This moment in time is recorded in a birth chart.

The birth chart is a chart of a time period, defined by heavenly stems and earthly branches of that year, month, day and hour, by which the background qualities of the path of destiny can be diagnosed and interpreted. This birth chart, also called the 'four pillars of destiny',[3] is used in Chinese astrology (*bazi*), but also in Chinese medicine, where it became known as the 'birth chart' used in acupuncture according to the heavenly stems and earthly branches.[4]

The first inhalation defines the foundation, direction and inspiration by which people go forward, grow, develop and decline until ultimately death arrives. At birth the way people will travel along their path of destiny is still unknown to them. They do not yet know which choices they will make, which circumstances will affect them, what will happen to them or what will be taken away from them. They do not know the level of health they will enjoy or what diseases they will meet. They do not yet know the challenges that life will offer them. Constitutional acupuncture is a method of knowing and guiding an individual's development on the path of destiny and can serve to prevent and cure disease.

THE CHINESE CALENDAR[5]

The emperor of China was considered heaven's earthly ambassador. He ruled his country and people in concordance with the cycles of heaven and earth to keep order in the natural development and heaven's influence on all life. Because of his upright *qi*, rituals and ability to occupy the proper position between heaven and earth, he was able to order his empire according to the universal laws of

---

3   Each period of time (year, month, day, hours) in the calendar is related to natural phenomena and cycles and is anchored in the qualities of the ten heavenly stems and twelve earthly branches.
4   The other name, used in the classics, is the five movements (*wuyun* 五運) and six qi (*liuqi* 六氣).
5   The first Chinese calendar was introduced around 2650 BCE.

heaven; he was the governor of the world,[6] and, as long as he organized his empire with humility and virtue, he had the heavenly mandate.[7] In his position between heaven and earth, he compiled the calendar as a representation of heaven on earth, a projection of natural principles based on celestial or astronomical cycles and the cycles of nature. In order to remain in harmony with heaven and to please the ancestral spirits,[8] the calendar with its astronomical calculations, cycles of seasons and other celestial elements had an important role in rituals and decisions.

The start of the flow of *qi* through the channels at the date and time of birth constitutes the personal framework through which the *shen* – the individual emperor of the human being with the body as his empire – is connected to its source.

SHANGDI

The name *Shangdi* equals heaven, it is the name of the Lord in the High, an ancient name that was common during the Shang Dynasty. *Shangdi* was considered the emperor of heaven who sent spirits and messengers to awaken life in this world. You may be used to the Chinese word *tian* for heaven. Like *Shangdi*, it too is a name to describe the supreme being in the sky (*tian*). It is often used in relation to the word *di*, earth; heaven and earth, the yin and yang of cosmic revelation.

The *Shangdi* story of the revelation given to me by my teachers goes like this: When there was no movement yet, yin and yang were in rest and there was peace; the world was in a mystical oneness. *Shangdi* determined that the poles of yin and yang started breathing again to manifest the world, to awaken the movement of yang as the sky above and the movement of yin as the earth below. A world had been created in the realm of dynamic dualities and opposites. The emperor of China was the ambassador of *Shangdi* and was the enlightened One on earth.

---

6   Just like in the body: The heart is the emperor of the body (world) and houses the celestial spirits (*shen*) to rule the body.
7   The emperors certainly did not always comply. Some were tyrants and dictators. The image is a metaphor of the good and based on mythology.
8   Heaven was seen as a judicial ethical power that could reward and punish. Sacrifices given to ancestors of the emperor were primarily meant to please heaven.

THE FOUR EMANATIONS IN THE *YIJING*[9]

The first hexagram in the *Yijing* or Book of Changes,[10] *Qian*, Heaven, is often translated as The Creative. I prefer the translation by Alfred Huang, who calls it The Initiative, which is less static. It describes an activity of doing to get things going, a force of action. It represents the potency and movement of a new beginning. The first four Chinese characters of the text about this hexagram are *yuan heng li zhen*.[11]

Before shedding more light on these words in regards to their translation and meaning, I would like to start with a general comment. These words collectively are often seen as the attributes of heaven. Some scholars describe the qualities of these characters as the virtues of heaven. I prefer to see them as emanations or as natural inner forces of heaven. Emanations are specific expressions flowing from a source or essence, but are mystically similar to their source. They are experienced differently, being on another level of manifestation, and are faces of heaven seen from different perspectives.

These natural inner forces of heaven are present during conception, when the *jing*-essence of the father and the *jing*-essence of the mother merge to create a new being with an inspired new *jing* that inherently carries the attributes of a life cycle. The effects of the emanations continue to nourish the being from the time we are born until we die – from the inside from the kidney area and from the outside through each new inhalation. One of my teachers taught me that the four emanations, along with heaven, are the archetypes of the five phases. They are the differentiation of the potential of the Oneness into the fivefold living form of existence.

The words *yuan heng li zhen* appear many times in different combinations in the *Yijing*. Their meaning and translation have been a subject of discussion for many years. The Daoist Master Alfred Huang translates these words as sublime and initiative (*yuan*), prosperous and smooth (*heng*), favourable and beneficial (*li*) and steadfast and upright (*zhen*).[12] Other teachers have suggested 'the original pervasive force benefits the pure'. Wu Jing-Nuan[13] translates this phrase from the oracle bones[14] as 'the origin' (*yuan*), 'a sacrifice' (*heng*), 'to profit' (*li*) and 'the

---

9   The *Yijing*, *I Ching* or the Book of Changes is the oldest Chinese classic that can be used as an oracle or as a wisdom book. It provides insight through symbols consisting of six lines, yang-closed lines and yin-open lines.

10 See Appendix II.

11 *Yuan* 元 means original, beginning, *Heng* 亨 means gift to a superior, proceed smoothly, *Li* 利 means beneficial and *Zhen* 貞 means divine, correct, firm.

12 Huang 1998.

13 Wu 1991.

14 In ancient China, oracle bones of animals were used for divination. They bear the earliest form of Chinese writing.

divination' (*zhen*). However, the phrase *yuan heng li zhen* – as far as I know – has not been mentioned in the oracle bones. They do appear in combinations as *yuanheng* and *lizhen*, but not as one phrase with separate characters.

HEXAGRAMS[15]

Hexagrams are symbols and as such have multiple meanings, making them challenging to explore and comprehend. An understanding starts with the awareness of the symbols of the *Yijing* and knowing the place of a hexagram in the context and order of hexagrams, as well as its structure, image and the qualities it represents, but, because of the texts added later, there is a possibility that people will think there is only one truth or meaning. That is not the case. It is precisely personal development and intuitive connection with symbols, based on knowledge and inner truth-finding, that determine the direction of the investigator of the *Yijing*.

Qian, Heaven, is pure yang. It expresses itself in time by being agile and is unstoppable. Constant transformation is its inner nature and the only immutable quality of the cosmos. I understand the natural inner powers of the manifestation of heaven – *yuan heng li zhen* – as the archetypal structure or blueprint of change and in that sense of all cyclical development in time. *Yuan heng li zhen* is the fundamental structure inherent in transformation, resulting in the repeating cycle of growth, blossoming, decline and death.

Qian is associated with the rising sun, the visible expression of heaven and the source of light and *qi*. It radiates to nourish all that exists and represents the centre of manifestation, the source of the purest yang *qi* which creates the world. The earth phase of the *wuxing*[16] is the subtle manifestation of heaven on earth, bearing the attribute of being able to transform and guide and nourish all there is.

The guidance of all transformations on earth and in humans is mirrored in the adaptation of the stomach pulse[17] to the different seasons in one year: fine and delicate in spring, like the beats of a fine hammer in summer, soft and feeble in late summer, small and rough in autumn and small and falling like a stone on the earth in winter.[18] Being a central linking bridge between heaven and earth, the stomach guides the transformations of all seasons and gives life to the cycles of nature in humans.

---

15 See Appendix II.
16 The five phases: water, fire, wood, metal and earth.
17 Superficial *guan* position or middle position of the right radial pulse.
18 *Huang Di Nei Jing Su Wen* Chapters 18 and 19.

THE DYNAMICS OF THREE

The oneness, the unnamed source of existence, that reveals itself as heaven and earth means that differentiation has taken place. Cooperation or conflict is inherently present in revelation. The one, the first or the unique implies that the second, the third and the many are present to acknowledge or reject the power of the one. The dynamics of dualities such as in yin and yang, heaven and earth, masculine and feminine seek dynamic opposition and balance to express life. They eventually find peace and tranquillity in wholeness, because they are temporary revelations showing different aspects of the same source and are mystically identical to each other.

People live between heaven and earth, stand on mother earth and reach for father heaven, and are subject to the cooperation and resistances of opposites. Humanity sees itself as separate from God, nature and so on, whereas in reality we are not only not different but we are god, nature and earth. This worldview is not separate but fundamentally inclusive. In modern Western culture we seem to focus more on taking positions and having conflict than on understanding the unity of existence.

Separation is also between you and me. You as reader and me as writer. This text is a human field between heaven and earth where we meet. It is even so that because of this text we create together our mutual space in which we exchange our *qi*, each having our own position of understanding. Maybe it warms your heart or leads to resistance or leads to changes of insight or maybe it confirms your own thoughts and concepts. In any case, we have two different positions and the relationship between us is the 'third' living entity in which our different beings merge. This happens even though these words were written down much longer ago. Yet this meeting leads to a living contact between each other. The relationship is partly determined by the content, but also by the cooperation of yin and yang, openness and closedness, activity and passivity, rigidity and flexibility of our beings within the text. Despite the fact that this text is printed on paper, it is a living entity that moves within you, the reader, and with which we communicate. This bridges duality and is a source of the experience of oneness.

TIME AND ONENESS

Most Western researchers agree that time has a beginning, and that it is measured from the cosmological 'big bang'. Time in yin–yang theory began when yin and yang started to breathe and make contact, giving rise to the idea of 'moments'. Past, present and future have emerged.

We seem to use past experiences and ideas about the future to create thoughts. Ideas, concepts and lessons are based on the past and build new concepts and future expectations and desires. Deep down, we know that thoughts are limited and that everything will eventually disappear. But, no matter what, most of us stick to the idea of eternity. Our past and future expectations help us to understand the world, sharpen the mind, create concepts and gain insight into physical, emotional and mental life. This designs our world, based on the flow of time which is so different from the oneness, in which there is wholeness, united without any motive or differentiation. In the oneness of heaven there is no past or future, no opinions and concepts, no yin and yang or heaven and earth. The oneness of heaven is a life-giving source, generating and supporting life in every living entity.

All life is united and connected to the same life-giving source, which is called God, heaven or *Dao* or some other name. But no name is enough. A name cannot be given because each name contains the opposite and creates differentiation. Experiencing the oneness of heaven is an immediate experience with unlimited possibilities, without sense of time. It is an experience without identification, effort, struggle, conflict or confirmation of past concepts. This experience comes from being completely free from motives or conclusions.

J.D. van Buren often started his lectures with the Universal Spark, which is an aspect of oneness. 'From the Universal Spark comes life-giving *qi* which is the result of contraction of the *qi* of the Waters of Life.' This is not a Chinese philosophical concept. It is more a theosophical way of thinking. It describes, in a wonderful way, the action and initiative of heaven. The Universal Spark (US) is the breath that creates everything that exists between heaven and earth. He continued to say that the US was eternal, always active. 'It has a giving part and a receiving part. The giving part is the emanation of heavenly life-giving breath as a result of the fragmentation of the US. The receiving part receives all experiences of all living entities. Experiences of how we move, think, feel, act and communicate. This makes us co-responsible for the quality of the US as life-giving source.'

We, as humans, contain this Spark of Life within our true self. It is through self-knowledge that we are able to connect to the origin of all that exists, namely heaven.

TIME AND DUALITY

'I'm so busy. When shall we meet?' … 'I have to check my schedule, see when I can.' We seem to have accepted that it is normal for the agenda to dominate life and that spontaneous encounters have become rarer. I don't know if you recognize this: During my holidays I often intended to organize my agenda differently once I returned from holiday and take more time for relaxation. But soon I felt the time pressure again when I returned to work. When learning to deal with it, I was asked if I was able to do nothing. At the time I didn't even understand the question ... Luckily, I really learned to enjoy 'doing nothing'. I don't mean to meditate or sit still regularly; doing nothing has no other purpose than doing nothing. It's actually a strange saying, because doing nothing has nothing to do with doing. On the contrary!

Time is often considered our enemy but it should be our friend. Besides doing nothing, we need time to think, to feel, to digest, to find our own way in society and so forth. Time is also an essential factor in periods when a lot is happening and when changes and adjustments are expected. We need time to process emotional shocks. We need time to enable us to relate to all changes in periods of individual emancipation and physical and psychological developments. We need time to heal.

In Chapter 39 of the *Huang Di Nei Jing Su Wen*, the Yellow Emperor begins with an unexpected fourfold statement about the practitioner's qualities before starting to diagnose a patient through questions, observations and touch.[19] It clarifies a few things about time in the world of duality we are living in. It states that it is important for the practitioner for diagnosis and thus treatment to verify the law of heaven in humans, which means within the twelve channels and six *qi*,[20] the five movements[21] and how planets and stars[22] have their effect on human affairs. The Yellow Emperor says he wants to have some realization about it. He continues that in our created world of yin and yang, it is important not to stick only with historical facts, but to bring the history into the now-reality of the present. This means that it is good to listen to the history of a patient, but the practitioner needs to translate this to what the history means for the present. Is the history an incentive to develop or is the patient frozen in the past, full of traumatic feelings due to guilt, shame, anger and so on? It emphasizes that it is crucial for treatment to observe and diagnose how people have been attached to the experiences of their past.

One translation states that practitioners must become one with the present, emphasizing the fact that what has been established in the past does not remain

---

19 *Huang Di Nei Jing Su Wen* Chapter 39 'On pain of various kinds'. This chapter has a peculiar start and is most important for practitioners.

20 Coming from the 12-year orbit of the planet Jupiter.

21 Coming from the five heavens: the green azure dragon, the red vermilion bird, the yellow dragon, the white tiger and the dark warrior heavens with the planets Jupiter, Mars, Saturn, Venus and Mercury, respectively.

22 The 28 star constellations or moon houses.

unchanged.[23] No change would be contrary to all cosmic laws. Change may be the only unchanging quality of life. In order to attune the past to the present, the rules, regulations, laws and so on of the past must be fully understood and the present must be viewed with a flexible mind, free from dogmas and rigidity.

> And those who are good in discussing the human body should be able to verify their theory on their own. Those who know how to speak about other people must have dealt with themselves sufficiently.[24]

This statement is a golden rule found in different forms in many philosophies and religions: You should treat others the way you want to be treated yourself. It also emphasizes the importance of self-knowledge.

The Yellow Emperor ends with:

> It is only when the above conditions are met that they [practitioners] can be regarded as having achieved the level of true understanding without ignorance and with an understanding of essential principles, which is called brightness.
>
> Thereby their understanding of the Way is free of confusion and the essential numbers can be known to their full extent. This is the so-called understanding.

By first understanding heaven's reflection in humanity, second the meaning of the past in the present and third that all humans are equal without exception, one is a bright practitioner!

Yuan heng li zhen as the natural inner powers of heaven, the four emanations and the first four words of the hexagram *Qian*, Heaven, are the revelation of the oneness in time and duality. Understanding the past, present and future, growth, blossoming, decay and death are guiding principles on the path of understanding the Way.

YUAN AND WOOD

J. Legge translates *yuan* as great and originating, R. Wilhelm as sublime, A. Huang as sublime and initiative. From other translators I have seen translations as head of a body, origin, beginning of a cycle, source, leader of goodness, impulse, beginning and great or grand (especially in combination with *heng*).

The emanation *yuan* is the breath of heaven in the East. It can be seen as a

---

23 Some scholars suggest, because of this statement, that the channel system needs to be adapted to the evolving human being of the present.

24 *Huang Di Nei Jing Su Wen* Chapter 39.

force on a more condensed level of manifestation than its source. *Yuan* is part of a cyclical movement rooted in the emanation *zhen* in the North and moves into the direction of the emanation *heng* in the South. The *qi* of *yuan* is described as the beginning of all things and beings, an initial cause, a creative principle, connected to the source of existence. In addition to all these aspects, *yuan* is a guiding principle. It is always active to adjust changes to everyone's personal *qi*. For instance, without the *qi* of *yuan* it would be impossible to convert food into *ying qi* for the channel network.

YUAN IN THE WUXING

Yuan is the archetypical foundation for all expressions of the phase of wood of the *wuxing* theory. It is the fundamental principle behind the movements of the East, the three *hun*[25] and the *qi* of the liver and gallbladder as well as the wood qualities of the lungs and large intestine in their functions as placed in the East of the Chinese hourly clock. In pulse diagnosis it can be felt as vital and gentle, coming up quickly, being lifted up and flexible.

HENG AND FIRE

There are many possible translations and even more interpretations found for *heng*. In the *Yijing*, *heng* is several times combined with *yuan*; *yuanheng* can have several meanings: to participate or accept or make a sacrificial offering, ready for presentation, meeting of good things, gift to a superior or connection to heaven. *Yuanheng* is the acceptance of natural sacrifices, an innate quality of every development in time and is the answer of humanity to the sacrifice of heaven. In essence, it is the sacrifice to experience and serve the oneness of existence.

SACRIFICIAL OFFERINGS

In ancient times the emperor's authority to rule the empire was given to him by heaven. The emperor took care of his country as a representative of heaven on earth, by showing respect to the source[26] of his authority and asking for reward for his virtue and good deeds through sacrifices in special temples. The most famous place for these offerings was the Temple of Heaven in Beijing where the

---

25 The wood aspect of the five *shen*. The five *shen* or *wu-shen* are the spirits of heaven: *shen* mind or 'spirit', *yi* intent, *po* animal soul, *zhi* purpose, will, and *hun* cloud soul.
26 Heaven and to ancestors representing heaven.

emperor held an important ceremony at the Circular Mound Altar[27] at winter solstice, the astronomical beginning of the year, to attune with the spirits of heaven in order to give good guidance for the coming year. No ordinary people were allowed to watch or attend the ceremony to make sure that everything that happened was completely pure.[28] The offering in winter is somewhat similar to a meditation technique where people, before going to sleep, leave the thoughts and feelings of the day behind and only bring into the night that which has been learned from it in its most essential form. This can then be a source of light for the energy of the next day after it has been purified overnight.

Sacrificial offerings with a direct purpose

Often people consulted the Book of Changes to seek advice on uncertainty about an important decision or a sense of obligation. Instead of trusting themselves or their intuition they would first bring sacrifice to heaven in order to come in tune with the will of heaven. Another example of purposeful offering is the sacrifice offered to the deceased aiming to create a sense of security. Many people are still fearful of ghosts (*gui*) as entities of the deceased. Therefore, money and food are given to the deceased during funerals to keep them busy and to prevent them from disturbing the realm of the living as ghosts. This type of offering is primarily motivated by desires of the self.

Sacrificial offerings in harmony with heaven

These are sacrifices that are part of and fit in with natural, often cyclical, developments in time.

In Beijing there are still those who go to pray for a good harvest or a fortunate outcome at the Altar of Prayer, which is part of the park of the Temple of Heaven where the ambassador of heaven on earth offered his thanks for the harvest of last year and prayed for good weather and abundant harvest for the upcoming season. The emperor's goal was not to achieve anything specific, but to avoid getting in the way of the natural course of events. In the body there are also natural sacrifices, such as when the deciduous teeth are sacrificed to allow the natural growth of the permanent teeth, as well as in nature when the leaves of a tree fall in the autumn as the moisture from the tree withdraws to allow the tree to survive during winter.

---

27 The Circular Mound Altar is built based on the number nine, the number that symbolizes heaven.
28 Later, in the Confucian time, heaven was seen as a power to reward virtues and good deeds but also to punish evil.

TRANSFORMATION AND ADJUSTMENTS

The text in the *Yijing* often refers to proper adjustments to natural development in time (*yuanheng*):

> Following the virtue of heaven, one should not appear as a leader.
>
> When Yang (Day) is predominating go forward, when Yin (Night) predominates retreat.

Hexagram 1

People like to stay in control. We find it difficult when circumstances force us to go in directions that are not easy. We sacrifice sleep, relationships, health and so on to continue with our plans and behaviour. We are so challenged to move, to want, to have and so forth, that we are not aware any more that times of activity alternate with times of rest. And when things really get out of hand we are ready to sacrifice anything to feel happy again. From these *Yijing* texts we might learn that we are able to live without the obsessive need to live up to expectations. Burnouts are often the incentive to look into our own forced behaviour. Then we are ready for change, to practise yoga, mindfulness or find a psychotherapist and maybe we start to adjust our life to the natural way of developing without any force.

SELFLESSNESS

The sages of the world mention that being selfless and acceptance of the flow of circumstances go hand in hand with a completely clear and awakened mind. Selflessness is the expression of the profound primordial spirit called *yuan-shen*. Striving for that condition will always fail, because striving is the opposite of selflessness. Nature is complete in itself, and equals heaven in its creative self-organizing dynamics. Being part of nature, humanity holds the key to the natural state of being through the acceptance of natural sacrifices (*yuanheng*) along with self-knowledge.

> Once upon a time there was a Chinese farmer whose horse ran away. That evening, all of his neighbours came around to commiserate. They said, 'We are so sorry to hear your horse has run away. This is most unfortunate.' The farmer said, 'maybe'. The next day the horse came back bringing 10 wild horses with it, and in the evening everybody came back and said, 'Oh, isn't that lucky. What a great turn of events. You now have 11 horses!' The farmer again said, 'maybe'.

The following day his son tried to break one of the horses, and while riding it, he was thrown and broke his leg. The neighbours then said, 'Oh dear, that's too bad,' and the farmer responded, 'maybe'. The next day the conscription officers came around to conscript people into the army, and they rejected his son because he had a broken leg. Again, all the neighbours came around and said, 'Isn't that great!' Again, he said, 'maybe'.

COMPLETION

As a character on its own, *heng* has different meanings: determination, fulfilment, success, opening, increase, prosperous, smooth, success, completion and development. These translations refer to the completion of development of what has been initiated and created by *yuan*. It describes the full expression of awakened life in a realized form, such as flowers and fruits, and as the ever-penetrating consciousness of the oneness of heaven in all existing forms.

Heng in the *wuxing*

Heng is the archetypical foundation for all expressions of the phase of fire of the *wuxing* theory. It is the fundamental principle behind the movements of the South. The *yuan-shen*, heart-*shen*, the *qi* of the heart, small intestine, heart constrictor and *san jiao* as well as the fire quality of the spleen as placed in the South of the Chinese hourly clock.

In the event that the *hun* (*yuan*) are relatively too active with regard to the *shen* (*heng*), there are symptoms such as restlessness, chaotic *shen*, daydreams, abundance of plans without executing them, confusion, frustration; when the *hun* are relatively too weak compared to the *shen* there are symptoms such as depression, difficulty in making decisions, lack of creativity and imagination, emotional instability. Phases of transformation and healing that take place through the collaboration of wood along with fire always involve sacrificing the old to give a chance to the new. As seen in the above cases, a new balance has to be found in which peace only arises when a part of the introverted or extroverted ego is 'sacrificed'. Often through trauma counselling and partly by giving up control along with regaining faith in the natural state and development of things, people find renewed balance. Treatment of *yuanheng*, the wood and fire collaboration, is a wonderful healing contribution to this process.

In pulse diagnosis *heng* can be felt as steady flow, coming up quickly, disappearing slowly (a hook-like pulse), round and of good sound.

LI AND METAL

Li combined with *zhen* (*lizhen*) means benefiting (*li*) from divination (*zhen*). In addition, it could mean that further divination is recommended or it predicts a favourable prognosis.

After the guidance of *heng*, the state of openness and acceptance of the natural development in life, the time seems ready to look into the future. However, the way of *lizhen* is not self-evident. The direction moves towards the emanation *zhen*, a deep source of existence.

Li on its own means beneficial, suitable, favourable, further development, furthering, harvest. It is the beneficial force or the force of gathering, the capacity to satisfy one's need, which is the result of the natural situation and development of each being.

In *Huang Di Nei Jing Su Wen* Chapter 1, the Yellow Emperor asks why people don't live as long as before. Qibo answers:

> … They followed the pattern of Yin and Yang … They lived their lives according to a regular pattern …[29]

After growth and maturity, the natural movement includes the inward movement. From the heat of the summer to the coolness of autumn, from the active *wei qi* at the surface of the body during the day to the cleansing and warming activity of the *wei qi* in the internal organs during the night, the *qi* moves inward, from yang to yin.

Part of the natural progression of yin and yang is to reap the benefits (*li*) of the harvest of life to gain insight, understanding and wisdom. The philosopher Mencius stated:

> If a man loves others, and no responsive attachment is shown to him, let him turn inwards and examine his own benevolence. If he is trying to rule others, and his government is unsuccessful, let him turn inwards and examine his wisdom. If he treats others politely, and they do not return his politeness, let him turn inwards and examine his own feeling of respect.[30]

The qualities of emanations *li* face the natural way of letting go. Only the essences of the inner harvest of experiences, whatever they may be, are carried

---

29 Lu 1990.
30 Mencius, Book 4A *Li Lou*(1), Chapter 4.

in and nourish the essence, as do the life fluids of the tree that withdraw into the roots to safeguard life against cold through the winter.

Letting go takes love
To let go doesn't mean to stop caring,
it means I can't do it for someone else.
To let go is not to cut myself off;
it is the realization that I can't control another.
To let go is not to enable,
but to allow learning from natural consequences.
To let go is to admit powerlessness,
which means the outcome is not in my hands.
To let go is not to try to change or blame another,
I can only change myself.
To let go is not to care for, but to care about.
To let go is not to fix, but to be supportive.
To let go is not to judge,
but to allow another to be a human being.
To let go is not to be in the middle arranging outcomes,
but to allow others to effect their own outcomes.
To let go is not to be protective;
it is to permit another to face reality.
To let go is not to deny, but to accept.
To let go is not to nag, scold, or argue,
but to search out my own shortcomings and to correct them.
To let go is not to adjust everything to my desires,
but to take each day as it comes and to cherish the moment.
To let go is not to criticize and regulate anyone,
but to try to become what I dream I can be.
To let go is not to regret the past,
but to grow and live for the future.
To let go is to fear less and love more.

Anonymous poem

LI IN THE *WUXING*

Li is the archetypical foundation for all expressions of the phase of metal of the *wuxing* theory. It is the fundamental principle behind the movements of the

West, the seven *po* and the *qi* of the lungs, large intestine as well as the metal quality of the bladder and kidney in their functions as placed in the West of the Chinese hourly clock.

In pulse diagnosis it can be felt as slightly larger than summer, but thinner, slower, peaceful, empty upwards and it disappears quickly.

ZHEN AND WATER

Zhen is translated as divination or to profit by means of divination especially when used in the combination with *li* (*lizhen*).

In the seasonal cycle of spring, summer and autumn *zhen* is related to the winter. In the cycle of beginning, growth, further development and harvesting it means maturity but also death. Other translations are: true, authentic, correctness, firmness, steadiness, steadfastness, perseverance.

The Chinese character for *zhen* is very close to the character *zheng,* which means upright. For this reason *zhen* is often translated as upright.

Zhen is the most authentic *qi* we own. It is hidden in the depths of our being and works behind our conditioned behaviour and reactions to the outside world. It is a determining force with a tendency to immutability. The authentic *qi* is the foundation of existence and is firm, true and steadfast. Some people relate this to the initial creative power of love.

Zhen resides in the foundation of water as a potential force and is expressed by the heart *shen*. The true self of the heart (*yuan-shen*) is the power at the origin of all processes of life, emanating from the source of life. *Yuan-shen* and *zhen* are the dual manifestation of the Universal Spark. Together they dominate and govern all vital activities.

The keys to open the gates of love are self-knowledge and self-respect, when they are the pivot of our actions to be upright, true to ourselves and authentic. Hidden therein lies the deepest source of our existence.

ZHEN IN THE *WUXING*

Zhen is the archetypical foundation for all expressions of the phase of water of the *wuxing* theory. It is the fundamental principle behind the movements of the North, the *zhi* and the *qi* of the kidneys and bladder as well as the water quality of the *san jiao* and gallbladder in their functions as placed in the North of the Chinese hourly clock.

In pulse diagnosis it can be felt as firm, deep, small and soft, not hard.

A FINAL NOTE

The Warring States Period (475–221 BCE) was a very interesting time in the history of China. It was full of contradictions, a period characterized by wars of different states. It ended when the state of Qin conquered the other states and founded the first unified Chinese empire with new military and bureaucratic structures. At the same time it was a period of abundance of new developments and new ideas; it is called the renaissance period of Chinese civilization with great thinkers like Mencius, Zhuangzi and other great philosophers. These men were focused on finding the way back to peace, back to balance and on restoring good order.

The scholars of the time, who composed the *Huang Di Nei Jing Su Wen*, as well as the later Confucians and Daoists, are believed to have compiled their theories, poems, thoughts and philosophies from older classical philosophies and documents of ancient China.[31] New insights arose during the Warring States, based on old insights from centuries before.

Contrary to popular belief that people were inherently bad, Mencius was the first to claim that people were good by nature. Till then it was believed that people needed to be punished and only educated according to moral standards. Mencius said that humans are destined to naturally have virtues such as benevolence, righteousness, propriety and wisdom. Education and further cultivation are necessary to support the growth of already existing virtues. Self-cultivation was seen as a responsibility and individual choice of everyone. The environment of humans influences the virtues, but Mencius emphasized that everyone is responsible for his or her own choices in life.

The first chapter of the *Huang Di Nei Jing Su Wen*, 'On the heavenly truth of ancient times', shows a major transformation from an old paradigm of dependency to a paradigm of self-responsibility. It describes the natural development of humans based on their innate true *qi*. Before the time of the *Huang Di Nei Jing Su Wen*, illnesses were explained as the product of ghosts (*gui*) entering the body and causing illness. In the first chapter of the *Huang Di Nei Jing Su Wen* people are held responsible for their own health and preventing illness by a healthy lifestyle and most importantly by protecting their authentic *qi*.

Although the sentence *yuan heng li zhen* is not mentioned in medical texts, the content and expression of these virtues of heaven are also hidden in the first words of the *Huang Di Nei Jing Su Wen*:

When one is completely free from wishes, ambition and distracting thoughts, indifferent to fame and gain, the true *qi* will come in the wake of it. When

---

31   E.g. the Book of Odes.

one concentrates his spirit internally and keeps a sound mind, how can illness occur?[32]

The Yellow Emperor in ancient times was born with divine talents; he was good at speech in his childhood, had a quick and perfect apprehension in his boyhood, and developed a polite manner and good character in his youth. He finally reached the status of heaven and became the Emperor[33] after growing up.[34]

Or:

The Yellow Emperor of ancient times, was bright and clever when he was born, good at talking when he was a child, had a modest style of doing things and an upright character when he was young; in his youth, he was honest and possessed a strong ability of distinguishing what was right and what was wrong. He became an emperor when he grew up.[35]

In his pure and rapid development as a child the Yellow Emperor is an example of the expression of the qualities of the virtues of the emanations *yuan heng li zhen* in humans. By the natural inner forces of heaven he became the son of heaven and a true example for everyone.

---

32 Translation: Bing, Wu and Wu (1997).
33 The son of heaven.
34 Lu 1990.
35 Translation: Bing, Wu and Wu (1997).

CHAPTER 4

THE FIVE HEAVENS

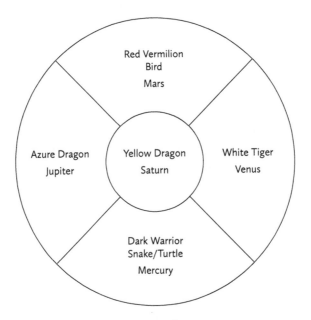

Figure 4.1 Five heavens

The four emanations, *yuan, heng, li, zhen*, emanate from heaven to take shape on earth. In the sky they reveal themselves as the four segments around a fifth central area.[1] The four compass points of the segments North, East, South, West are the four gateways through which the undifferentiated heavenly *qi* pours into the differentiated field of earth. The meaning of 'emanation' is that what is differentiated is mystically equal to the undifferentiated source. Different perceptions are due to the different directions and therefore the different viewpoints, which implies that unity in diversity can always be found and is accessible.

---

1 During the Warring States period, the Yellow Emperor was added as the central yellow heaven and yellow dragon.

The five different faces emanate on the physical realm with five different qualities that we have come to know as water, fire, wood, metal and earth. The ten great movements, ten heavenly stems, twelve earthly branches and twelve channels are the linking fields of influence between the subtle and the more dense realms of existence. The more clearly and unambiguously the intention and direction of an acupuncture stimulus moves the *qi* in the connecting fields, the better the message is received. Constitutional acupuncture therefore only uses a few acupuncture points per treatment.

THE HEART-*SHEN*

The emperor (or once an empress)[2] was seen as an adept ambassador of heaven while the empire was thriving. With the help of advisers who understood the orbits of the stars and planets, the son of heaven aligned the calendar of the seasons and months with heaven by means of rituals. He made sacrifices in imperial ancestral temples to keep the cosmic order and to please the emperors of earlier dynasties to bring order, happiness, prosperity, peace and harmony all year round. Of course, there were accidents, wars, floods and the like, and subsequently, it was the emperor's duty to bring prosperity through complementary worships of heaven, gods and forefathers. This was not always the case in the past, as emperors, being human, were prone to power conflicts, fights, humiliations, self-interest, hatred, jealousy and other human conflicts.

The place and function of the heart-*shen* in the body is comparable to that of the emperor. The heart-*shen* rules all that is called 'being' or 'self'. It receives the mandate of heaven to rule its 'empire': the physical, psychological and spiritual aspects of being. The *yuan-shen*, the primordial, pre-natal *shen*, can be seen as the undifferentiated collective space on the vertical axis in which it communicates with the cosmic yin and yang of heaven and earth. At birth, the *yuan-shen* withdraws and the *wu-shen* appears, the five acquired post-natal *shen*. These activate sensations through the senses, the power of desires and will and gives the opportunity to develop self-awareness. The undifferentiated wholeness changes into a differentiated state of the personality. Yet the pure undifferentiated is always accessible to every human being as a point of reference of truth for actions, thoughts, feelings and behaviour.

On the horizontal human level, the heart guards health throughout the changes of the 'seasons of life', such as infancy to toddlerhood, childhood to adulthood and old age. The stillness of the heart is the reference point that

---

2 Wu Zetian, the famous empress of the Tang Dynasty.

guides the five *zang* through these periods of possible introversion, extraversion, happiness, sadness and so forth. 'The heart-*shen* is the supreme commander, sovereign, monarch, master of the human body, it dominates the spirit, ideology and thought of man',[3] and above all, it is the *shen* that guides the *qi* and maintains all transformations and natural processes of life. Whatever method the Chinese medicine practitioner follows, the heart-*shen* must always be given the first attention so people can coincide freely with this reference point of truth, authenticity, wholeness and health.

LAW OF ANALOGY

In the Western world we learn to think, explain and understand according to the law of cause and effect. For instance, a burned skin (an effect) happens when the sun (the cause of the stimulus) has been shining on it for too long. Chinese philosophy and medicine is, to a great extent, built on the law of analogy, which is characterized by the interdependent interaction of differentiated elements, even when elements appear to be unrelated. Heaven has a sun and a moon, humans have two eyes, the left eye related to the sun, yang and the constitution, the right eye to the moon, yin and behaviour.

The equivalent interrelationships between the elements determine the outcome of the relationship, rather than one causing the other. The cosmic model of yin and yang, heaven–earth–human with subdivisions such as *shen qi jing* accomplishes the totality of existence through the interdependence of its elements because, according to the law of analogy, all parts of the whole are jointly responsible for the whole. This notion implies that the five heavens do not radiate *qi*, causing an effect, but are energetically deeply connected to the five phases of the existence of nature and humans.

The law of analogy is different and somewhat unusual for people, but both the law of analogy and the law of cause and effect are wise ways of thinking. The paradigm of the law of analogy makes humans co-responsible for the existence and maintenance of life, meaning that the impact of acupuncture treatments contributes to the well-being of patients as well as nature and humanity as a whole.

---

3   *Huang Di Nei Jing Su Wen* Chapter 8.

THE FIVE HEAVENS WERE EACH ASSIGNED AN ANIMAL AND A COLOUR

Humans consider themselves superior to animals, but in (Chinese) mythology, animals are considered to be beings who, unlike humans, naturally follow the flow of heaven and in that sense take up the mandate of heaven. The different characters of animals associated with the influence of the different heavens on humans illustrate the unity of the mandate in the diversity of existence.

Colours are fractions of light. The subtle radiance of light is received by the eyes, the gates of the *shen*, which form the link between the unity of the undifferentiated light of heaven and the differentiated level of earth and humanity.[4]

The green-azure (*qing*) heaven, the dragon, eastern heaven, wood

Green-azure is the sparkling colour of the eastern sky on a clear morning. *Qing* and the power of the dragon of the eastern heaven represent vitality and the sparkling *qi* of spring, the morning, and the creation of life in general.

The dragon bears a different symbol in Western culture than in Eastern culture. In the West, the dragon is associated with the serpent of paradise or a beast primarily interested in wealth and virgins. Unlike this dangerous beast, the dragon in the Eastern culture is considered a powerful animal that brings good luck and whose breath offers life. Wise and generous, dragons are considered the ancestors of emperors, the ambassadors of heaven on earth.

The orbit of the ruling planet Jupiter around the sun takes about twelve years.[5] The twelve served as model for the twelve earthly branches, the twelve zodiac signs, the Chinese hourly clock and the twelve main channels. The aspects of the eastern heaven draw attention to the vital underlying forces of an organized integrated wholeness, such as the health and flow of *qi* in the channel system.

The World Health Organization defines health as follows: 'Health is a state of complete physical, mental, and social well-being and not merely the absence of disease or infirmity.'[6] In other words, the path to health is the path that restores the state of wholeness and integrity, which includes the free flow of *qi* in the pathways of the channels. Any obstruction in the form of chaos or stagnation in the system requires the use of the channels and points related to the eastern heaven.

---

4 The relationship between eyes and light is special and different from the other senses. Sound is a vibration of the air and is received by the ear, the gates of the *jing*, the densest form of *qi*. The mouth and nose fall even more into the area of the earth and humans. The senses of taste and smell are activated by particles in the air that attach themselves to droplets and moisture.
5 11.86 years.
6 WHO Constitution, available at www.who.int/about/governance/constitution.

All aspects of wood[7] operate in the atmosphere of the eastern heaven and initiate changes and movements through free flow of vital *qi*. This expresses itself in creativity, ambition, authority, kindness, strength and vitality. When this *qi* stagnates or is otherwise disturbed, the vital *qi* tries to find a way out to restore the order. Often this adjustment of expression comes in the form of passive or active anger. The healthy way would be through the power of love and connection.

The vital *qi* of the green azure dragon heaven is reflected in the *jing well* points and their function to remove and disperse obstruction of *qi* in the channels and vitalize *wei qi* and *ying qi*.

The red vermilion bird heaven, southern heaven, fire

Red is the colour of the South and the summer. The red colour vermilion is a red pigment which is found in the mineral cinnabar. Refining cinnabar is complicated and therefore known as an essential factor in Chinese alchemy to find immortality. Originally, alchemy was engaged in the use of science of chemistry and magic to convert base metals into precious metals. With the use of cinnabar, alchemy eventually became a process of inner purification of the body and the being, with the aim of achieving immortality or self-transcendence. Cinnabar is a yang force that corresponds to solar forces. Both provide the means for transformation that takes place more easily with heat and thus with the power of the South and summer.

The bird is seen as the only non-mythical animal that can escape the gravity of the earth and thus symbolizes the metamorphosis from an earthly to a heavenly level.

The red planet Mars offers the opportunity to feel and have emotions. The fact that feelings exist is connected to a heavenly principle and is closely related to consciousness. Perceptions that result in movements and sensations are the fundamental characteristics of emotions that make humans human.

The red vermilion bird heaven and the planet Mars represent the transcendent potential of experiences and feelings, through which human spiritual experience can be perceived independently of the material world. These experiences bring the danger that people 'fly away', become vague and unrooted. It is therefore recommended to make spirituality practical in everyday life by actively making the choice to be present in the moment and stimulating awareness through authenticity. This is regulated by cooperation and good alignment of

---

7   Wood in the *wuxing* is liver and gallbladder, but the lungs and large intestine, besides being metal, are in the East of the Chinese hourly clock and therefore considered wood as well. The division *jué yin* belongs to wood like all other *qi* related in one way or another to the East.

the phases fire, earth and water. Without these vehicles and active presence, people may disappear into an imaginary world that appears real to them.

All aspects of fire operate in the atmosphere of the southern heaven. Warmth initiates transformations and movements in numerous directions. Because of the ever-present duality of yin and yang, such as up–down, inside–outside, conscious–subconscious, intelligence–intuition, active–passive, there is always the chance of imbalance and conflict. A natural balance is crucial to keep the expression of the fire of the southern heaven healthy. Then presence may arise resulting in, for example, inspiration, passion, focus and diversity and feeling alive and awake. A disturbed balance easily leads to rising *qi* and heat and underactivity of the central fundamental consciousness. It easily causes excess fire in the form of overexcitement or mania as well as heartburn, constipation, migraine or burnout and feeling down, depression and overall exhaustion.

The transformative and health promoting *qi* of the red vermilion bird heaven is reflected in the *ying spring* points to balance fire-water in the channels and calm emotions.

The yellow dragon heaven, central heaven, earth

The central yellow dragon heaven is placed in the centre when links are made to the five phases with the Yellow Emperor in the central position. Another name for the Yellow Emperor was the 'emperor with the four faces'. He occupies the centre of the universe, allowing him to observe everything that happens around him.

In some traditions, yellow was valued as a colour that only the emperor was allowed to use. It represents central strength, supreme power, royalty and prosperity from heaven.

Chinese dragons in mythology are depicted as snake-like beasts with four legs and no wings. They are mystical beasts that derive supernatural powers from the subtle spiritual realm. They fly without wings. They symbolize strength and power, leadership in evolution and change.

According to legend, the Yellow Emperor (Huangdi 2698–2599 BCE) was turned into a dragon at the end of his life.[8] He ascended and joined the heavenly

---

8   The Yellow Emperor is considered the ancestor of everyone and sometimes people called themselves 'children of the dragon' to indicate the special experience or desire for the union of heaven and earth. The symbolic significance of the mythical Yellow Emperor has not always been the same over the centuries. The origin of the name and its mystical side have always been the subject of debate. Yet he can be seen as the divine sage and an example to all. His appearance symbolizes the union of heaven and earth and the power given to him who received the mandate from heaven on earth. Cultural customs and esoteric and medical writings are said to have come from him, the *Huangdi Neijing*. For some he was the Immortal and the example of the existence of the mandate of heaven that can exist in a living being as a source of unity and authenticity.

emperor (*Shangdi*) in his residence around the North Pole Star[9] and the seven stars of the Great Bear or Big Dipper. By his returning to the source, the conjunction of earthly *qi* and heavenly *qi* was completed, yin and yang coincided and merged. Sacrificing his original expression on earth, the world of forms and cycles of time, allowed for transformation and regulation in a different form and in a different realm. The initiative of transformation implies a meeting of yin and yang. No dark without light, no autumn without spring, no taking without giving, no enlightenment without ignorance and confusion.

As the essence of yin and yang meet in the centre and embrace each other in the yellow dragon heaven, it contributes to transformation, harmony, balance and order, just like the associated planet Saturn.

All aspects of earth operate in the atmosphere of the central heaven. Earth initiates changes and movements through seeking harmony between heaven and earth, yin and yang. The agent that makes transformation possible is dampness because it brings together the properties of the other four phases. The right amount of dampness is created by a good balance between dryness and moisture, movement and rest, cold and heat, solid and liquid. The right degree of dampness stimulates transformation, growth and development and establishes a stable, calm, solid central place of trust. Transformations become difficult when there is a 'central' *qi* stagnation. It leads to physical and psychological feelings of heaviness, thoughtfulness, pensiveness and a lack of growth and development.

The harmonizing *qi* of the yellow dragon heaven is reflected in the *shu stream* points. They replenish *qi* and remove damp, especially in cases when people suffer from abdominal digestive illnesses. On the yin channels, *shu stream* points are also *yuan source* points, regulating, vitalizing and guiding the *qi* in the channels and internal organs.

The white tiger heaven, the western heaven, metal

The planet Venus may appear in the East, just before sunrise. It is then called the morning star. During another part of the year when it sets in the West just after sunset, it is called the evening star. Its name is the Great White or the Golden Planet because of the bright light that is compared to the reflected light on metal weapons. In the Chinese paradigm, the rising of Venus in the East foretells virtue, and as an evening star setting in the West, it is primarily indicative of friction and struggle.

The character of the white tiger is yin in relation to the yang of the dragon

---

9   The North Pole Star appears to be the centre of the sky and always visible to people living in the northern hemisphere. The other star constellations rotate around the North Pole Star. It is therefore seen as the home of *Shangdi*, the highest emperor or the emperor of heaven.

of the eastern heaven. The white tiger receives the yang life-giving light source and internalizes it through yin power. The yin tiger protects against evil by regulating and thereby strengthening the internal, creating pure inner strength. He shows strength and is the leader of all animals, always on the alert in the West to detect and repel attackers such as ghosts and demons that rise at sunset.

All aspects of metal operate in the atmosphere of the western heaven. They initiate change and movement through introversion, introspection and insight. Healthy internalization requires a distinction between useful and useless and a sharp and clear vision, along with sensitivity to the needs of society and the self. When this *qi* is disturbed, the vision is blurred and the relationship is broken. It easily causes perceptions of separation, punishment, anger and feelings of injustice.

Survival depends on the white tiger heaven of the West. It is reflected in the *jing* river points that cleanse and regulate the flow of *qi* in the channels and protect them from external pathogenic factors.

The dark tortoise and snake heaven (dark warrior), northern heaven, water

With regard to the northern heaven, it is common to see images of the dark tortoise along with a snake curled around the tortoise. Sometimes it is depicted with a dark warrior standing on top of the tortoise's shell.

The dark colours are related to the North where the sun never shines. The tortoise combines the close bond between heaven and earth in one being: Its dark shell is round from above, and seen from below it appears as a square, the symbols of heaven and earth, respectively; the shield is strong with remarkable mystical designs. Along with the fact that this animal also seems fearless and can grow very old, it made people look at tortoises with great respect. The tortoise therefore represents the animal of longevity.

The coiled snake symbolizes alertness and control of unconscious hidden instinctive forces.

The dark warrior standing on the tortoise's back shows his control over fear, instincts and emotions and his ability to transform and transcend these forces for the better and sustain life. He transcends and understands heaven and earth and is a source for all revealed life.

The orbit of the planet Mercury is too close to the sun to be seen often and easily. Mercury is seen as the hidden substitute for the life-giving breaths of the sun, the original yang. Mercury's light and powers are deeply hidden. It represents the hidden generative, creative *qi* of kidney yang and *Ming Men*, known as the fire of the kidneys. It represents the hidden life force behind all shapes and forms.

All aspects of water operate in the atmosphere of the northern heaven. They initiate changes and movements through withdrawal and gathering forces. They cultivate any development in favour of the continuation of the life cycle so that the hidden heavenly *qi* may reveal itself at the appropriate time. It results in a nourishing *qi* that manifests in wisdom, authenticity, sexuality and talent.

The hidden *qi* of the dark tortoise heaven is reflected in the *he sea* points that revitalize and replenish the *qi* in the channels.

CHAPTER 5

DYNAMICS OF MOVEMENTS[1]

DYNAMICS OF THE GREAT MOVEMENTS

Table 5.1 Five heavens and correspondences

Heavens	Azure Dragon		Red Vermilion Bird		Yellow Dragon		White Tiger		Dark Warrior	
	Wood Heaven		Fire Heaven		Earth Heaven		Metal Heaven		Water Heaven	
Planets	Jupiter		Mars		Saturn		Venus		Mercury	
GM	1 Earth +	2 Metal −	3 Water +	4 Wood −	5 Fire +	6 Earth −	7 Metal +	8 Water −	9 Wood +	10 Fire −
HS	*Jia*	*Yi*	*Bing*	*Ding*	*Wu*	*Ji*	*Geng*	*Xin*	*Ren*	*Gui*
Years ending with	...4	...5	...6	...7	...8	...9	...0	...1	...2	...3
Phases	Wood		Fire		Earth		Metal		Water	
Organs	Gb	Liv	S.i.	Ht	St	Sp	L.i.	Lu	Bl	Ki

The five heavens and five planets are expressed in forces known as five movements. The yin and yang manifestations of these five movements give rise to the ten great movements that dynamize ten heavenly stems. The dynamics between these forces determine the rhythm of developments in nature, of which humans are a part. It may seem to us that the *qi* of humans is independent of the *qi* of the earth and nature, but this is far from the truth. We are an intrinsic part of the energetic field of the earth, through which we resonate and participate with the frequencies of the different great movements. The *qi* of the five heavens and planets, ten great movements and ten heavenly stems are in constant motion

---

1   Like the five *shen*, the great movements and heavenly stems are pretty weighty topics because of their connection to the subtle world.

and interaction, working together to create the right conditions for growth and development.

Each time period of a particular year, month, day and hour is defined by a combination of a great movement and a heavenly stem.

An example: the year 2021

- The heavenly stem is *Xin*, the organ lung, the great movement water. This is written in short: '*Xin*, lung in water'.
- The white tiger heaven gives rise to the heavenly stem *Xin* which relates to metal and lung.
- The dark warrior heaven gives rise to the great movement water that dynamizes the heavenly stem *Xin*.

The great movements influence atmospheric forces and the development of the climate. Each year has its own individual climatic colouring that can be considered normal for that particular year. Great movements are called great because they define and determine all cycles on earth and in humans, making the great movement of the date of birth one of the most important.

Since they describe every development on earth, we can conclude that the development of people, their temperament, behaviour and typology, like any other developmental cycle, is determined by the great movements. The interconnection and balance between the great movement and heavenly stem determine the qualities and characteristics, strengths and weaknesses in the physical, emotional, mental and spiritual realms of a person and thus determine health and disease.

Dynamics of active and passive great movements and the effect on the five phases

The sequence of the five heavens starts with the eastern heaven which is associated with wood. The eastern heaven represents the vital *qi* that arises from an organized, integrated wholeness. The sequence of the great movements starts in the centre with the great movement earth, which marks the beginning of life on earth and receives the emanation of the unity of heaven at the centre of earthly existence. Earth is followed by the great movements metal, water, wood and fire, and each phase has its own particular role and place in the cycle.

The first great movement earth dominates years ending with 4, such as 2004, followed by the great movement metal dominating the years ending with 5, water 6, wood 7 and fire 8, for instance the years 2005, 2006, 2007, 2008 respectively. The first five great movements then repeat themselves to complete the number of ten great movements. Years ending on 9 belong again to great movement earth, 0 to metal, and so on.

The odd numbered great movements are considered yang and active, the even numbered yin and passive: Therefore, the first great movement earth is yang and active, the second great movement metal yin and passive, the third water yang and active and so on,[2] with each great movement having an active phase and a passive phase, always in a rhythm of five years apart.

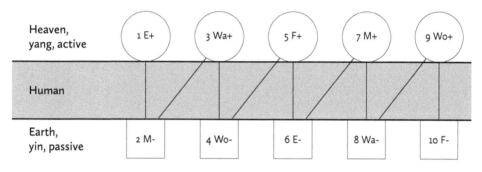

Figure 5.1 Active and passive great movements

When the master of the year is excessive it will invade the element which it can subjugate and at the same time insult the *qi* by which it should be controlled itself. When the master of the year is deficient, it will not be victorious itself, it will be insulted by the subduing element. When the master is victorious itself, it will only be lightly insulted.[3]

This quote clarifies a number of things: Every year is dominated by a great movement that can lean towards activity or passivity and is being influenced by other great movements.

When the great movement earth is active (first great movement, e.g. 2004), this activity tends to subdue the great movement water via the *ke*-cycle.[4] This

---

2   This concerns the number order of the great movements and not the ending numbers of years.

3   *Huang Di Nei Jing Su Wen* Chapter 67; the topic of insufficient and excess great movements is discussed in detail in Chapters 66, 67 and 69 of the *Huang Di Nei Jing Su Wen*. The classics use the words insufficient and excessive; this book instead uses passive and active to emphasize more or less action. Excess and insufficiency describe the surplus or deficient amount of *qi* of the great movements.

4   The *ke*-cycle (relationship grandmother–grandchild, e.g. wood controls earth) is known as the destroying cycle or controlling cycle. In our language both terms may have a negative meaning, but to maintain healthy development, this protection of limits of the five phases by the *ke*-cycle is necessary and indispensable for the correct order and containment of the five phases. Together with the *sheng*-cycle (generating or nourishing cycle, relationship mother–child, e.g. fire nourishes earth), the *ke*-cycle ensures a healthy balance between the five phases.

can lead to insufficiency of water in general and of the kidney *qi* especially, because the *ke*-cycle operates from yang to yin and vice versa. Climatologically it may lead to more moisture and rain. In addition, the great movement earth tends to deny or insult the great movement wood, which in turn affects the amount and quality of wind and growth in general.

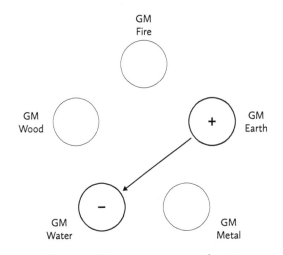

Figure 5.2 Great movement earth active

When the great movement earth is insufficient (sixth great movement, e.g. 2009), the great movement wood and especially the *qi* of gallbladder and liver become stronger. The great movement wood then tends to subdue the great movement earth even further. This leads to more wind, and plants flower but bear less fruit. The other great movements follow an identical relative pattern, depending on their active or passive character.

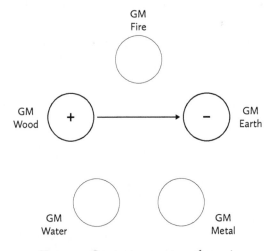

Figure 5.3 Great movement earth passive

Table 5.2 Active and passive great movements and climatic effects on *wuxing*

	Great Movement	Active / Passive	'Climate'	Years Ending With[5]
1	Earth	Active	Excess Damp, Subdues Water	4
2	Metal	Passive	More Heat and Fire	5
3	Water	Active	Excess Cold, Subdues Fire	6
4	Wood	Passive	More Dryness and Metal	7
5	Fire	Active	Excess Heat, Subdues Metal	8
6	Earth	Passive	More Wind and Wood	9
7	Metal	Active	Excess Dryness, Subdues Wood	0
8	Water	Passive	More Damp and Earth	1
9	Wood	Active	Excess Wind, Subdues Earth	2
10	Fire	Passive	More Cold and Water	3

Each year has a different nature according to the great movement that domi-nates that particular year.

For example, a year dominated by the active great movement water (e.g. 2016 or 2026) tends to subdue the great movement fire (*ke*-cycle). In such a year, it would be normal for the *qi* of water to be clearly present while the *qi* of fire is not developing sufficiently. A cooler and wetter climate can be expected.[6]

For the channel system, it means that the *qi* of water and the kidneys tend to be more active and the *qi* of fire, particularly the *qi* of the heart, is subdued and tends to become passive and insufficient.

An *innate* tendency for the great movement water to be active and stronger and the great movement fire to be passive and weaker is present in people born in years with an active great movement water, e.g. 1956, and people born in years with a passive great movement fire, e.g. 1963. These people should take good care of the heart *qi* in years like 2016 and 2026. These years challenge the *qi* of the heart in all layers of its existence, such as heart-*shen*, senses, blood, love, joy, happiness, intimacy, eyes, communication, sleep and so on.

In the same manner, we can apply this concept to past problems, accidents or illnesses of our patients by comparing the great movement of that particular year/time/moment with the great movement that dominates the year of birth.

---

5   See the 'Important Note' section in Chapter 2.
6   These 'deviations' in the climate are not called pathological or perverse *qi*. They are called excess *qi* when characteristics of the year are abundant and powerful and are called insufficient when the characteristics are scarce and weak. Pathological or perverse is *qi* that is unexpected and misplaced for that year.

What happened in the past does then not seem so coincidental but fits into the relationship between the energetic configuration of the moment and the personal birth chart.

The great movements define all cycles on earth and in humans

To clarify the dynamics, we continue to use the example 1956, active great movement water and passive great movement fire: The active great movement water not only affects the kidneys and bladder, but all *qi* that relates to water, such as the *jin yé*, the division *tai yang*, the gallbladder and *san jiao*. The passive great movement fire can affect the heart, small intestine, *san jiao* and heart constrictor, as well as the divisions *shao yang*, *shao yin* and spleen.[7] Strong active great movement water and weak passive great movement fire may result in kidney overactivity, leading to strong willpower or strong sexual desire along with insomnia, panic attacks or confusion of the mind. The passive great movement fire might lead to reactive excess of fluids, more oedema, cysts or reduced abundance of rising *qi* which can cause low blood pressure.

Developmental stages

Great movements have an important role in developmental stages, regardless of the date of birth. For example, the great movement earth is important for processes of identification, individuation and emancipation. During the early years of life, it controls strong physical growth and first development of self-preservation. It has a very important function during puberty, when children desire to become more independent of their parents. The great movement earth is involved in every identity issue and needs to be supported in people who cannot persevere, who are said to have no backbone.

The great movement metal is important in periods when people need structure. This is meant metaphorically and also literally, for example when bones need to become firmer.[8] The great movement metal is involved in turning inward for self-development and self-knowledge or showing an interest in psycho-emotional bodywork.

The great movement water is involved in the development of sexuality and gender, authenticity and in finding a purpose in life.

The great movement wood is involved in the development of individual

---

7   See the chapters in this book on the earthly branches.
8   The bones are controlled by the kidneys, which, as we will see later in the chapters on earthly branches, are connected to metal. Bone growth in childhood or after fractures is controlled from the heart and the heart constrictor and spleen: Heaven (fire) creates earth (spleen) which creates humans (kidneys). The white colour of bones and the solidity of the inner structure of bones are controlled by metal.

independent actions of the ego, along with the sense of freedom of movement and the development of assertiveness.

The great movement fire is active in the developmental stages in which feelings of intimacy and relationships are developed.

It should be noted that, depending on the dynamics between the energetic configuration of a person's birth chart and stages of development, some stages of development can be easier, while other stages of development can be a challenge.

> A female patient, born in 1942 (active great movement wood), experiences serious identity problems in 2019 along with lack of sleep and exhaustion, digestive issues and pains all over her body. In this case, the innate tendency of the active great movement wood to become excessive subdues the great movement earth. This pattern was emphasized in 2019 (passive great movement earth), which resulted in an even stronger great movement wood subduing the passive great movement earth easily. This was exacerbated by her behaviour as well as circumstances, but everything together reinforced her innate tendencies and contributed to the identity crisis. It would have been possible to treat all symptoms separately, but using a constitutional approach by treating and balancing the great movements helped her to be free of the symptoms.[9]

Summary

- Date of birth defines strengths, weaknesses and tendencies (constitutional *qi*).
- The *qi* configurations of the past, current or future dates combined with the date of birth provide insight into the influence of the prevailing *qi* on the constitutional *qi*.
- Apart from governing/defining time periods of year, month, day and hour, great movements also govern/define/influence periods and stages of personal development.

DYNAMICS OF HOST AND GUEST MOVEMENTS

Five elements take turns and each element will have ruled once towards the end of the fifth year, and so, the process will start from the very beginning within a cycle. Atmospheric forces spread according to the four seasons already

---

9   The treatment principles are discussed in Chapter 17.

established. This goes on like a ring with neither beginning nor end. The same applies to each quinate period.[10]

The 10,000 things come into existence through the transformation of *yuan qi*, the five movements define the entire heaven.[11]

Table 5.3 Relationship of guest to host movements

Years with Great Movement Earth (active and passive[12])					
Unfavourable destroying relation	20–1	03–04	15–06	27–08	08–11
Guest movement	Earth	Metal	Water	Wood	Fire
Host movement	Spring/ wood	Summer/ fire	Late summer/ earth	Autumn/ metal	Winter/ water

Years with Great Movement Metal (active and passive)					
Favourable destroying relation	20–1	03–04	15–06	27–08	08–11
Guest movement	Metal	Water	Wood	Fire	Earth
Host movement	Spring/ wood	Summer/ fire	Late summer/ earth	Autumn/ metal	Winter/ water

Years with Great Movement Water (active and passive)					
Favourable generating relation	20–1	03–04	15–06	27–08	08–11
Guest movement	Water	Wood	Fire	Earth	Metal
Host movement	Spring/ wood	Summer/ fire	Late summer/ earth	Autumn/ metal	Winter/ water

Years with Great Movement Wood (active and passive)					
Equal relation	20–1	03–04	15–06	27–08	08–11
Guest movement	Wood	Fire	Earth	Metal	Water
Host movement	Spring/ wood	Summer/ fire	Late summer/ earth	Autumn/ metal	Winter/ water

---

10 *Huang Di Nei Jing Su Wen* Chapter 9.
11 *Huang Di Nei Jing Su Wen* Chapter 66.
12 Active means that the influences are more active and come sooner in contrast to the passive great movements.

Years with Great Movement Fire (active and passive)					
Unfavourable generating relation	20–1	03–04	15–06	27–08	08–11
Guest movement	Fire	Earth	Metal	Water	Wood
Host movement	Spring/ wood	Summer/ fire	Late summer/ earth	Autumn/ metal	Winter/ water

Host movements

The great movements determine all cycles on earth and in humans, including the cycle of the seasons. The five great movements are reflected in the five seasons: spring, summer, late summer, autumn and winter. The seasons are called host movements because the rhythm, sequence and qualities and expression of the seasons are more or less stable.

Guest movements

'Normal' deviations from the five seasons/host movements are determined by the great movement of a specific year. This is because the great movement of the year defines the first guest movement that visits the first host movement. The guest affects the host, just as the host in a house is affected by the different energies of their guests. As a result, the seasons differ from each other each year. The spring can be colder, the summer wetter, the autumn can last longer or the winter can be windier than normal. The question is justified, whether these seasonal fluctuations are pathological. Constitutional acupuncture defines pathological or perverse *qi* as *qi* that cannot be expected based on the forces in the Chinese calendar. The colouration of the five seasons in a given year is determined by the five guest movements.

The first guest movement in a year dominated by a great movement earth is earth. The first guest movement in a year dominated by a great movement metal is metal, followed by water, wood, fire and earth.

The sequence of the guest movements, attuned to the great movement of the year, develop in parallel and in the same order as the host movements, but change from year to year because the cycle of the guest movements in a new year always begins with a movement corresponding to the great movement of that year.

As a result, the guest movements influence and modify the 'normal' characteristics of the seasons. The nature of these changes is determined by the relationship between guest and host movements.

Unfavourable destroyer[13]

In years that end with 4 and 9, the great movement and consequently the first guest movement are both earth. The relationship between guest and host movements is called unfavourable destroyer due to the reverse *ke*-cycle relationship. For example, in the first period the guest movement earth affects the host movement wood of spring. It is to be expected that the seasons develop with powerful climatic tensions. Strong seasonal deviations such as periods of prolonged heat or rain, cold or the like are to be expected during these years. This is considered normal and not pathological or perverse *qi*. In fact, the system is expected to be challenged rather than remain untouched during those years.

People born in years with an unfavourable destroying relationship of the five seasons often seem to need times of great tension and dramatic happenings in order to develop and learn. In this way, they seem to achieve true inner transformation.[14]

Favourable destroyer

In years ending with 5 and 0, the great movement and consequently the first guest movement are both metal. The relationship between guest and host movements is called favourable destroying due to its *ke*-cycle relationship. The seasons are out of balance due to the impairment of cosmic influences. The effect of a favourable destroyer relationship is comparable to the unfavourable relationship, but less intense.

People born in years with a favourable destroying relationship of the five seasons can cope well with stress. During stressful times they show their strength and individuality, which makes them act stubbornly, relying on their

---

13   In the classics other names may be used: Unfavourable destroyer = Disagreement; Favourable destroyer = Celestial form; Favourable generator = Favourable transformation; Equal = Celestial concordance; Unfavourable generator = Small opposition.

14   This and subsequent texts on the relationship between seasons, date of birth and emotional–mental development were not described in the classics, but are the result of years of observations in clinic. It is not about whether my observations are complete and always recognizable. You may have other observations. Understanding the impact of the relationships of the host and guest movements on human *qi* may help us understand and treat others better. Discovering this phenomenon was an eye-opener for me. I became softer and more humble. These characteristics of both host and guest movements will be active all year round from 20 January onwards. However, a nuance must be made. While the general relationships between the guest and host movements are relevant for the entire year, each one of the five seasons will have its own particular quality due to the different *qi* involved. For example, a year ending with 4 is characterized by an unfavourable destroyer relationship. In the spring, the guest–host movement relationship will be earth subduing wood, which will have a different quality and effect than in autumn, when water is subduing earth. Therefore the quality of the unfavourable destroyer relationship will be different for people born in the spring season to people born in the autumn season. It is beyond the scope of this book to go into this subject in detail, but I am convinced that, through vigilance and research, you will notice the differences over time.

own understanding, intelligence and self-confidence. They prefer to focus on cosmic influences and abstract areas, such as religion, philosophies, inner understanding of life, mathematics and so on, as long as it serves earthly practicalities and does not become too vague and woolly. They are used to inner conflicts and may seem calm on the outside, yet have a strong and turbulent inner life.

Favourable generator

In years that end with 6 and 1, the great movement and consequently the first guest movement are both water. The relationship between guest and host movements is called favourable generating due to its *sheng*-cycle relationship. It is expected that the climate will develop harmoniously and that the seasons will naturally flow into each other. Strong and long-lasting deviations from the normal development of the seasons are of a pathological nature. For example, if spring is too dry or too warm for a longer period of time, this will lead to immediate complaints and illnesses in people with a weak condition. Stronger people are more likely to fall ill some weeks or months later. Whether they are considered strong or weak depends on the quality of their *jing* and *wei qi* as well as the strengths and weaknesses of the *qi* in their birth chart.

People born in a year with a favourable generating relationship of the five seasons are accustomed to feeling balanced and nourished. Even when they feel overwhelmed by difficult circumstances, their deepest emotional layer remains harmonious and stable. They can recover through their own efforts or know when and who to ask for help. In times of stress, it helps them to be encouraged to recognize this.

Equal

In years ending with 7 and 2, the great movement and consequently the first guest movement are both wood. The relationship between guest and host movements is called equal. The seasons are expected to develop smoothly without any resistances. However, if too many equal *qi* are present, it can lead to excess or stagnation, depending on the nature of the *qi*. For example, too much earth easily leads to more moisture, rain and stagnation and too much fire to abundant heat, rising *qi* and so on. Prolonged deviation from the normal pattern of development, for example if rain or heat lasts too long, is considered pathological *qi*.

People born in a year of equal *qi* of the five seasons seek stimulation and challenge. They get bored quickly when there is a lot of routine and not enough 'spice'. These people like rhythm and habit, but greatly appreciate a certain freedom within the restriction of habits.

Unfavourable generator

In years ending with 8 and 3, the great movement and consequently the first guest movement are both fire. The relationship between guest and host movements is called unfavourable generating due to its reverse *sheng* relationship. The seasons are expected to develop with a certain resistance. Earthly developments will be determined by cosmic influences, which may result in obstructions in the development of seasons with critical intensities. This is considered normal. The influence of the sun, moon, star constellations and climatic changes are felt more intensely.

For people born in years of an unfavourable generating relationship of the five seasons, it is normal to take time to digest. Life is experienced as a resistance that has to be dealt with. These people are used to the way in which they can develop through feeling and dealing with resistances. Reassuring them that these resistances are expected challenges gives them peace of mind. They gradually might learn that time is their friend. As they develop trust in the power of time, they learn to build confidence to do what feels right to them. Once decided, they wholeheartedly follow their decision.

CHAPTER 6

DYNAMICS OF THE GREAT MOVEMENT EARTH[1]

Studying mysticism is studying the self;
and studying the self is forgetting the self;
forgetting the self is being one,
enlightened by all things.[2]

Heaven and earth exist in the subtle world of ideas as opposed to the dense world of phenomena which we can directly observe and investigate scientifically. Heaven is the image of the eternal creative principle and earth of the ever nourishing. They are eternal principles, without birth or death, with neither beginning nor end.

Heaven is eternal and earth is lasting
How can they be eternal and lasting?
Because they do not live for themselves
That is how they can be eternal[3]

These subtle essential principles cannot be perceived directly by the human senses. It is through the heart-*shen* – the intermediary between the subtle and dense worlds – that humans can perceive the subtle vibrations of heaven and earth. Manifested, phenomenal forms such as the planets, stars, moon, sun and earth are emanated reflections of the original essences.

---

1   Born in years ending with a 4 and 9 like 1994 and 1959, after the Chinese New Year.
2   My mother Sjoe.
3   *Dao De Jing* Chapter 7.

EARTH

So, what is the significance of earth?

If heaven represents the blue sky, earth is the planet earth. If heaven is repre-sented in the manifestation of all yang, as the subtle cosmic *qi*, earth represents the manifestation of yin, as the physical denser substances within the totality of the universe. If heaven is time, earth is space. If heaven is represented by the sun and stars, earth represents the moon and planets. How do we translate these immense concepts of the yin and yang of the cosmos into our observable and treatable reality?

THE FLOW OF THE FIVE SEASONS/HOST MOVEMENTS IN ONE YEAR PROGRESSES THROUGH TIME AND GENERATES SPACE

The five movements are called *wuxing* – literally meaning five movements:[4] wood, fire, earth, metal and water. Wood occupies the East and reigns over the *qi* of spring, fire occupies the South and reigns over the *qi* of the summer, metal occupies the West and reigns over the *qi* of autumn and water occupies the North and reigns over the *qi* of the winter.

Wood governs birth and first growth, fire blossoming and heat, metal decay, constriction and dryness and water death, storage and cold. The earth occupies the centre between the other four phases, serving as a landing area for the emanated bright light of heaven. It thus forms the stable platform upon which the subtle and denser manifestations of the other four phases can unfold. Following this concept, the earth receives and responds to heaven and creates the conditions for the developments of the other four movements.

In the fivefold cycle of the great movements, earth is placed between the two yang movements of wood and fire and the two yin movements of metal and water. Yin and yang meet in the great movement earth, showing respect and support to heaven and earth to guide all other movements through inte-gration, fertilization and transformation. Nourishing, nurturing, receiving and responding are all expressions of earth. In the cycle of the five movements earth is nourished by fire and nourishes metal.

---

4   *Wuxing* is often translated as five phases or five elements. *Wu* 五 means five. The character depicts the interaction of yin and yang. There is also an earlier character depicting four sides and a centre. The character *Xing* 行 means movement or phase. *Wuxing* depicts the flow of life between heaven and earth. Heaven is yang, earth is yin, the five 'moving stars' or planets move between heaven and earth: Jupiter for wood, Mars for fire, Saturn for earth, Venus for metal and Mercury for water. The flow of life on earth expresses itself according to the movements in heaven.

According to the creative principle, heaven creates earth which generates humans and humanity. The water of the earth receives, the fire of the earth generates. In other words, heaven is being received by the yin of earth, the yang of earth generates humans and humanity. The fusion of water/yin and fire/yang within earth creates moisture which is needed to transform heavenly *qi* and attune it to the level of human consciousness and physicality. Moisture is the medium through which latent heavenly forces can be transformed into concrete, physical reality and transformed into *qi* of the (meridian) channel system. People receive and respond to input from heaven, nature and food that is then transformed by the yin and yang of the earth.

After creation has taken place, humans/humanity stand(s) between heaven above and earth below. Heaven and earth represent yin and yang, above and below, superior and inferior, outside and inside. Humanity is influenced by heaven and earth and responds to its experiences of these. We must endure and reap the benefits of the energetic dance between yin and yang and ideally avoid conflict with heaven and earth. In a sense, humanity is in the centre of opposing and cooperating forces and has the opportunity to learn to recognize these very forces within and to use them for the individual and collective good through love and wisdom, with the aim of reunification and togetherness, the attributes of heaven and earth.

FIVE GREAT MOVEMENTS AND THE *WU-SHEN*

Although the *Huang Di Nei Jing Su Wen* describes climatic and seasonal influences only, we previously discussed the influence of the five great movements on developmental stages such as personal development of the ego, behaviour, and physical and psychological growth of children and adults. The movements, in combination with the heavenly stems, operate between the subtle realm of heaven and the denser realm of earth, physicality, *qi* and *xuè*. This hinge between heaven and earth is comparable to the influence of the *wu-shen*, which, among other properties, transform the subtle reality of heaven into expressions of the concrete physical existence of the earth and humanity.

Unbalanced, disturbed great movements go hand in hand with problems in the expression of the various *wu-shen*. Treatments therefore must focus on both the great movements and the *wu-shen*.

The translation of *shen* as 'spirit' is problematic, because spirit means something different in Western culture than in Eastern culture. In the West, the spirit has a Christian/religious connotation, which indicates a religious attitude and personal experience of it. Spirit is opposite to the physical material world. In

Eastern thought, there is no opposition of spirit and matter. Instead of separation there is unity between the two. Spirit and matter are the different sides of the same coin, like yin and yang. Yang is more subtle and lighter; yin is denser and heavier. It is wonderful when these thoughts are recognizable to everyone but, because spirit has a certain religious meaning, I have chosen not to translate the word *shen*. The *wu-shen* are the heart-*shen*, *hun*, *po*, *yi* and *zhi*.

The *shen* of the earth: *Yi,* intent and purpose

The *yi* is the *shen* associated with the spleen. It processes, harmonizes, transforms, integrates and transports *qi* in order to exchange it with the self and the environment. Its qualities are expressed in intellect, learned memory, ideas, imagining, opinions, cognitive mind, conceptual thinking, mental work, processing, integration, 'digestion', transformation, consciousness, ability to focus and pay attention, implementing thoughts and so on.

A stagnant *yi* means that people have difficulty processing information. It results in poor memory and slow thinking, producing *ying qi xu* first and finally heart-*shen qi xu*.

An insufficient *yi* leads to distraction and difficulty concentrating, resulting in a lack of empathy and sympathy. These people find it difficult to give and/or receive.

Yi stagnation and insufficiency are common in children who are overloaded with intellectual knowledge and lack creative stimulation and playfulness. Treatment of the *yi* alone is insufficient if their capacity for creativity and playfulness are not addressed at the same time.

Excessive *yi* is associated with obsession for the past. It physically leads to decreased blood flow and clotting due to blood stagnation.

The most important point to treat *yi* issues is Bl-49, *Yi She*. It stimulates memory and concentration and restores the emotional and mental purpose of life. It can be used in cases where people are stubborn, obsessive and unable to be receptive. St-40, *Feng Long* and Sp-3, *Tai Bai* are used when people feel foggy in their head due to *yi* issues.

The *qi* of the small intestine, specifically the duodenum,[5] also belong to the *yi*. Discerning food and dividing it into pure and impure, useful and useless, is the first stage of processing information in the broadest sense of the word. It can be influenced by treating acupuncture points on the small intestine, the stomach and *ren mai* channels, e.g. St-21, *Liang Men*, St-36, *Zu San Li*, St-39, *Xia Ju Xu* and Cv-13, *Shang Wan*, Cv-12, *Zhong Wan* and Cv-10, *Xia Wan*.

---

5   The duodenum is governed by the stomach *qi*.

The heart and *yi*

The Chinese character for *yi* 意 consists of two parts. The lower part is the radical for the heart, the upper part radical means sounds or musical note. It means that intentions and purposes are directed by and vibrate from the heart. *Yi* is the vibrating intention of the heart that expresses itself in all movements, behaviour and speech. The heart acknowledges the vibration as being part of its own nature and sings the song of the self. Consciously cultivating a harmoniously attuned song of the self is a choice that we can all freely enter into. Healthy communication from the essence of the self in an open connection with others requires a balanced function of *yi* in alignment with the heart.

Lack of guidance and nourishment from the heart manifests in a single-minded focus on intellectuality as dogma and strong ego-oriented activities.[6] In those cases, the heart should be treated first. The main points are Bl-44, *Shen Tang*, Ht-7, *Shen Men*, Ht-6, *Yin Xi*, Ht-5, *Tong Li*, especially when the *yi* insufficiency comes with anxiety, insomnia, depression and/or heartbreak (also where there is blood deficiency/*xuè xu*).

> The Heart holds the office of Lord and sovereign. The radiance of the spirits (*shenming*) stems from it.[7]

The heart is the sovereign of the centre, the ruler of the Forbidden City with the authority to govern information from all the sense organs. With the help of its servants, such as the *yi*, the heart constrictor, blood and channel system, the sovereign responds and radiates to every part of the body and beyond, where it, together with the *yi*, nourishes and nurtures.

The essence of the *yi* is expressed in intuitive thinking and feeling, which has a wider meaning than mental thinking and emotional behaviour. It imparts virtue, dedication, engagement, empathy, sympathy and creative thinking. It is a unified whole that shows itself as the connecting *qi* that moves from the heart to every part of its empire (the body) to align every movement, thought, emotion, speech or action with the authentic self. The *qi* of the heart and *yi* reach out and report back to the heart and the inner self so the heart-*shen* and body can come into unity.

In Chinese medicine the earth is associated with thinking and intellect. The more one focuses solely on intellect and acquiring knowledge, without the use of intuition and intelligence, the more this leads to blockages and chaos. First, this occurs in the *qi* and organs related to the earth and subsequently in all other *qi*,

---

6   J.D. van Buren has often stated that this imbalance of the *yi* can be a cause of cancer due to a reverse flow of *qi* from the spleen to the heart resulting in a chronic stagnation of earth.

7   *Huang Di Nei Jing Su Wen* Chapter 8.

because healthy earth is necessary for all transformative processes in the body. Therefore stagnation of the earth affects the whole body. Blockages and chaos arise from a lack of flow, lack of integration, insufficient transformation arising from an underactive uninspired foundation within the heart.

A healthy interaction between the great movements fire and earth is a prerequisite for the correct functioning of earth and the *yi*. Together they lead to intuitive thinking and belonging, which in turn lead to spontaneity, originality, creativity and unique and independent self as an expression of heaven.

> When something takes charge of the beings, we speak of the Heart.
> When the Heart applies itself, we speak of Intent.
> When the Intent becomes permanent, we speak of Will ...[8]

The heart is the covenant with the self. The door to this promise is opened by full interest, dedication, integrity and surrender, which leads to integration of information and action. However, there is a danger that a person inflates the ego and strives for worldly honour only, becoming entangled in desires whereby the quintessence of the heart is lost.

IDENTITY

The great movement earth is the landing area for the light of heaven and the heavenly mandate. It is the vital centre that harmonizes, integrates, fertilizes and transforms the cycle of seasons in nature and the developmental stages of the body and psyche in humans. The heavenly mandate is causal and authentic and manifests itself in inner and outer values of the self in relation to the ego, society, colleagues, acquaintances, peers, work and so on. The self is the bridge connecting the origin of the essence of life with its expression into the world. The mandate and the self, with their innate and acquired abilities in addition to one's own experiences and interpretations, make each person unique. In essence, each human being has this unique pre-natal heavenly energetic network that is separate from the movements of the ego, and it is this aspect that is addressed as the self-healing ability. This makes a healthy balance of the active great movement earth an important factor in finding health.

The passive great movement earth is responsible for perceiving and understanding the influence of personal and social identity on the self and society.

---

8   *Ling Shu* Chapter 8, my notes from a class with (Father) Claude Larre.

The self respects and supports interaction and reflection with heaven when the great movement earth is in balance. People can then act with virtue. The passive great movement earth has a receiving, yin character. People with this energy in balance are able to receive and respond with care and like to serve, even when they are extrovert in behaviour. The passive great movement earth is more balanced if it remains responsive instead of taking too much initiative. This also applies to the active great movement. The well-balanced great movement earth results in social connectedness and a firm sense of belonging.

To be content with what you have and what you are
Guards against confusion.
To cease with sufficiency avoids exhaustion
Those who practice 'contentment and sufficiency' long endure.[9]

BELONGING AND BECOMING

The healthy path of belonging is to be taken with great attention, dedication and awareness, *without* focusing on a goal. It gives the feeling that things 'happen' automatically and effortlessly and develop naturally. With belonging, there is no desire, no becoming, only a direction is outlined. Due to attentive involvement and awareness in the process of development, this path is an experience of unity and is only possible with little use of willpower and personal interventions.

A balanced great movement earth means that the activity, the path and the goal are implicitly connected in unity. People feel integrated in themselves and in society, authentic, loyal to their own temperament, character and identity. They are drawn to processing information that can serve as a guide to experiencing the world in a coherent way. The great movement earth is disturbed through selfishness, self-centredness or personal and socially motivated intentions. Modern society is full of these motives, such as greed, possessiveness, the need to keep everything under control, maintaining grudges, the desire to have contact with everyone through social media and so on. This means that the great movement earth is easily out of balance and health seems in these times hardly possible.

A TYPICAL CASE

Mrs A has a persistent headache that comes from the neck, especially aggravated when she wakes up early. The neck feels tight, the head feels as if there

---

9   *Dao De Jing* Chapter 44 (Ming 2016).

is a blanket over it. In addition, she frequently experiences a mild autumn depression.

She has had a good, fulfilling job for many years, but would like to change jobs. The routine of her current job no longer presents enough challenges. She is capable of hard work and has strong willpower to succeed in any project she embarks upon. She is a team player at work and also takes care of three teenagers. She regularly has job interviews but is always being rejected. She thinks that's fine because she didn't find the jobs very interesting anyway. When I ask what kind of job she is looking for, she comes up with suggestions based on what her friends and family expect of her and what she can offer to others. When asking what she really wants, she looks at me in surprise. She doesn't know ... 'I've never thought about that.'

Her life is completely dedicated to serving her partner, children, employees, customers, parents and friends. She had no idea what she could do for herself. For that reason, she only looked at jobs she already knew, without considering where she belonged.

First treatment principle: Strengthen and balance the great movement earth.

After a few treatments, she found a new job and her pain and depression disappeared.

THE CHALLENGES

In a mystical sense, solving a great movement earth imbalance is the greatest challenge in life we will ever face: being whole and dissolving the experience of separation. This means that the power of desire needs to be reduced. Desires, thoughts and experiences are stimuli to achieve distant goals and pull us away from the essence of the self. With the sense of belonging, the ego is still active, but engages with what is present, rather than what may be desired. The secret to this challenge is to be aware of the path that is unfolding instead of reaching for the distant goal of wholeness.

Because of the relationship between earth and heaven, earth possesses creative qualities and offers people the opportunity to live, nourish themselves and others well, and communicate with people with a sense of freedom.

People born with the active great movement earth like to initiate and be part of what is initiated. They have a strong sense of 'I am'. Their decisiveness might make them impatient to wait for the right time and the right circumstances. They like to take on responsibility, serve and care for others, unfortunately sometimes without even tuning in to whether people want to be helped. They may suffer from a desire to stay in control. People born with the passive great movement earth have similar characteristics, but from a yin perspective, usually with a more wait-and-see and responsive attitude. Insecurity can cause them to withdraw inwardly, or they can cover up negative feelings and display modified behaviour or overpositioning.

The great movement earth enables one to work hard without getting tired. People may find it unbearable to be sick. They often mistake illness for failure. If they cannot resolve the disease themselves quickly, this often leads to (medical) intervention. As an unfortunate result, they may lose contact with their inner strength and become increasingly dependent on the care of doctors, therapists and medicines, and lose touch with their hearts even more. Because of the preference to intellectualize (yi) rather than listen to their feelings and the implications of this behaviour, treatment and focus on the intuition of the heart may lead to sudden healing.

SHORT- AND LONG-TERM SOLUTIONS

People use short-term solutions to quickly fuel a weaker active or passive great movement. These solutions seem to work fast, but in the long run deplete the qi of this weak great movement. Sugar is a well-known short-term solution for fatigue due to a sugar dip. People feel better quickly, but the dip is even deeper shortly after. The long-term solutions for sugar dips are more beneficial: for example vegetables, nuts or unsweetened cottage cheese. The qi builds up slowly but for a longer period of time, but this approach does require more discipline and perseverance.

When people suffer from illness and seek advice and treatment, it is important to get to know and understand their short-term solution behaviour. The dynamics of the birth chart may often be the cause of weakness of great movements. For instance, people born in 1974 are affected by an active great movement earth in the birth chart. There is a tendency that this active great movement subdues the great movement water, which then leads to water short-term solution behaviour when the great movement water becomes too weak. The innate weaker great movement water is easier to treat compared to the person's pursuit of great movement earth short-term solutions, because the earth active great movement is one of the stronger innate aspects of the birth chart. It takes longer to cure people who show weakness and imbalances in their own constitutionally strong aspects.

People may also show short-term solution behaviour unrelated to the birth chart. This may be caused by trauma, surgery, environmental and social problems or hereditary circumstances. Treatments targeting the great movements make the transition to long-term solutions easier for patients, but they should be reminded and guided.

Short-term solutions for balancing the great movement earth:

- too much attention to nutrition
- too much sugar or other refined carbohydrates
- relying on approval and sympathy, as well as being competitive; this strengthens and supports the ego in the short term, but nothing could be further from the truth in the longer term
- demanding attention and reaction; people with a weakened great movement earth may feel increasingly weaker and insecure inwardly, to the extent that they start to doubt themselves. The more this happens, the more they may seek approval. In order to become aware of a sense of 'I am', they become opinionated, critical or place themselves in a victim role. Unfortunately, confirmation by opposition or victimization seem to be the only ways to confirm the right to exist. It is the responsibility of the practitioner to observe this behaviour and see it as a signpost for treatment of the weakened great movement earth.

Long-term solutions for balancing the great movement earth:

- especially the positive development of a stronger identity and individuality without feeling the need to inflate the ego. This requires positive affirmations along with an open learning attitude and being able to take responsibility with commitment and patience. The basic idea is openness to reflect, positivity and the willingness to change if necessary
- the above qualities go hand in hand with a wish to serve others with empathy and the willingness to give up the expectation that one should always feel good and happy in order to experience a compassionate connection in togetherness.

When the great movement earth is weakened, it leads to symptoms and diseases such as headache with a heavy head feeling, abdominal distension, insecurity, dietary problems, blood diseases, scoliosis, chronic fatigue syndrome, cysts, stagnation of *qi* and food, sinusitis and so on.

CHAPTER 7

DYNAMICS OF THE GREAT MOVEMENT METAL[1]

NOURISHING AND PROTECTION

For a healthy life we need an identity, nutrition, freedom and social embedding. The metal emanating from the emanation *li* gathers the requirements to build a healthy body with solid structure, physical strength and resources (*jing qi*), and the ability to defend against dangerous, impure and vicious attacks from the outside world.[2] The ability of metal to gather the beneficial is one of the conditions which enables human beings to build up protection (*wei qi*) against pathogenic factors. When this condition is met, there is inner strength to communicate with oneself and the world in a healthy way.

The great movement metal forms the structure and substance of the physical body and thus aids the constitution and re-constitution of the *jing* and *wei qi*. The *jing* manifests itself in the nature of the physicality, nutrition of the body, the removal of waste products, and so on, where it is insurmountably dependent on the gathering function of metal.

Babies and toddlers are mainly *po* (metal). Their *jing* is built, in large part, by perceiving and receiving caring, physical touch, through which the body guarantees the safe home base of the *jing* and *po*. This builds their freedom and security, which enables healthy breathing and an open way of communicating with the world. Unfortunately, the reverse is also true: Children are neglected or blocked in their development by too much care and attention. Stronger children, in particular, have the strength to resist the limited space and freedom that some caregivers offer. This strength to resist can reveal itself through illnesses such

---

1 Born in years ending with a 5 and 0 such as 1995 and 1960, after the Chinese New Year.
2 External pathogenic factors can be caused by variations in climate, weather and seasons, but also socio-emotional impulses. They are abnormal or excessive conditions that disrupt the normal flow of *qi*.

as eczema, asthma and hyperactive behaviour. Insufficient or excessive care in childhood is of course not the only cause of these diseases/symptoms.

The gathering quality of the emanation *li* is a prerequisite for the spiritual-psychological growth of consciousness

This statement requires further explanation. What do I mean by spiritual-psychological growth and consciousness and what is the contribution of *li*?

'Spiritual' can be briefly summed up as the path of connection and strength to the source of life and consciousness or, as one of my teachers said, 'that which is good for the spirit'. 'Psychological' is anything that has to do with the mind and which affects human behaviour. Consciousness is the ability to experience and perceive; in other words, it is an awareness of the world, including yourself. Consciousness receives the echoes and imprints of experiences from within and without. Growth can generally be summed up as an increase in size, quantity and/or complexity.

Mature, spiritual-psychological growth of consciousness implies that people are able to keep themselves collected, despite the abundance of impressions from within and without, so that they remain integrated in themselves as well as with their environment. People will have achieved authenticity and simplicity because they have been able to release unnecessarily built-up psychological patterns. The function of integrating the useful by distinguishing it from the useless is indispensable for recognizing and acknowledging the influence of *qi* from within oneself and from others.

INTERACTION

The great movement metal manages the continuous movements that take place between the inner and outer world. People respond to information received by the senses, digest the just-eaten food, process air in the lungs, and so on. The great movement metal is the intrinsic part in all these processes. It means that interaction between people and the environment comes under pressure in the event of a distortion in the great movement metal.

The active yang great movement metal protects against external pathogenic or excessive incidents by utilizing information received from the senses and *wei qi*. It distinguishes information into good and bad, pathogenic and healthy. It functions by strengthening the inside and defending the body externally against outside invaders by activating the *xuè*, *jin yé*, *qi* and *wei qi*.

The passive yin great movement metal is responsive and focuses on the inner support of the body. It supports the structure of the vital elements of the body such as the bones and fascia and ensures their healthy functioning supported by the hereditary and acquired *qi*.

DYNAMIC DUALITIES

Dualities such as inner–outer, ego–environment, up–down, good–bad and so on are not only perceived through the separate forces of these entities, but precisely through the vital connections and movements between them. Inhalation, exhalation, expansion, contraction, intense and dull are some of the vital expressions of interaction. The energy exchange between dualities is always changing and never constant in nature, being a true example of the expression of life.

In relationships, each partner has his or her own position and builds the relationship through changes in intensity, attention and commitment. Dualities express their qualities of relationship through the vital flow and exchange of energy between the two poles, which is/can be influenced by receptivity, flexibility and the degree of perceiving each other and adapting to the flow of interactions perceived by both. The vitality of dualities is best reflected in the way the two communicate within the field they evoke, taking into account that the interaction and communication is never stable but flows in tides of intensity. The way people function in the field of dynamic dualities is strongly determined by the function of the great movement metal. This means that when dualities are addressed, the great movement metal should always be included as the interactive resource connecting them. The health status of the great movement metal must be explored and treated, if necessary, before treatment of dualities such as yin and yang, like and unlike *qi*,[3] ascending and descending *qi* can be embarked upon!

THE GREAT MOVEMENT METAL, *PO* AND *JING*

For communication, the great movement earth (identity) needs the great movement metal (interaction), which in turn functions in close relation to the great movement water (integration). It can be compared to the earth and the seven *po* which, together with the *jing*, form the communicative body as in body language, facial expressions and other bodily gestures, and provide the physical and physiological maintenance of the body through nourishment, waste excretion, respiration and assimilation.

The quality of actions of the great movements earth, metal and water, *yi*,

---

3   These are methods of constitutional acupuncture that will be discussed in Chapter 17.

po and *jing*, determine the psycho-physical expressions of people, such as a weaker or stronger stamina, firmer or weaker posture, flexibility, stiffness, easy or inhibited movements, transformative or stagnant development of emotions and so on. Vital for the well-being of the psyche are the relationships between these great movements and the human resources that stem from them. This is reflected in the close relationship between identity of the great movement earth with the *yi*, the exchanges with the world of great movement metal with the *po* – the animal soul, and integration and authenticity of the great movement water with the *zhi* – the will, and *jing*-essence.

The great movement metal and the *po* are both intermediaries between the perceived and the self.

ENTRIES AND EXITS

The body makes contact with and protects against the outside world in various ways. Breathing, which animates the *po*, is a superior life-giving form of exchange between an organism and its environment. The senses that perceive touch, temperature and pain, which occur as early as the second week of pregnancy and with the mouth being the first sense of touch, protect against injuries from heat or cold and so on. The senses in general are indispensable for supporting and maintaining a balanced relationship with the surrounding physical world. The nose is the gateway for the breath of life.[4] Smells easily lead to feelings of like and disgust and have a strong influence on various kinds of emotions. Smells may awake hunger or aversion, pleasant or terrible memories and may arouse sexual urges. Even though all senses report to the *shen*, the nose and the tactile sense appear to be by far the most important senses for self-perception.

The *po* stand for the seven openings in the head through which information from the environment enters, making people aware of the world, and their desires and emotions.

> *Po* is connected with the idea of brightening, for with the emotions the interior (of the personality) is governed.[5]

Emotions are reactions to impulses from the outside world and accumulated thoughts, which are unpleasant when they lead to stagnation or chaos. Emotions, even challenging ones, are experienced positively when they are accompanied by

---

4   The lungs store the breath and the breath houses the *po*. When the lungs are exhausted, the nose becomes blocked and breathing is reduced.

5   Needham 1962.

free flow or *qi*. The inner perceptions and experiences are made possible through the intervention of the seven *po* and the great movement metal.

The seven *po* are also associated with the waxing and waning of the bright white light of the moon. The changeability of the expression of the light of the moon coincides with the idea that the seven *po* control waxing and waning, growth and decline on all levels, such as the increase and decrease of emotional intelligence, the increase and decrease of spiritual-psychological growth of consciousness, the increase and decrease of mental and physical strength. Those increases and decreases can occur independently of each other. As people age, the growth of emotional intelligence, vulnerability, introspection and protection can refine and expand the mind and spirit, while, at the same time, the *po* decrease physical strength. This calls for a nuanced treatment of the different aspects of the seven *po* and the great movement metal and thus for insight into development of emotions such as worry, regret, guilt, blame, shame, anger, resentment, nervousness, jealousy, fear and so on.

ILLNESS AND RESPONSIBILITY

The Chinese character *po*, *Bai Gui*, is translated as white ghost. *Bai* means white, the radical *Gui* means ghost.

Gui (ghosts) and *po* are not the same. The entities that are attached to and stay with the earth when people die are called *po*, but might act like ghosts (*gui*).[6] *Gui* act independently and autonomously and can cause disturbances upon entry, which usually show a sudden change in behaviour. For centuries, perhaps still now, illnesses were seen as the result of *gui* entering the body, leading to the advice to eliminate pathologically perverse *qi* from the body. This view changed with the appearance of the text of *Huang Di Nei Jing Su Wen* Chapter 1:

> I am told the people in ancient times could all survive to more than one hundred years old, and they appeared to be quite healthy and strong in actions, but the people at present time are different, they are not so nimble in actions when

---

6   There are three types of ghosts (*gui*), which are all irrational, independent and self-governing: the wandering ghost, the hungry ghost and the sexual ghost. The names describe the kind of desires they want to fulfil by invading a person who allows that ghost the opportunity to do so. Wandering ghosts mostly become attached to this world after a sudden accident; they desire to find their suddenly lost home. Hungry ghosts desire to finish unfinished, often emotional issues. Sexual ghosts are attracted by people who are open for physical love and are attached to this world as a result of missing their loved ones.

they are only fifty, and what is the reason? Is it due to the change of spiritual principles or caused by the artificial behaviour of men?[7]

Qibo's answer was a major shift in thinking at that time. It was normal to investigate old scriptures of ancient times to educate people in the current times. In this chapter Qibo speaks about the people of the past and how they took on responsibility by living in accordance with nature. In the years before the *Huang Di Nei Jing Su Wen* was composed, people took much less responsibility for themselves and for their own health. During the Warring States Period,[8] the legalists tried to establish a better government by creating political and administrative structures. They were not interested in cosmology or ethics (as the Confucianists were). The will of the legislator was dominant and people were punished when they showed private opinions. This idea is echoed in the *Huang Di Nei Jing Su Wen* when it speaks of the ill *qi* that has to be expelled.

In Chapter 1 of the *Huang Di Nei Jing Su Wen*, Qibo answers with a completely different view on life, making people responsible for themselves:

> When one is completely free from wishes, ambition and distracting thoughts, indifferent to fame and gain, the true *qi* will come in the wake of it. When one concentrates his spirit internally and keeps a sound mind, how can illness occur?

Concentration of the spirit internally is determined by the power of the emanation *li*, the seven *po* and the great movement metal. They govern the interaction between people and the surrounding world by which people may manage the way of keeping good health and true *qi*.

TREATING THE *PO*[9]

The main point to treat *po* issues is Bl-42 *Po Hu*, the *po* door, door of vital fluids. It accesses the *po* very deeply, reconnecting them to the essential being, soothing the *shen*. Needling helps to rediscover the preciousness and quality of life. The reaction to treatment might be that the patient starts cleansing through all openings. This should not last longer than five days. This treatment can be supported by Bl-43 *Gao Huang Shu*, vital region *Shu*, *yu* of vital centres. It tonifies all deficient conditions and nourishes people in their autonomy from their mother figure. Other points that work on the seven *po* are Lu-1, *Zhong*

---

7   *Huang Di Nei Jing Su Wen* Chapter 1, second century BCE.
8   475–221 BCE.
9   This subject is discussed further in Chapter 19.

Fu, Lu-2, *Yun Men*, Lu-3, *Tian Fu*, Lu-7, *Lie Que*, Lu-9, *Tai Yuan*, Bl-13, *Fei Shu*, Liv-4, *Zhong Fen*.[10]

SHORT- AND LONG-TERM SOLUTIONS

Short-term solutions for balancing the great movement metal:

- the tendency to collect things, just for the sake of collecting; people may become possessive and greedy
- the tendency to define and structure things
- the need to meet people for social confirmation, e.g. showing off and talking extensively about future plans or asking lots of questions. Being refused or rejected is strongly avoided
- people quickly often justify themselves because they do not tolerate criticism easily
- the strong need for time and space for oneself at regular intervals, although insecurity sometimes makes it difficult for people to focus and temporarily shut themselves off from others. This may sometimes be offset by stubbornness, a big mouth and aggressive behaviour
- greedy for *qi*, patients leave the practitioner with an empty and tired feeling
- the strong need to feel safe and at home with familiar habits, even dogmatic.

Long-term solutions for balancing the great movement metal:

There are roughly two long-term solutions to keep the great movement metal healthy. One is more physical and the other is more personal-social. When people are in balance, they protect themselves with appropriate strength, even if that means taking a defensive position or going against someone's strong opinion from time to time.

- Maintain health by providing physical strength and structure to the body through regular exercises and fresh air, in combination with a healthy diet. A balanced great movement metal provides a healthy *wei qi*. Not only do people feel better after exercise or other physical activity, they

---

10 Lu-3 and Liv-4 balance *hun* and *po*.

also get stiff and tired without it. It will then take a certain discipline and courage to get moving again.
- People can learn to focus on adequately fulfilling their needs without being over the top. They can find a balanced way to communicate with the outside world while still nourishing the inner world, alternating outward behaviour and presence with time for introspection.

Professions typically related to the great movement metal involve the collection of material or data. This allows the objective world to be integrated with the subjective inner being which leads to a better understanding of the world.

When the great movement metal is weakened, it leads to symptoms and diseases due to lack of structures; physically, in bone structures and joints, blood cells and organs, and figuratively, weakness of structure is seen in behaviour and emotions. Physically, the lack of strength in structure may lead to fatigue, weak muscle nutrition, weakened *wei qi*, arthritis, blood cell malformations and cardiac arrhythmias. The lack of inner psychological structure causes complaints such as nervousness in groups, overcompensation for deep fear and strong feelings of commitment.

CHAPTER 8

DYNAMICS OF THE GREAT MOVEMENT WATER[1]

It is said that the Universal Spark is a result of contraction of energies out of the waters,
the Waters of Life.
Life is not our lives, but what has gone before.
The Universal Spark has a giving part and a receiving part.
It contains terrific energies, which when fragmented will make life.
Everything that lives in the universe is made living thereby.
On the other hand, it receives the experiences from all those living entities,
that are being returned to the Universal Spark,
which grows in strength of energy,
increasing its evolution and the rate of vibration.[2]

PATH OF LIFE

When the eyes first open and breathing begins, babies intrinsically identify with the affirmation of existence and the living entity (baby) makes contact with the inner and outer world within the fields of the great movements earth and metal. When the baby is healthy, they can breathe, eat, drink, defecate, urinate, sleep and learn to protect, nurture and love.

At birth the cosmic *qi* (*da qi*) enters the body in the lungs and connects with the human *qi* derived from nourishment (*gu qi*). During the first breath, the kidney *qi* grasps the *qi* of the lungs and roots it in the moving *qi* (*dong qi*) in the

---

1 Born in years ending with a 6 and 1 such as 1996 and 1961, after the Chinese New Year.
2 Oral teachings from J.D. van Buren.

area between the kidneys, close to *Ming Men*, the door of life or gate of fate.[3] In this precious moment, the fate and destiny[4] of the newborn child are defined. It is the great movement water that connects the newborn child with their origin in the place between the kidneys. The personal destiny is therefore important for anyone looking for authenticity.[5]

Fate is the insurmountable. It is based on the uncontrollable, unchanging order of heaven, the circumstances and conditions to which everyone is subject. It includes the flow of time, date, culture and place of birth. Fate shapes everyone differently. This is partly due to the time of birth which creates a dynamic configuration of *qi*. That specific moment can be captured by the heavenly stems and earthly branches, the time dividers of the Chinese calendar, that is, a birth chart.

The combined experiences of all individual fates form a collective field in which all human beings carry and pass on the collective *jing* of humanity. In this sense, healing of an individual contributes to the healing of the collective.

Destiny is based on a personal purpose and an idea. It is determined by choices and transformations, by personal interventions on the path to the future. After all, everyone approaches the challenges of life in their own unique way, including the human responsibility to shape life as a growing, learning and conscious decision-making being.

From birth, the individual path of destiny lies ahead. It is rooted in the kidney region from which the deep function of the *san jiao* moves the *qi* upward to distribute it across the body and the twelve channels. The being, imbued with the *qi* of destiny, can be personalized and attuned to it.

THE UNIVERSAL SPARK AND THE SEED OF GOODNESS

In the context of the Universal Spark, J.D. van Buren stated that it is a human's responsibility to return the purest form of personal *qi* to the Universal Spark by thinking, feeling, speaking and doing correctly. In this way, he continued, humans contribute to the quality of the Universal Spark. I don't know about you, but this statement still occupies me and I often wonder what he meant by the word correct. Is correct related to the five virtues of Confucius: *ren, yi, li,*

---

3   *Nan Jing* Question 66. The moving *qi* between the kidneys is the root of life and the root of the twelve main channels and is called the original *qi*. Translations are Lu 1990 and Unschuld 1986.
4   Fate is what happens regardless of your efforts. Destiny is what belongs to you and what happens when you commit to grow, learn and take risks.
5   The development *along* the destined path of life is guided by the great movement wood and the three *hun*. The origin of the path of destiny is within the great movement water and is influenced by heredity, the moment and place of birth, upbringing and the choices people make.

zhi and *xin*?[6] Or is it more personal and less moral? In my experience, correct means that thinking, feeling, speaking and behaviour are in line with each other and also with each and everyone's personal roots. Human virtues are often imposed from without, but they become living entities when discovered and nurtured within humans themselves.

In order to govern properly, monarchs consulted extensively with their counsellors and happily invited philosophers to exchange views with them. The philosopher Mencius was one of them. On his travels he spoke with various kings and addressed them in very clear terms, pointing out to them misconceptions and imperfections in their thinking, conduct and policy according to the five virtues. He spoke, like Confucius, of humanity and moral standards within the context of heaven's superiority, but moreover he discerned the innate human seed of goodness that is present in every human being from birth. He stated that in the development of natural personal tendencies it is extremely important to carefully guide the potential of that seed through virtues.

In my opinion, the seed of goodness equals the deeply hidden human universal spark, the expression of the essence of existence. Together with the *jing, qi, shen*, the human universal spark or seed, rooted in the emanation *zhen*, is the reference and expression of one's true nature, in which virtues and truth resonate. Its vibrations are the basic frequencies to which people can align their thinking, feeling, speaking and acting. It is an unnameable place in human beings, yet it is the basis of the righteousness of action, regardless of personal preference.

CHALLENGES

The pattern of birth–breathing–grasping–rooting basically happens to everyone. This is in contrast to the time and place of birth and sociocultural-psychological circumstances. In addition, the stems and branches birth chart is composed of many cycles, so much so that you can assume that each birth chart is unique with its different qualities of the *qi* of hours, days, months, seasons, years, star constellations, lunar and solar aspects, abnormalities in climate and so on. Then there is the absence of opposite qualities. The winter is cold and warmth is absent, the night is dark and light is absent. How all of this affects individual experiences depends on the innate strengths and weaknesses of each individual.

The configuration of *qi* at the time of birth is the beginning point of the journey of personal development because personal imbalances and personal

---

6   *Ren*: benevolence, compassion, humanity; *yi*: selflessness, rightness, honesty, uprightness; *li*: propriety, good manners, ceremony, worship; *zhi*: knowledge, wisdom; *xin*: integrity.

strengths and weaknesses generate the tendency to evolve and rebalance. Active great movements that become more active, or passive great movements that become more passive, sooner or later may lead to imbalance and disease but, before that happens, the innate self-healing power within leads people to attempt to restore balance through healthy or unhealthy choices. Which is chosen doesn't matter at first, as long as there is some acceptable balance created. Simply put, everyone faces the challenge to calm the innate (over)active elements and support the (under)active or passive ones. For example, there is a specific challenge for people born with the great movement water. The appeal of society may take them away from their inner being, as does the fear of dealing with psychological trauma. They push the ego outward, away from its authenticity. For these people, the challenge of self-reflection and inner healing is evident, essential and almost inescapable.

Diagnosis and treatment according to heavenly stems and earthly branches is about understanding the innate challenges of the individual and the way they are managed along the path of life. It is at the heart of the work of stems and branches practitioners to diagnose and align treatment to the patient's personal responses to life's challenges posed by the moment of birth, upbringing, heredity, authenticity, circumstances and choices made. The birth chart, pulse and body diagnosis, along with the medical history, are the most important tools to determine the impact on health of personal conditions and (un)conscious choices.

For each practitioner, meeting the challenges of the great movement water is essential, regardless of the practitioner's birth chart. In order not to risk misdiagnoses and inappropriate treatments because their own challenges are projected onto patients, the practitioner must refine their own *qi* and maintain as much autonomy and authenticity as possible, while not harming a vibrant (*shen*) connection with the patient.

EXERCISE

The Universal Spark is the result of contraction (emanation *li*) of the energies from the waters of Life (emanation *zhen*). Bringing together the essences of experiences is a similar movement but on a different level of existence. It promotes the spark of authenticity.

Every day before bedtime you look back on the past day. With mindfulness you bring the essence – the deep meaning and function that an experience entails – within the consciousness field of the self. It is important to focus only on the basic essential meaning, so that the actual experiences can disappear.

Experiences don't need to be forgotten, but holding and nurturing experiences results in living in the past and this exercise is about presence in the moment. You leave behind all the experiences, including those that moved you or others, with the belief that you did your utmost and that your behaviour was well intentioned. The *qi* of the night, in which everything withdraws to a point of rest and turnaround, does the job. The essences merge with the peaceful cavity in the self where thoughts do not disturb. Without social intervention and personal obsessions, the will can relax and authenticity sprout.

When you wake up you tune in to the *shen*-ming of the heart and essence of the kidney-*jing* to meet the day with renewed pure *qi*. Over time, the place of truth-finding and authenticity may manifest in you and it usually becomes clear that 'right and wrong' are relative terms.

I wrote this text in a romantic cottage on one of the Dutch islands. I looked out over meadows, in the distance a rotating mill, which I know is still being worked, grinding grain. There are sheep and horses that defy the cold of winter. I write my book here and to get inspiration I take long walks through the forest and the dunes or on the wide beach. What is the essence of this experience for me to be here and to write? The place itself is wonderful. There is the silence of the island and the concentration of winter. It is significant for me to write, that I am here more than forty years after I started studying Chinese medicine and philosophy and putting into words what I have experienced on this path. It is important to me, because these experiences as a human being, as practitioner and as teacher, in combination with what I have learned over the years, are being put into words on paper. This is so different from oral teaching. Writing helps me to further organize my feelings and thoughts. It brings me closer to myself and thus contributes to the meaning of my life. The essence is the feeling that it contributes to who and what I am on my path of life. Moreover, I hope this book adds to the skills of colleagues and benefits patients. With these thoughts I will soon fall asleep, forgetting the day but with the certainty of enrichment during the night.

ZHI, WILL AND WISDOM

> The heart of compassion is the start of humaneness (*Ren*); the heart of shame is the start of righteousness (*Yi*); the heart of modesty and yielding is the start of propriety (*Li*); the heart of right and wrong is the start of wisdom (*Zhi*).[7]

---

7   The four hearts of Mencius 6A6. Translations (Dutch) Borel 1931, van der Leeuw 2008.

Humanity is the heart of man, righteousness is the path of man.[8]

According to Mencius people needed to be nourished to let their nature flourish into virtues. Compassion, shame, modesty, yielding and the heart of right and wrong are the human instruments for processing the five virtues. The seed of goodness is the true, authentic *qi* founded deep in the great movement water. It is the potential force of righteousness and truth-finding of the heart-*shen* and the key to wisdom (*zhi*).

The innate good nature of the human heart and humaneness comes from benevolence and love. However, the human will has its own plans and usually focuses on other goals. Desires and beliefs are difficult to avoid and can seduce people to take other directions. The personal often deviates from the path of love, humaneness and inner cultivation, making attunement with righteousness difficult.

The reference point of righteousness is situated within humans. Laws and legislations are outward projections of what is anchored in people themselves: the power of the will, the will of power and wisdom. The path from will to wisdom stems from realization and possibly therefore through reconciliation with the fact that the personal will may and can be equal to the love of heaven.

The unity and wholeness of heaven is balanced, pure and without conflict or opposition. Human actuality between heaven and earth exists in the world of duality, connection, communication, agreements and disagreements. Due to the moving dynamics between opposite forces of yin and yang, people are by nature in motion, unbalanced and fallible. It makes people human, searching for balance on the path of trial and error, of losing and winning, of learning and becoming knowledgeable and wise. Inner cultivation is the path of return to the state of wholeness and non-duality, not as a goal but as a way of experiencing and understanding the 'self' in its connection with all of life.

While on a walk, my father told me a story he once read in a book about the nature of the spirit and a mystical gong. It happened in an ancient city far away where the gong of the temple was struck by people who wanted to learn their virtue. The gong resonated with the pureness of the virtue of the spirit of the person who struck the gong. Most of the time the sound was muffled, but often unexpectedly it could make a powerful and full sound. The story was about a brave man who, on a journey of inner cleansing, finally captured the heart of a beautiful woman by the most beautiful bright sound that emanated

---

8   Mencius 6A11.

when he struck the gong. I can't quite recall the whole story, but I do remember the conversation with my father afterwards and the lessons we learned from it.

The clear, full sound of compassion[9] resonates in the harmonious vibration of the unbound gong. Compassion moves those who receive, feel and share the feelings of passion. The true vibration of the gong tunes every being to the source of compassion. It is controlled from the outside by the moral compass of society and from within by the sense of righteousness. The principle of humanity means love for others, not only for yourself, and righteousness means correcting yourself and not the other. The source of compassion is the purity, peace, harmony and unity of inner righteousness.[10] The purity of unity, once broken by duality, heals through compassion that bridges dual forces.

As a practical example: Children are one with their mother until the unity is broken by birth and the cutting of the umbilical cord. After that, children have a lot to learn to become independent beings with free will, a journey where failure is a source of growth and development. It is precisely through trial and error that children gradually learn to stay authentic and become independent and autonomous. As they grow older, they also start to do naughty things and push the boundaries, sometimes causing them to be punished or rejected. The competitive world is calling. Parenting and guidance by caregivers and teachers may lead to morally and socially correct behaviour, but competition and punishment, as necessary as it sometimes is, disconnect people from their authentic source[11] and limit their ability to become independent beings with free will. The distance to authenticity can be bridged by an empathetic atmosphere and a compassionate bond to teach children the art of living with authenticity.

SHEN-YI-ZHI

When the Heart applies itself,
We speak of Intent.
When Intent becomes permanent,
We speak of Will.[12]

---

9   Compassion means suffering together – in Greek and Latin passion means suffering – which connects compassion with empathy. However, empathy, like sympathy, is rooted in a feeling; it is not the activity of sharing. Compassion is that active sharing of a common passion.
10 To avoid any misunderstanding, I would like to emphasize here that the source of compassion and righteousness is Love, the basic principle of life.
11 *Zhen*, true authentic *qi*, is peace, unity and harmony and in essence pure and without conflict.
12 *Ling Shu* Chapter 8. Translations are Wu 1993, Larre and de La Vallée 2004.

Shen-yi-zhi determine the orientation in life.[13] The *shen* receives, coordinates and integrates information. The understanding of information functions in cooperation with processing and analysis by the *yi*. Predispositions, knowledge, new ideas, concepts and purposes are born. The direction of intentions and conclusions of the mind are determined by the *zhi*. It determines the inner strength, the perseverance, the intensity to realize ideas, ideals and ambitions. It might lead to deep understanding and anchoring of what has been learned. However, the *zhi* is usually facing outward with a will that directs *qi* based on desires, passions and daily routine.

Too strong outward orientation may lead to overwork and fatigue, stubbornness and wilfulness. In the long run, this conduct leads to depletion of the great movement water and the *jing*. Treatment should focus on strengthening the *jing* and reducing the drive.

My preference for reducing the outward facing, beside treating the great movement water, is Ki-4, *Da Zhong*, great bell, especially when it is accompanied by lumbago, constipation, stabbing pain in the back, fear and warm soles of the feet. Another option is sedation of Ki-2, *Ran Gu*, blazing valley, especially if wilful behaviour is accompanied by occipital headaches, dry mouth, attacks of acute diarrhoea, high blood pressure, night sweats and/or restless legs.

The result of the inward orientation of the *zhi* can lead to guiding the *qi* based on authenticity, self-awareness and processing experiences. Too strong inward orientation may lead to aloof behaviour and possibly depression. A long-lasting inward orientation exhausts the great movement water and the will. It results in lack of will, vitality, authenticity and a fear to move.

Besides treating the great movement water, I prefer acupuncture points like Bl-52, *Zhi Shi*, lodge of the will, Ki-4, *Da Zhong*, great bell and Ki-5, *Shui Quan*, water spring.

Bl-52 strengthens the willpower and determination. It works well with depression where the will to try and get better is absent. It provides the will to live.

Ki-4 strengthens the *shen* and the will (along with Ki-5) and calms emotions when people are exhausted and depressed from chronic insufficiency of the kidneys. It can strengthen the will and/or soften driven-ness. It may be used

---

13 The heart is the foundation of the character *zhi*, 志 wisdom (similar to the character *yi*, 意 intention). The top part of the character *zhi* shows a small plant rising straight from the earth. It looks like a picture of a phallus, very straight and firm. The character *zhi* symbolizes an unmistakably clear direction of growth with a secure rootedness in the heart.

with disorientation, somnolence or when people want to keep aloof. It works on the ancestral *qi* of the kidneys and is the main point for fear.

Ki-5 is the 'will' point of the body: It commands the body to heal and reinforces the power of water, especially when there is fear of moving forward, when people feel blocked as if something stops them from moving.

Insufficient heart-*shen* and insufficient *qi* can lead to insufficiency of the *zhi* because the heart-*shen* guides the *qi* that gives strength to the *zhi*. These insufficiencies display in symptoms such as no will to live, no motivation, no orientation, and so on. *Zhi*, on the other hand, directs the *qi* and leads the heart-*shen* to interact with the *jing*. Because of this coherence of *shen* and *zhi* functions, *zhi* insufficiency always leads to *shao yin* imbalances and should be treated accordingly by points like Ki-9, Ki-16, Cv-23.

THE DYNAMICS OF THE UNDIVIDED

From the first breath, the individual undivided *yuan-shen*[14] and pre-natal *jing qi* undergo transformations into personal divided post-natal *jing qi*, *wu-shen* and the twelve-channel system.

The expression of post-natal conditions is usually overshadowed by post-natal will, striving and desires due to life's challenges. The *wu-shen* function in a world of duality to give direction to life. But there is another, more mystical side to the spiritual sources, which can be important for diagnosis and treatment of patients, as well as for self-cultivation.

The existence in duality is so steeped in opposites of affirming the good and rejecting the bad and achieving goals and 'performance' that it is complicated to imagine the source of duality: the heavenly non-dual world, in which love is not the opposite of indifference or hatred and righteousness doesn't choose between good and bad. In the non-dual state, love and righteousness are of their own and the world is characterized by 'what-there-is' rather than good or evil, straight or crooked, negative or positive. This state is called the natural state in which all is accepted as it is, without labelling experiences and observations. Sometimes it is seen as going where the wind blows, but nothing could be further from the truth. Being completely aware of what 'is' (in the present) involves an increase in belonging and a decrease of desire and becoming.

---

14 *Yuan shen* is the original undivided *shen*, born from the source of life. The *wu-shen* are the divided five *shen*, the five spiritual sources heart-*shen*, *yi*, *po*, *zhi* and *hun*. After birth, they collaborate in an integrated way.

The heart-*shen* can tune into the influx from heaven – intuition – when there is being and belonging. This state is best described as a state of 'withdrawal and gentle resistance to action' in order to be open to impressions, presence and involvement.

All great movements and heavenly stems and earthly branches enable understanding of the natural state, yet the great movement water is the personal gateway to it.

SHORT- AND LONG-TERM SOLUTIONS

Short-term solutions[15] for balancing the great movement water:

- the tendency to be opinionated and individualistic; this may lead to dogmatism and being overcritical
- the tendency to be perfect and determined
- seeking short-term solutions in general
- obsessively wanting to find deep meaning and understanding
- to compensate for fear and insecurity people may become greedy and possessive
- the tendency to be dependent on sexual desires and confirmation.

Long-term solutions for balancing the great movement water:

The long-term solutions are not so easy. There is a danger that confirmation leads people to consider themselves knowledgeable and wise. In the end, this belief stagnates *qi* and *xuè*, more than it gives freedom. It suppresses further inner cultivation. It may also get in the way of a balanced sexual experience, but moreover it often leads to quite serious symptoms and illnesses because one is unaware of this situation that stagnates the flow of *jing*. Unfortunately, the severity of diseases and disorders seems to be the only way to surrender the inflated ego.

- accept things as they are, without struggles, desires or competition
- no vanity, selfless, silent obedience
- belonging

---

15   Short-term solutions describe behaviour that temporarily repairs and satisfies a shortcoming of a great movement. In the long run, they exhaust that great movement in question. The behaviour does not necessarily have to be 'wrong', but it is not desirable for that person with that specific great movement in the birth chart (long-term solutions are beneficial).

- upright, veracity, truthfulness
- cultivate authenticity
- typical professions: journalists, scientists, researchers, but also, for example, multi-talented artists.

A weakened great movement water leads to symptoms and disorders such as back pains, skin diseases, rheumatoid arthritis and so on. The corresponding aspect in these disorders is consistently a deep uncertainty and inadequacy of the essence-*jing*, compensated for by an active outward-looking presentation or by withdrawal and shyness. Of course, the deeper the disease, the more serious the problem, but due to the relationship with the great movement water, diseases may affect the authentic original *qi*. This can lead to serious illness in the long run. The prevention of an insufficient great movement water is therefore crucial.[16]

---

16 The difference between insufficient water phase and insufficient great movement water is the possible extent of the insufficiency in multiple *qi* belonging to water, such as *jin yé*, gallbladder, *san jiao*, bladder and kidney. These correlations are further explained in the chapters on the earthly branches.

CHAPTER 9

DYNAMICS OF THE GREAT MOVEMENT WOOD[1]

I once met a lama who recently meditated for three years, three months, three days and three hours.

I asked him about loneliness, being separated from his friends and brothers and sisters.

'What was it like to be alone for more than three years?'

He looked at me and said: 'Why do you think I was alone? I was not.'

'But you were alone in your cave, weren't you?'

'I was never alone;

In meditation I was connected with everything and everybody, with all my brothers and sisters, I was never on my own at all.'

Because the undivided is divided, life connects the separate parts with each other, distances are bridged, relationships are established and changes in circumstances can occur. The great movement wood connects and integrates individual components into a network of interacting parts. The interaction allows movements between the different parts to take place and goals to be pursued. The body is such a wholeness in which the free flow of fluids, *qi* and *xuè*, the various organs, tissues, limbs and so on together form a network that pursues health, 'a state of complete physical, mental, and social well-being and not merely the absence of disease'.[2]

The limitations of form are transcended by the *qi* connecting the seemingly separate parts of the body. This is true for the physical body, the more subtle bodies and human consciousness, which itself is part of the consciousness of

---

1   Born in years ending with a 7 and 2 such as 1997 and 1952, after the Chinese New Year.

2   WHO Constitution, available at www.who.int/about/governance/constitution.

the wholeness of families, peer groups and friends, sociocultural groupings, even of all of humanity. Group awareness, intuitive alignment between people, making spontaneous choices are just a few examples of the boundlessness of life we call *qi*.

The degree of cooperation and integration depends on the consciousness initiated by the great movement wood through the manifestation of the emanation *yuan*. The original creative principle, the onset of movement from the beginning, remains constantly active. It initiates, guides and creates all changes and movements such as breathing, adaptation to light and dark, cold and warm, meeting others, digesting food and so on. For example, when someone suddenly wakes up at night due to a loud noise, *qi* is initiated, activated and positioned. Consciousness tries to connect and integrate with the world. The eyes and ears are opened, the mind begins to think, the body begins to communicate, and so on. The degree and speed with which this happens shows the degree of alertness of the great movement wood. The same is true for blood pressure adjustments when people change positions or for flexibility of mind and body when there is a sudden threat. Disturbances in the great movement wood as a result of stagnations, weaknesses, insufficiencies, accumulations, unnatural ascending and descending of *qi* and so on influence the integrated free flow of *qi* and thus the natural order and freedom of movement in the broadest sense of the word. The underlying denominator of seemingly unrelated complaints such as high blood pressure, insomnia together with difficulty waking up, rigid behaviour, stiff muscles, glaucoma and so on is the health and balance of the great movement wood.

MOVEMENT

> *Wu Ji*, as a single state, is remained changeless, an undifferentiated unity, void and without form. It was beyond existence. Only when Time intersected Space was there the division into two, the creation of a duality and the birth of change. It is represented by the *Tai Ji* symbol.[3]

Movement is an alteration of place in time. This is an acceptable definition in the physical world, but it is less applicable to the non-physical world where movements are hard to perceive. Non-physical movements such as time, intuition, thinking and feeling, visions, planning, inspiration and imagination are

---

3   J.D. van Buren.

examples of subtle manifestations whose inner movement need not be directly observable. There may not be a visible displacement, but invisible to physical perception the mind moves in time and place. Thinking about the past moves the mind to the past. The mind is no longer fully in the present. Thinking about the future moves the mind to the realm of expectations. Intuition moves and changes impressions and imagination moves the mind into a suggested world different from reality. The mind transforms the current condition by 'alterations of place in time'.

This implies that obsessions and trauma from the past as well as imaginary thoughts and expectations that are not fulfilled may cause stagnated or chaotic movements and transformations of *qi* that may cause diseases, often also with physical complaints. The great movement wood initiates those movements of *qi* that are necessary to experience the movements of the present again and direct the consciousness to order it.

The movements and changes of interaction between people and with the self makes *qi* perceptible for sensitive and trained people. It creates new conditions, new relationships, new points of view, visible and invisible, but not imperceptible.

THREE

The birth of the new is symbolically represented by the number three (*san* 三).

The *Dao* gives birth to One;
One gives birth to Two;
Two gives birth to Three;
Three gives birth to the 10,000 beings[4]

In this chapter of the *Dao De Jing*, Laozi presents the beginning of existence. Heaven, as the first manifestation of *Dao*, is symbolized by a centre of the circle, evoked out of an infinite space. Number two is the differentiation known as yin and yang, heaven and earth, that induces the movement of *qi*.

Symbolically, the number three is depicted as a circle with a central point. Here, we have the circumference, the centre and the field in between as represented by the radius. Thus three stands for three in one, the trinity, the subtle initiator of birth and first appearance of life and its flow is said to be present in every human being. Examples of the symbol of three are manifold: Father,

---

4   *Dao De Jing*, opening text from Chapter 42, translated from Kluwer 1995.

Son and Holy Spirit; Atma, Buddhi and Manas; Brahma, Vishnu and Shiva; *jing*, *qi* and *shen*; the three *hun*; lower, middle and upper burner and the three *dan tien* with the three spirits. Similarly, the first three great movements earth, metal and water form a trinity, a functional coherence that gives structure to the flow of life.

A teacher once taught me that after the first three great movements have been formed, it is as if the breath is held for a moment, a moment of stillness and reflection, before the fourth great movement wood expresses the vital *qi*.

The cycle of great movements begins with the great movement earth: The idea or impulse of heaven manifests a reflection on earth as the self with an identity that receives the mandate of heaven. The great movement metal is the second in line. It guides the *qi* of heaven into duality and leads the collaboration between two opposing forces as inner and outer world. The great movement water is the conclusion and grasps the heavenly impulse, rooting it in the essence of the human being. Together, these three great movements function in unity.

The centre of the circle represents the potential that might acquire a field of expression; the radius, symbolizing the field within the circumference, represents the nature of the living potential. This is limited by the circumference of the circle, the actual relationship of the revealed potential with its expression in the present place and time. For example, the potential, the great movement earth of the practitioner, is the knowledge of the field of the profession, wisdom, experience, the ability to have and share compassion, intention and willpower. The relationship between the practitioner and the patient is the nature of the living potential and belongs to the great movement metal. The quality of interaction has a major impact on the nature of the treatment, the mutual trust and the outcome of the treatment. The treatment itself is limited by the given circumstances and gives space to the actual character and skills of the practitioner (great movement water).

From the other side, the patient's demand for health is the potential, the relationship between the patient and the practitioner is the nature of the living potential and allows treatment to focus on diseases, symptoms and discomforts in any form.

The nature of the cooperation of the first three great movements – earth, metal and water – determines the direction of the treatment: formal, mechanical, using protocols such as formulas or acupuncture point combinations, TCM, *Zang Fu*-related, herbs, Japanese acupuncture, constitutional acupuncture and so on. I have no judgement on any form of treatment, though of course I have a preference, but dogmatic thinking and assuming that there are methods that surpass others only says something about the flexibility of the speaker's great movement metal. Treatment is about finding the right alignment and exchange, meaning that the fourth great movement is involved and *qi* – movement and change and thus life – can do its job.

I have noticed that when the potentials of the practitioner and patient, the nature of the relationship and the focus of the associated actual treatment harmonize, immediately after the needles are inserted patients hold their breath for a moment as if the mind and body are waiting and getting ready to receive changes. A short moment of silence occurs, including in the pulse, just before changes appear. The resulting changes and free movements of *qi* due to the collaborating forces of the first three great movements ultimately depend on the health of the fourth, the great movement wood.

YUAN IS ROOTED IN *ZHEN*

Health requires free flow of *qi* of the great movement wood. This mainly depends on the health and balance of the deep function of the *san jiao* which is related to the emanation *zhen*.[5]

According to the *Nan Jing*, the free flow of *qi* of the *san jiao* determines and harmonizes the free flow of all *qi* throughout the body. The *san jiao* ascends the moving *qi* between the kidneys and in addition controls the movements and changes in the three burners and the five *zang* and six *fu*. Of course, the organs are controlled by the *san jiao*, but I think that the numbers five and six are mentioned for a reason. Paul Unschuld translates the first sentence of Chapter 38 of the *Nan Jing* as follows: 'The depots are but five; only the palaces are six. Why is that so?'[6]

The deep function of the *san jiao* constitutes the human attunement between heaven and earth. It establishes the flow of *qi* between the moving *qi* between the kidneys – *dong qi* – and with the totality of being and enables the original authentic *qi* to flow throughout the body.[7]

The yang number five refers to the yang-life-essence of heaven in all yin

---

5   This is discussed further in the chapter on the earthly branches. The *san jiao* belongs to the fire phase, but in the Chinese hourly clock and the cycle of the earthly branches, it belongs to the water phase based on the emanation *zhen*.

6   Unschuld 1986.

7   *Nan Jing* Chapter 66: The moving *qi* between the kidneys is the root of human life and the root of the twelve channels, and that is why it is called the starting original *qi*. The *san jiao* is a special organ that transmits the original influences. It is in charge of the flow of three influences (heaven–earth–human or ancestral *qi-ying qi-wei qi*, the three true influences) for distribution among the five *zang* and six *fu*. The starting or original is an honourable name of the *san jiao*. This is why the places where the *qi* of the *san jiao* is housed are called the starting or *yuan source* points. When the five *zang* and six *fu* are diseased, the *yuan source* points may be addressed for treatments.

forms, including humans. It refers to the cooperation of the five great movements from heaven that describe and determine all phenomena; in other words, how Life is expressed in the Form.

The yin number six represents the yin-form-principle of earth and humans which houses the yang-life-essence of heaven. Six represents the six directions and the six *qi*, the nature of the relationship of earth and humans with heaven. The relationship between humans and heaven enables human life to attune through the six channels to the six climates, the six directions, and spiritual principles of heaven.[8]

The *san jiao* regulates the free flow of *qi* and therefore the state of all that is represented by five and six and thus in addition to the five *zang* and six *fu* the health of all life and all forms.

ACUPUNCTURE POINTS THAT FUNCTION IN LINE WITH THE DEEP FUNCTION OF THE *SAN JIAO*

The deep function of the *san jiao* is fulfilled by the *ren mai*. *Ren mai* points on the lower abdomen are especially suitable.

Sj-2, *Ye Men*, fluid door, with Sj-3, *Zhong Zhu*, middle island, open the possible blockage between the kidneys, liver and *qi* in the abdomen.

Sj-4, *Yang Qi*, pool of yang, promotes the function of *chong* and *ren mai*, strengthens the human relation to *yuan qi* and tonifies the *san jiao* function in the abdomen. Sj-4 strengthens the function of the *san jiao* to be the envoy of original *qi*.

Sj-6, *Zhi Gou*, branch ditch, asks the *yuan qi* to fill the channels. This point spreads the *qi* and clears obstructions. Along with Sj-2 it irrigates the body. It can be used with Bl-64, *Jing Gou*, capital bone, when the *san jiao* is insufficient, especially since Bl-64 nourishes the liver. This combination restores the free flow of *qi* at all levels.

Liv-3, *Tai Chong*, great surge, regulates the liver *qi* and builds fluids in the liver. This point is especially important for the authentic vital *qi*, which, liberated by *san jiao*, guides human life on its path of destiny.

---

8 Foot *tai yang*–hand *tai yang*; foot *shao yang*–hand *shao yang*; foot *yang ming*–hand *yang ming*; foot *tai yin*–hand *tai yin*; foot *jué yin*–hand *jué yin*; foot *shao yin*–hand *shao yin*.

THE THREE *HUN*: GUIDING PURPOSES
AND ONWARD MOVEMENT

There are three different *hun*, but they always act in concert. One may be more accentuated than others, but they never appear alone.

The most physically orientated *hun* focuses on physical movement and communication. It connects with the outside world through the focus on pleasures and the pursuit of passions. It is involved in growth and procreation. When the physical impulses from the environment are too overwhelming, damage to this *hun* may lead to frequent illness and growth retardation in children.

The second *hun* focuses on social interaction based on feelings such as sympathy, empathy, emotional sensations and moods. An impairment of this *hun* causes reduced sense of shame or, conversely, an intense sense of shame. People may shamelessly talk about private topics, which is, however, accompanied by hidden nervousness and insecurity. Intense feelings of shame are reflected in the difficulties people experience in navigating life; a relationship or not, work that feels authentic, a happy life that matches their wishes are some of the issues that preoccupy them. Shame is an emotion that prefers to be invisible. It is only later in life that it may become clear that shame may be at the root of feelings of failure. And, even then, shame likes to remain invisible behind all kinds of compensation mechanisms.

The third *hun* focuses on self-development and improvement of virtues that lead to purity of the mind and intuitive communication. Pointless and silly behaviour may be due to the ill condition of the third *hun*. It looks like dementia, and it maybe is, but it is based on a *hun* issue.

THE THREE *HUN* FOLLOW THE
ZHI-WILL OF THE HEART-*SHEN*

The three *hun* are the spiritual sources that correspond to the great movement wood. The direction, activity and focus of the three *hun* affect the great movement wood which as a result may become excessive, insufficient, uprooted or stagnant.

In *Ling Shu* Chapter 8 it is stated: 'That which faithfully follows the *shen* in their coming and going denotes the *hun*.' The *shen* desires, the *hun* follows.

The three *hun* have no purpose of themselves but follow the will of the heart-*shen*. The heart-*shen* integrates and gathers the three *hun* when it reaches outward to the world or inward to the self. However, the three *hun* move and direct the *shen* as well and are therefore important in guiding the developmental path of destiny that arises at birth. The subtle energetic exchange between the three *hun* and the *shen* is decisive for a smooth course and onward movement on this path.

When the heart-*shen* reaches out, the *zhi* commands the *qi*, for example the eyes focus their attention on something unexpected and the three *hun* follow the desire to see something. The heart-*shen*, being open and looking outward and inward, receives the image. The *hun* govern the grasping, the attachment, the confirmation of the focus, the purpose by which they direct the *shen* to turn outward and determine the movements, planning, life dreams, encounters that are needed. When they direct the *shen* to turn inward, they determine the relationship with intuition, inspiration, imagination, visualization, sensitivity and having ideas.

When the three *hun* are overactive in relation to the *shen*, people dream a lot, they become more chaotic and have many plans that do not lead to success. In the end, it often leads to frustration and resentment.

When the three *hun* are underactive in relation to the *shen*, people feel depressed, apathetic with a lack of creativity and imagination, have no vision or plans and find it difficult to make decisions.

When the three *hun* descend, the *qi* becomes slower, the focus of the consciousness is more on the form, material, external world and the five senses. The *qi* becomes 'harder', less flexible and resistant to change.

When the three *hun* ascend, the *qi* opens and cultivates the three *dan tien*. This movement gives the opportunity to achieve agreement and unity between thoughts, feelings, speech, actions with openness and flexibility to change. However, there is the danger of uprooting and becoming ungrounded.

I prefer to treat the *hun* issues prior to treatments of great movement wood issues.

Bl-47, *Hun Men*, hun gate, is used for depression, frustration and long-term resentment. It helps to plan one's life and find a sense of direction in purpose.

Liv-4, *Zhong Feng*, central blockade, middle seal, balances the *hun* with the *po*.

Liv-3, *Tai Chong*, great surge, is used when the *hun* are too active due to stagnation.

Liv-5, *Li Gou*, drain of the calf, is used with fear, nervousness, depression.[9]

---

9   To avoid depression or confusion, J.D. van Buren advised using this point in conjunction with Gb-37, Gb-40 or Gb-41.

Lu-7, *Lie Que*, broken sequence, is used in cases of emotional tension caused by unsettled *hun* which manifests in tense shoulders, shallow breathing and feelings of oppression in the chest. It calms the mind, releases the *qi* of emotions and settles the *hun*.

Ki-21, *You Men*, hidden gate, helps people to face fears and move on with life.

Ht-1, *Ji Quan*, highest spring, reestablishes the connection between individual and greater (collective) consciousness.[10]

SHORT- AND LONG-TERM SOLUTIONS

There are two types of great movement wood expressions:

1. Physically lethargic people with a great deal of mental activity.
2. Overactive people with an inordinate desire to feel life's challenges.

Short-term solutions for balancing the great movement wood:

- multitasking talents; people don't find peace doing just one thing at a time
- boastfulness
- need for stimulation from the outside world
- excessive focus on starting new ideas, concepts and activities along with the fight for justice.

Short-term solutions may lead to (subdued) anger, resentment and manipulations.

The excessive desire to feel life's challenges is expressed in:

- living fast like a steamroller, but dying young
- going out every night
- a strong desire to drive fast cars
- impatient behaviour and the desire to make decisions.

Long-term solutions for balancing the great movement wood:

---

10 The three *hun* represent and connect with universal and collective consciousness.

- gentleness along with flexibility and adaptability allowing for smooth development
- focus on growth in general, without exerting pressure
- commitment, feelings of love and dedication
- the quality of thinking; to be able to sit quietly and consider something
- creativity as initial force for communication, education, expression and so on
- righteousness as inner virtue (not as an ethical principle for correcting others)
- rituals: seriously performing rituals in any form brings people into contact and attunement with the authenticity and preciousness of the creativity of the *shen*. A ritual reveals what is essentially and truthfully already present in the *shen*. It strengthens and intensifies the interconnectedness of the *shen–hun* relationship. Important in this regard is the discussion in Chapter 3 on *yuanheng* in connection with the acceptance of natural sacrifices and the oneness of existence.

Especially with the great movement wood, the practitioner must have some degree of persuasion to enable the patient to understand the development and severity of their complaints. People with great movement wood issues can have their own (stubborn) ideas of what is needed. Only when the patient trusts the practitioner is there dedication and loyalty to the approach proposed by the practitioner. Then, any trust gained is strong and lasting. Clarity and honesty are keywords for a good relationship. This process can sometimes take some time, which unfortunately can make diseases more serious.

CHAPTER 10

DYNAMICS OF THE GREAT MOVEMENT FIRE[1]

The moon has many faces, she plays the game of birth and death.
The sun has only one face, but knows when to hide.

The *shen* (the mind or spirit) is a very elaborate subject. For more information about this, I would like to refer the reader to the many books and articles that have been written about it. This chapter discusses only a few aspects of the *shen* that are important for understanding the great movement fire to which it is related.

The heart-*shen* has outward and inward movements; it reaches out to the surrounding world and its own inner being. It does this down to the smallest detail, with which the wholeness of the *shen* recognizes itself, partly connected with its source, partly with its projection in the surrounding world and partly with the impressions of life that return to the heart. The given and received impressions of the heart-*shen* are congruent with the giving and receiving parts of the Universal Spark discussed in Chapter 3.

THE HEART-*SHEN* AND *ZHI*-WILL

Sensations arise from the inner and outer senses experienced in the heart-*shen*. These evoke wishes, intentions, ideas and opinions in the *yi* which the *zhi*, will, chooses to express and realize. Wishes and will, *yi* and *zhi*, cause action, direction of *qi* and movement to achieve a goal. Thought becomes part of the will when the will and one's wishes focus on what is desired.

A thought process is attracted by the power of time, as thoughts directed, for instance, to the future distract from experiencing the now. Willpower, combined

---

1 Born in years ending with an 8 and 3 such as 1998 and 1963, after the Chinese New Year.

with wishes, expresses the longing for something that is not yet owned but can be realized. It drives people to push their limits and possibilities. Together, the will, thinking and *shen* determine the inner strength, perseverance and intensity to achieve set goals. Later we will discuss how the great movement fire and the kidneys – which house the *zhi* – can induce people to overwork and burn out.[2]

When the heart applies itself, one speaks of intent (*yi*).[3]

This sentence indicates that the *shen* takes the initiative to action, which, in turn, is guided by intention.

When purpose is permanent, one speaks of will (*zhi*).

When persistent intention establishes the goal, one speaks of will. In other words, the will carries out the activities determined by intentions arising from the initiative of the *shen*.[4]

When the persevering will changes, we speak of thought.[5]

This means that the mind is controlled by the will. This is extremely important, as people are characterized by free will and the ability to think and be aware of the free or limited qualities of that will. The will (*zhi*) is the source of thought. Thinking is usually attributed to the phase earth, especially thinking in circles when something seems to have a life of its own and cannot be stopped, but thinking is actually controlled by the will. That is why the power of the will for real change and healing is so important. Understanding survival strategies, such as thinking that hard labour is required, but realizing that working too hard is actually a strategy for preventing someone from seeing themselves in the mirror, helps in the process of healing. Treatments of the great movement fire and especially of the willpower of the kidneys, *zhi*, can be very supportive in releasing survival strategies that have come into play. Relaxation of the will is therefore a prerequisite for calming excessive thinking – on the understanding that the will itself is directed by the heart-*shen*!

As the heart-*shen* experiences sensations, the will and desires (including

---

2   See Chapter 21 on the heavenly stem *gui* and Chapter 17 on the concept of unlike *qi*.
3   *Ling Shu* Chapter 8.
4   It should be remembered that a heart that is full of desires and passions changes the quality of the blood, that changes the intent (*yi*) and the will (*zhi*).
5   *Ling Shu* Chapter 8.

those of social and personal interest) become focused on action and movement, allowing the will to create confusion or to put people under pressure, because the power of the will and the desire for power are incredibly compelling. To overcome this vicious circle of overloaded cyclical movement of *shen–yi–zhi–shen*, one should begin by calming the *shen* as the initiator. The will of the heart is able to strengthen or weaken, purify or pollute the body/being and, although existing complaints may indicate an excessive will/*zhi* is present, one should start by diagnosing and treating the heart-*shen*.

SELF-AWARENESS

Self-awareness and self-cultivation belong to the domain of the heart-*shen*. This path requires attunement to the heart-*shen* and may lead to a balanced, undisturbed heart-*shen*. However, there is another force on the watch that can disrupt this path: the identity and ego[6] are perceived and felt by the heart-*shen*.

The more important the ego becomes, the more likely the pure *qi* of the heart-*shen* is being disturbed by an overwhelming great movement earth. It results in an increase of intentions, willpower and desires. Then people may deviate further and further from the path of the original *shen*, the earthly representative of heaven. In concrete terms, this implies that the meaning of life is determined by the achievement of set goals and performance objectives and less by subtle, religious or spiritual inclinations.[7] The vertical relationship between humans and the subtle invisible realms loses out to the horizontal, more practical or 'realistic' realms.

THE INTEGRATED *SHEN*

The *wu-shen* is the integrated collaboration of the five different spiritual sources: the heart-*shen*, the *yi*, the seven *po*, the *zhi* and the three *hun*. The heart-*shen* is an integral part of this fivefold system.

In the events of the course of time and place, the heart-*shen* and the great movement fire nourish the *yi*, the great movement earth, intention, ego and thus the will. In integration, the *wu-shen* functions integrally with all aspects of the *shen* and mutual differences of the five phases are recognized as part of the process of healing and wholeness. It can be more or less assumed that integration leads to health. When the integration is broken, the different parts

---

6   Great movement earth.
7   When spiritual development is the stated goal, it stems from the ego's desires as well.

of the *wu-shen* are highlighted, but not integrated. This can lead to stagnation, underactivity, overactivity, cold and heat and so on, and subsequently illness.

> Take, for example, children who generally have an integrated *shen* due to their playful nature. Let us look at a boy of about ten years old. His imagination, willpower and sense of self are integrated. He likes to play, is a creative and happy child. However, the school requires a different attunement because he must adapt to the large group in the classroom and the protocol of the curriculum. It is then understandable that problems arise in the area of the great movement metal and the seven *po*, such as respiratory and/or skin disorders, or behavioural problems such as 'disobedience' and 'absence'. Because coordination and alignment with the environment is unsuccessful, the power of physiological instincts can become excessive or insufficient. This can be accompanied by disturbance of the senses, especially the ears and eyes and a blurred mind, involuntary movements or apathetic behaviour. In such cases it is important not only to treat the great movement metal, but also to focus on the integration of all spiritual sources: The alignment between *hun* and *po*, *shen-yi-zhi*, *po* and *jing*, *shen* and *po* and so on. Usually, the school situation cannot be changed, nevertheless the space, time and attention given to the child to learn to cope with the limitations the world demands may be managed.

COMPLETION

The great movement fire, related to the emanation *heng*, is about completion. It is the final stage, the peak experience.

For a better understanding, I would like you to consider for a moment what the word completion does to you. What does completion mean to you? How do you relate to completion? As it gets closer to completion, does it make you happy, does it cause stress or relaxation?

Usually, the concept of completion is part of a hierarchical way of thinking. It is based on better and worse, more and less, win and lose, superiority and inferiority. Something is not yet finished and must be finished, otherwise it is not complete. Finishing and continuing to the end is generally more positively valued than dropping out, although the latter often yields better opportunities for learning. Often the path leading to completion is seen as work or something that is sorely needed to achieve the goal, forgetting that the path that people are journeying on *is* real life.

The perception and experience of completion is relative. After all, something that is completed will still disappear in the long run. Moreover, something that is perceived as complete is generally separated from other aspects of existence and in that sense is incomplete. Completion exists in a limited field, such as the 'I am' that feels complete, even though the ego is separate from other egos. And that's a good thing, because we cannot function in our existence without a separate ego. On the path from completion to wholeness, from separation to integral wholeness, we can become more aware of ourselves in the world of abundance and open up to express the innate love and compassion we all possess to bridge the seemingly insurmountable distance between people. That is the process and path of individuation and maturity hidden in the *shen* and the great movement fire.

CREATIVITY

Realizing the greatness and smallness of the ego is an essential step towards equality and identification with the ever-abiding presence of the life principles of love and compassion. Love that is divided, for example something like 'out of love for my country I fight others', is incomplete and divided love. Undivided love is life's eternal ability to reveal itself in the attunement and guidance of every creation and is not concerned with contradictions and feelings of good and bad. Strangely enough, we seem to grow more and gain more self-knowledge through adversity than prosperity. That is no excuse to justify setbacks; but the fact is that setbacks, like prosperity, are also expressions of undivided love.

Love flows when expressing creativity, which is therefore a way out in adverse circumstances and offers healing when *qi* stagnates.

Creativity is emphatically about the process and not about the end product of the creative act. Being 'in' the process by being open to intuition and having the courage to make 'mistakes' is indispensable for the creative power of love. Being in the present, staying attuned to the possibilities of all those different moments of Now, without the will that drives towards completion, makes creativity unique and complete in itself. Making music, painting, giving an outstanding speech, a perfect 100-metre run or treatments in which everything matches come from being present in the moment, which is neither new nor old and is changing constantly.

The experience of the creative power of love not only brings joy and pleasure, it may cause grief and pain. It is accompanied by a different sense of time and the feeling that it is correct and reliable despite the pain. Recently, I had to say goodbye to a dear friend who was to die that day. When we looked each other in the eye for the last time, he said with tears in his eyes: 'Weird, this is sad and at the same time so beautiful.' The experience of love evoked beauty in which the sense of time had disappeared. It was good.

Creativity is so often described as the ability to shape something. This is in contrast to the creative power of love, which is like swimming in the stream of a flowing river. You will be taken into the speed of the current. Every moment is different and every moment is new and requires renewed attention. There's no room to look back or look far ahead. The process develops and one moment flows into the next. The experience of this form of creativity is almost always described as inner peace and the feeling of being carried along by something that cannot be mentioned.

Creativity based on the creative power of love is based on knowledge, techniques, methods and science, flexibility, recognizing patterns and details, skills and thinking about ideas and the like, but comes to completion only through attentive awareness. This means that there is no focus on a possible future outcome, only presence.[8] This form of completion causes the great movement fire to be an ever-penetrating awareness, independent of time and space.

THE DYNAMICS OF INTEGRATION AND SEQUENCE

Creativity based on the creative power of love arises in the perception of the moment but, above all, by integrating the properties of the other great movements: earth, ego and identity; metal, communication between the ego and the environment; water, the natural state and the dynamics of the undivided source, together with openness; and wood, flexibility to change and move. The combined integrated five great movements thus form the living dynamics, in which each great movement contributes in its own way in collaboration with the other.

Functioning in sequence towards a target has a different effect and meaning. Sequence means progression from one element to another. This means that there is a beginning that can lead to an end. It starts in the great movement earth and flows successively in the great movements metal, water, wood and fire. The seed grows in the spring through heat, sunlight, nutrients and water, and the young plant eventually flowers with seeds in the summer. The completion in the great movement fire is then based on past actions and experiences. Time, thoughts, will and desires determine the nature of completion.

The successive development of great movements is the most common. As an example: Someone in the company has an idea and intention (great movement

---

8   Nevertheless, you may have an opinion about the performance afterwards.

earth) that is being thought through and brainstormed (great movement metal). It is set against the bar of the mission statement (great movement water), after which departments are put to work (great movement wood) to develop the idea and implement it in the company (great movement fire).

Both forms of completion – integrated and targeted – have their pitfalls. People who have an imbalance in the great movement fire usually focus more on the end goals, performance and perfection. Without the integration of the properties of the various great movements, people are quickly at risk of burnout, because the purpose seems more important than their own health. Conversely, people who live mainly through the integrated form of creativity often cannot adapt to the values and habits of society. This path may be accompanied by uncertainty, fears and nervousness that may to some extent be offset by the styles of behaviour and lifestyle.

When a burnout arises due to excessive will and desires, the advice is to get creative in any way, as long as the process remains in the foreground and the result is not the goal. This form of creativity relaxes people so that they can return to experiencing joy and happiness in the moment. Somehow, the necessary inner drive and desire to be creative arises automatically when people regain playfulness. And the nice thing is that people appreciate this, because it also quickly turns out to be a fun tool to work on their own health. They will listen better to the signals within themselves and live a more integrated life. It often works to remind people of what they liked to do as a child and ask them to pick it up again.

The treatment of the insecure, nervous artist is more complicated because authenticity and stubbornness usually prevail. It can sometimes help to ask people to focus more on techniques and other forms in which the order of actions is important. Another more subtle way is to suggest that someone is indulging in the creation that wants to manifest by simply being a channel for that creation and focusing less on identification with the final product.

Both forms of creativity coexist and each has its own meaning and importance. The practitioner's advice should be consistent with the treatment of the great movement fire.

To treat the *shen* I prefer acupuncture points like Ht-7 and Ht-5 but the following points are even more important:

Si-5, *Yang Gu*, yang valley, brings mental clarity and discernment. It calms the *shen* and soothes restlessness.

L.i.-11, *Qi Chi*, crooked pond, in cases of *shen* disturbances due to heat transfer to the heart-*shen*, with symptoms such as agitation, manic disorders, chest tightness, and disconnection from cosmic intuitive *qi*.

Bl-62, *Shen Mai*, extending channel, in cases with yang daytime problems with symptoms such as sadness, mental fatigue, antisocial behaviour, mental instability due to a lack of rooting.

Ki-6, *Zhao Hai*, shining sea, is a point of light and a source of life. It is used in cases with yin night time problems with symptoms such as anger, paranoia and panic attacks. It calms and benefits the *shen*, soothes fears. It allows people to look at themselves and circumstances more calmly and easily.

Gv-24, *Shen Ting*, temple of *shen*, calms the *shen* in general. Advisable with frequent crying, fear, insecurity and depression.

Gv-23, *Shang Xing*, superior star, in cases where the 'vision' is disturbed. This can be literal eye conditions or figuratively when people give up on their goals. Usually this is also accompanied by frontal headache, sinusitis and nasal congestion. This point has a balancing effect on the *qi* of the small intestine, the heart, the *shen* and the great movement fire.

SHORT- AND LONG-TERM SOLUTIONS
Short-term solutions for balancing the great movement fire:

- the need for confirmation by opinions, belief systems, concepts, ideals
- the need for stimulation of the great movement fire by coffee or other food that activates fire, also done by a lot of talking and lust that is aimed at satisfying lust
- people feel unmotivated, frustrated and dissatisfied. They make up for a lack of stimulating experiences by expressing frustration and dissatisfaction. There may also be a tendency to be constantly active and have a busy schedule
- lack of awareness of the importance of the practical, realistic side of life may make people feel isolated. This feeling can be offset by self-pity, excessive rationalization, and/or a tendency to carry out practical things to perfection
- because the head requires more attention than the heart, people especially

desire heart-to-heart connections. People can appear cold and rational to one person, while they are described as warm and sensitive by the other.

Long-term solutions for balancing the great movement fire:

- the integrated form of *shen* and the great movement fire facilitate observation in silence with a peaceful mind. Creativity happens from freedom and is based on intuition and intelligence of the heart rather than intellect of the mind
- *qi* imparts vibrations and animates the forms. From the authenticity of the being, the great movement water and the *jing* nurture and maintain the forms and the essence by reproduction. The *shen* perceives everything, is connected with everything and is the source of understanding and insight. Understanding in general, self-awareness, awareness of the environment, interest in mental-psychological processes all contribute to the health of the great movement fire, as long as it originates from enthusiasm and enjoyment instead of compulsion
- rituals: seriously performing rituals in any form brings people into contact and attunement with the authenticity and preciousness of the creativity of the *shen*. A ritual reveals what is essentially and truthfully already present in the *shen*. It strengthens and intensifies the interconnectedness of the *shen–hun* relationship. Important in this regard is what was discussed in Chapter 3 about the *yuanheng* emanations in connection with the acceptance of natural sacrifices and the oneness of existence.

A weaker great movement fire leads to nervousness and insecurity. This is often hidden behind socially desirable or tough behaviour. Symptoms and diseases are, for example, migraines, headaches, neck and lower back issues, mouth ulcers, eye issues, confusion with stress, high blood pressure and so on.

CHAPTER 11

TREATING GREAT MOVEMENTS

Treat the ill person not the illness.

J.D. van Buren

Constitutional acupuncture focuses on people and not diseases. The totality of the human being at every level is taken into account in diagnostics and treatment in order to find a new balance in which the self-healing capacity of the entire system is given a new chance. The personality, sleep and eating pattern, social interaction, age, passions, work and so on are compared diagnostically with the innate and acquired possibilities in which the *jing-qi-shen* and the birth chart are central.

For treatments, channels are chosen that match the pulse and body diagnosis, history and other information about the patient and the constitutional birth chart. Next, points are chosen that treat the imbalances, but of course that also focus on treatment to cure unpleasant symptoms and diseases. In acute life-threatening conditions, constitutional treatment is combined with acupuncture points that protect life. For constitutional treatments, mere knowledge of the relationship between acupuncture points and syndromes and diseases is not sufficient. A constitutional approach requires good training in pulse and body diagnostics and a nuanced knowledge of the energetics of acupuncture points. Labelling people with a disease is not preferred because it can hinder the mutual exchange of human contact. Being biased by protocols and rules on the treatment of diseases leads to reduced sensitivity and a limitation of understanding of the underlying causes of complaints and diseases.

This is not to say that other forms of acupuncture are not good. On the contrary, I appreciate the effectiveness of many forms of acupuncture. However, this book is about constitutional acupuncture, where many colleagues feel at home and attract patients who appreciate them and their form of treatment.

The art of constitutional acupuncture is the art of treating the present based on history and the influence history has in the present with knowledge of the *qi* balance of the future with the prospect that diseases can be prevented. One of my teachers told me the following story: There used to be a wise man in every little village where people went every three months for advice. They were given advice on breathing, *qi* exercises, eating habits, herbs and sometimes they received acupuncture treatments. If they got sick, the wise man had to treat them for free.

Constitutional acupuncture is based on the time of a patient's birth and on the configuration of *qi* of the present and the future. This makes each treatment unique. If I learned one valuable thing from my teachers, it is that every con-sultation is a new consultation. Even though I have known the patient for over thirty years and I know the birth chart and pulse by heart, every consultation is a unique and precious moment for the patient and me. It is always about the imbalance of *qi* at *that* time, at *this* place and what internal and external forces have revealed themselves and can be expected. It is indeed an art form that takes into account everything and everyone who has influence over what is present and what has taken place. It's like playing and listening to a good piece of music in which all the instruments and layers of music make the concert.

In advance I would like to emphasize that the classifications and treatment proposals discussed below are suggestions and not protocols.

Rule of thumb:

- Born with a passive great movement: The advice is to decrease the activity of the active great movement first and nourish the passive great move-ment with acupuncture or moxibustion.
- Born with an active great movement: The advice is to first tonify the passive great movement.
- Always compare and solve the unbalanced *qi* of three great movements in the triangle of 'subdue and revenge'.

BIRTH CHART WITH PASSIVE GREAT MOVEMENT: DECREASE THE ACTIVE GREAT MOVEMENT

A gentleman born in 1985 with a passive great movement metal and an active great movement fire suffers from intestinal problems, chronic back pain and epicondylitis. He is a workaholic, has a difficult social life and feels frustrated and isolated due to insecurity and nervousness. The physical complaints indicate problems in the large intestine organ and channel, which is confirmed by further case history questioning and pulse diagnosis. In Chapter 17 we discuss that, in this case, choosing acupuncture points on the large intestine channel balances the great movement metal. However, there is more to this case. The great movement fire subdues the great movement metal by fire short-term solution behaviour, that overactivates the great movement fire. The great movement fire short-term solution behaviour is frustration, based on feeling weak and insecure, offset by workaholic behaviour. It must first be transformed into fire long-term great movement behaviour before the great movement metal can be addressed with lasting results. A treatment on the large intestine channel will certainly be successful but only for a short time. It is necessary to first treat the balance of the great movement fire. When behavioural change and increase in self-esteem have occurred, this usually leads to a significant reduction in complaints, caused by less suppression of the great movement metal, in this case the complaints of the large intestine *qi*.

A special case was another male patient, with similar problems and also born in 1985, who seemed to apply the fire long-term solutions well. While training for a marathon, his back and intestinal complaints continued unabated. Setting the goal of running a marathon and the intense training that came with it, which only later turned out to compensate for his past feelings of inferiority, made the *qi* of the great movement fire excessive, subduing the great movement metal over and over again. Only after a few treatments of the excessive great movement fire, once a month, did he share his past inferiority complex. He began to calm his desire for confirmation and viewed his training as a ritual. He tried to enjoy running alone for no other purpose than to entertain himself. The complaints disappeared and he completed the marathon.

BIRTH CHART WITH ACTIVE GREAT MOVEMENT: STRENGTHEN THE PASSIVE GREAT MOVEMENT

People born with an active great movement in the birth chart are challenged to keep the active great movement in shape and certainly also to curb the risk of overactivity. Even more important are the consequences of the activity of the great movement on the next great movement in the *ke*-cycle; experience has shown that the passive great movement easily becomes too passive and insufficient.

People born with an active great movement wood often enjoy physical exertion. They participate in sports, walking, yoga, *qigong* as long as the physical is addressed. However, the work of trainers and coaches who mentally guide people also falls under the great movement wood. They are involved in structuring and initiating change by awareness and personal growth.

The active great movement wood may subdue the great movement earth. Rather than taking it easy with the great movement wood behaviour and being less active, one often prefers to strengthen the great movement earth by looking for earth short-term solutions. This often leads to the search for approval and competition, as a result of which the great movement earth is temporarily active. Other symptoms of short-term solution behaviour are when people seek out worrying situations, repeat questions or defend and discuss their own point of view over and over again. It can lead to a very tense situation between the great movement wood and earth, as wood likes to combat the great movement earth. A vicious circle has then arisen. You do not solve this condition by only treating the great movement wood. It must go hand in hand with a dramatic change of short-term solutions towards long term in order to balance the great movement earth.

'SUBDUE AND REVENGE'

The dynamics between great movements can include three great movements. Let's look at the previous example in this chapter of the great movement wood that subdued the great movement earth. The great movement metal, the child of the great movement earth, is able to stand up for its mother. There are two options. Specifically, the great movement metal can be activated by short- or long-term solution behaviour but it is always with the aim of subduing the great movement wood. In the name of its mother, it takes 'revenge' on the overactive great movement wood.

During short-term solution metal behaviour, people might seek refuge in structure rather than allowing processes to develop, or dogmatically record every meeting they have. The long-term metal solution – for example, exercising regularly – seems a healthy choice, but it maintains the increased tension between the three great movements because it is an unnatural solution to the tension between the great movement wood and earth. This may cause various illnesses in the long run. For instance, when the dryness of the great movement metal prevails, the free flow of *qi* of the great movement wood can stagnate. The raised activity of the great movement metal evokes possible overactivity in the *qi* of the large intestine, lungs, bladder and kidneys.[1] It may lead to illnesses such as kidney stones, cystitis, lumbar disc problems, constipation, migraine, persistent sadness due to difficulty processing loss and/or waking up prematurely.

When triangle problems appear – I have called them 'subdue and revenge issues' – short-term solutions should be changed to long-term solutions,[2] but above all, the activity of initial active great movement should be lessened.

When a person is born with the passive great movement metal (for example, in 1965) the great movement fire is more active. This is reflected in increasing desires, more focus, active social life, strong opinions and belief systems and so on. Instead of strengthening the passive great movement metal by short- or long-term solutions, the person's great movement water may seek control over the great movement fire. This usually results in stronger willpower and authenticity.

In this situation, complaints initially arise in the passive great movement metal and the liver *qi*[3] with diseases such as herpes simplex, muscle problems, *wei qi* issues and so on. In the long term, there will be more complaints due to the tension between the great movements water and fire, such as high blood pressure, headache, bladder and prostate issues and so on. The most difficult challenge for these people is the change in behaviour: to adjust appreciation for the comfortable sense of strong will and authenticity (great movement water) and balance the passive great movement metal through inner spiritual enrichment and silence. The result of a balanced passive great movement metal is natural calmness in the great movement fire causing less desires, less strong opinions and less dependence on social life.

---

1   See the chapters on earthly branches.
2   With the great movement water there is a slightly more problematic process. Water short-term solutions become a purpose in themselves. Setting a goal as such activates the great movement water and keeps it going for a long time. In the end, people may collapse from burnout.
3   See Chapter 13 on the heavenly stem *Yi*.

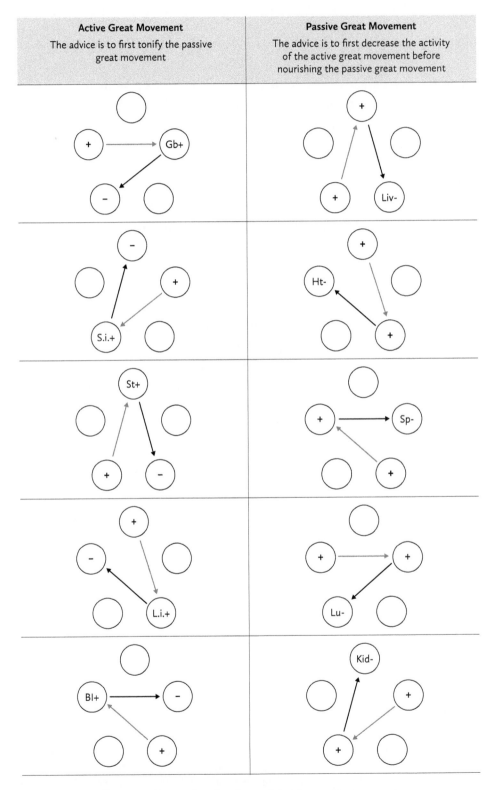

Figure 11.1 Dynamics of active and passive great movements

CHAPTER 12

DYNAMICS OF THE HEAVENLY STEM *JIA* 甲[1]

When I first heard of heavenly stems and earthly branches, I was amazed at those names. Heavenly combined with stems[2] and earthly with branches? The answer turned out to be a metaphor. On the blackboard J.D. van Buren drew an inverted tree with roots in heaven. 'This is what it's all about,' he said, without further explaining. It took a while, but eventually I understood.

Trees have a life that is complementary to that of mammals. They feed on carbon dioxide, water and salts that are transmuted into sugars. The flow of *qi* and liquids in the stem and branches allows the leaves to reach the sunlight, from which they receive the energy to transmute the sugars made into starches and proteins for growth and development. During this process they release waste – oxygen – into the air. Mammals need this and provide trees and plants with their waste material – carbon dioxide.

Like water, heavenly *qi* flows down from the inverted tree of eternal life. The eternal essence of life provides the life nutrients for all living essences through the ten heavenly stems that define and describe temporal life on earth and in humans. The twelve earthly branches are the revelations through which nature and (human) life on earth can come into contact with the eternal essence of their existence. There is exchange and, for people, the ability to respond – literally 'responsibility': offering and contributing to life through the earthly branches by aligning actions, thoughts, feelings and speech. These offerings are the nutrients for the life-giving heaven. Heaven offers to nourish matter and bring forms to life through the heavenly stems. The heavenly stems are dynamized by the five

---

1   Born in years ending with a 4 such as 2004 and 1974, after the Chinese New Year.
2   In the context of trees it is more usual to use the term 'trunks' – it has been a puzzle to me that the name 'stems' was chosen as that would normally be used for plants but not for trees. I do not know why 'stems' has been used rather than 'trunks'.

heavens and ten great movements. The deep *qi* of the earthly branches[3] express the human essence that attunes to nature and to the heavenly origin of all.

JIA 甲, THE FIRST HEAVENLY STEM

Jia is the first of the ten heavenly stems. The quality of *Jia* is shown in the yang of wood, the gallbladder.

The wood quality of *Jia* is based on the emanation *yuan* and the green azure dragon heaven.

Yuan is the initial cause, the creative and guiding principle, and is closely related to the source of existence. It is the origin of movement, growth, guidance and inspiration. The green azure dragon heaven, the heaven of the East, embodies the vitalizing principle behind every form of life.

The Chinese character *Jia* shows the force of breaking through, of being straight, vital and firm.

Jia represents the first expression of life on earth, the beginning of all things and beings. It represents the activity of heaven that manifests as waves of intuitive inspiration that seem to come out of nowhere. Its property shows in the conscious initial power to promote and develop thoughts and awareness by which ideas transform into the practical physical manifested world.

The image of the character *Jia* is twofold. First, it is the image of a new shoot, a bud or a root in its protective shell; second, it represents the shoot on the point of breaking through the protective shell or ground. Any kind of protection is associated with the heavenly stem *Jia*, such as the protective function of nails or the mindset to raise an emotional shield of protection.

Breaking through, described as 'yang moves in the East', is the activity of spring and the vitality of the light of sunrise. The nature of the heavenly stem *Jia* expresses itself in small shoots and flowers at the beginning of spring, just emerging from the ground, also in the first rays of light that fall on the land in the morning and in newborn babies opening their eyes and making first contact with their parents.

---

3   See the chapters on earthly branches.

THE GREAT MOVEMENT EARTH AND THE HEAVENLY STEM *JIA*

The Great Movements are the dynamics of the heavenly stems.[4]

The relationship between the great movement earth and the wood aspect of *Jia* is an example of the reverse *ke* or *wu*-cycle. From the point of view of the initiating/wood element of this combination, the earth that 'covers' the wood carries the dynamic of resistance that movements evoke because conflicts and contradictions are the resistances in which life has a dynamic opportunity to express itself. It is precisely the limitation of form – matter – that gives life the opportunity to gather and develop. In some traditions, the reverse *ke* or *wu*-cycle is called the 'law of friendship': The earth allows the wood of the tree to break open the earthly cover and reach for the light, take root and initiate creation.

The great movement earth is the dynamic force behind the heavenly stem *Jia*. People born with this combination may develop a strong sense of identity, purpose and direction in life with transformative and protective abilities. Due to the yang moving quality of *Jia* and the harmonizing quality of the earth aspect, people are able to change seemingly immutable rules and circumstances with strength and creativity. To realize and implement these transformations, people with '*Jia* in earth' need the help of other people.

When the combination of the great movement earth and the heavenly stem *Jia* develops too strongly, people can be seen as compelling and opinionated. When too weak, they are more vulnerable, with the feeling of being easily exhausted and depressed, both due to a lack of self-confidence.

HEAVEN MEETS EARTH MEETS HUMAN

The following acupuncture points work in harmony with the creative actions of '*Jia* in earth' and therefore fit well with a treatment in that context:

Window of sky points, which link heavenly *qi* with the *shen* aspect of the self: Bl-10, *Tian Zhu*, St-9, *Ren Ying*, Th-16, *Tian You*, S.i.-17, *Tian Rong*, S.i.-16, *Quan Liao*, L.i.-18, *Fu Tu*, (L.i.-17, *Tian Ding*),[5] Gv-16, *Feng Fu*, Cv-22, *Tian Tu*, Pc-1, *Tian Chi*, Lu-3, *Tian Fu*.

---

4   J.D. van Buren: 'Dynamics are functions and forces that initiate activity and change.'
5   L.i.-17 is not always seen as a window of the sky point, nor is it named in the classics, but its name suggests otherwise, and the point works as such.

To link heavenly *qi* with the *jing* aspect of the self, one may use Bl-40, *Wei Zhong*, Gb-30, *Huan Tiao*, St-30, *Qi Chong*, Gv-4, *Ming Men*, Gv-1, *Chang Qiang*, Ki-11, *Heng Gu*, Liv-12, *Ji Mai*, Sp-12, *Chong Men*, Cv-4, *Guan Yuan*, Cv-6, *Qi Hai*.

Cv-8, *Shen Que*, spirit gate. The *shen* reaches a point of balance. It tonifies yin in general and therefore supports yang; it opens and warms the channels and fills the *chong mai*.

Cv-12, *Zhong Wan*, central venter, a point of concentration of *qi* in the central area of the abdomen. It is the front *mu* point of the stomach and *san jiao* (middle burner) and the *hui* point of the *fu*. It tonifies all yang.

Cv-17, *Dan Zhong*, chest centre. Sea and *hui* point of *qi*, front *mu* point of *san jiao* (upper burner) and of the heart constrictor.

Cv-4, *Guan Yuan*, gate of *yuan qi*. Tonifies *yuan qi* and roots people in their base. Tonifies, moves and holds *xuè*. An entrance point for the lower *dan tien* in men.

Cv-6, *Qi Hai*, sea of *qi*. Point of a strong concentration of yin *qi* and reunion of yin and yang *qi*. Supports the root of life; regulates and maintains the metabolism of *qi* and *xuè* in general. An entrance point for the lower *dan tien* in women.

ACUPUNCTURE POINTS THAT INFLUENCE THE ACTIVE GREAT MOVEMENT EARTH AND THE HEAVENLY STEM *JIA*

At this point in this book, it is important to note that J.D. van Buren recommended that in treatments according to heavenly stems and earthly branches, the practitioner should stay away from directly needling a patient's 'own essential' *qi* and preferably opt for related *qi*. This is in line with the ancient concept to treat yin with yang or vice versa, to treat the healthy *qi* instead of the ill *qi*. For example, complaints on the yang, outside, of the elbow are treated on the yin, inside, of the opposite knee, or complaints of the right shoulder are treated with points on the healthy left shoulder. He advised not to address the birth *qi* directly, but indirectly via the *qi* that is 'missing' in the birth chart, which is usually weaker. A person born with '*Jia* in the earth', reflected in the *qi* of the gallbladder, is therefore not treated with gallbladder points, but for example with spleen or liver points.[6] This should of course correspond to pulse and body diagnosis.

People who are born with a different combination of great movement and heavenly stem and have problems in the realm of 'Jia, Gb in earth' can be treated with gallbladder points.

Gb-34, *Yang Ling Quan*, fountain of the yang mound, combines the earth quality of the great movement earth and the wood quality of the heavenly stem *Jia*. For teaching purposes, Gb-34 is called the 'stem point'.[7] The main channels each hold their own stem point in which the heavenly stems and great movements unite.[8]

Gb-34 voices and aligns the *qi* of the great movement earth with the heavenly stem *Jia* within the gallbladder channel. It can be applied to people with identity problems or in cases where people face difficult personal choices, as happens in divorces, changes in work or study, and so on. Gb-34 brings people back to themselves when they are carried away by emotions and when people are confused and uprooted with rising *qi* resulting in symptoms such as nausea, headaches and anxiety. The treatment can be supported by Sp-3, *Tai Bai*, supreme white, and S.i.-4, *Wang Gu*, wrist bone, if needed.

Gb-34 is a *hui* point that moistens all muscles and tendons that enables people to move freely (wood). The outcome of the treatment may be compared to a farmland that is moistened in the spring to ensure that life starts to sprout. Vitalized and supple muscles and tendons determine the way humans express themselves as living and moving beings. People become stiff in the muscles and psycho-emotional movements when the amount or quality of moisture decreases.

Gb-34 gives strength[9] and coordination and balances the expression of personality and identity and is therefore useful to treat insecurity and fear of other people. It is also used with fullness of *qi* superficially, which occurs when people have problems with the external world.[10]

---

6   The spleen shares the same great movement (earth), the liver shares the same phase in the five phases (wood). This topic is further discussed in Chapters 17 (on 'like qi and unlike qi') and 22 (on 'four possibilities'), discussing that acupuncture points of the gallbladder are relevant for people born with '*Yi*, Liv in metal' and '*Ji*, Sp in earth'.
7   The name 'stem point' is not of classical origin.
8   The stem points are Gb-34, Liv-4, S.i.-2, Ht-9, St-41, Sp-3, L.i.-1, Lu-5, Bl-65, Ki-2.
9   Immediately after treating Gb-34, the kidney pulse may feel insufficient and deeper (active great movement of earth subdues water), but within 15 minutes the kidney pulse usually recovers, regains strength and becomes distinct and healthier than before.
10 See Sp-21 in Chapter 18 on the heavenly stem *Ji* for internal issues.

Sp-4, *Gong Sun*, grandfather grandson. In *Grasping the Wind*[11] it is stated that the family name of the Yellow Emperor was Gong Sun. This might refer to the connecting quality of the *Luo* point Sp-4 to balance the earth (yellow) phase, when used with the *yuan source* point St-42, *Chong Yang*, rushing yang. It could also refer to the progression of life: The grandfather has passed on life to his offshoot, his grandson. This is a symbol of heaven revealing *qi* in the *chong mai*, of which Sp-4 is the opening point. *Chong mai* is the bridge from heaven into the post-natal life of humans. It provides the post-natal *qi* pattern based on pre-natal existence. This is the core quality of the central heaven, the great movement earth with the green azure dragon heaven and the heavenly stem *Jia*.

A ten-year-old boy, born in 2004, small and thin for his age, enters my room with his mother. He looks pale, has a dark blue area under his eyes, but he looks pretty sporty. He doesn't look at me or shake my hand. He sits quietly in the chair next to his mother and seems angry that he needs to be there. His mother shares a long story that comes down to the following: He is a very intelligent child with hypersensitivity; he uses Ritalin for attention deficit hyperactivity disorder. Many clinicians have seen him and the diagnosis varies from PDD NOS (pervasive developmental disorder, not otherwise specified) to Asperger's syndrome. In fact, the doctors don't really know. His communication is hesitant and he is very scared, tired, but enjoys sports and does this very intensively. He barely eats and is very picky. On further questioning it appears that health problems were evident from the very beginning of his life: He was often very ill and regularly visited paediatricians. He now attends school only occasionally.

His mother's pregnancy appeared to have been very restless, especially during weeks 20–24, and she experienced many complicated emotional states during other weeks as well. With pulse diagnosis, it is particularly apparent that the *jing*, stomach, spleen and other earth pulses like liver and small intestine are very insufficient.[12] When the great movement earth is affected, it has an impact on all earth in general.

It is tempting to share more about this patient and the given treatment, but I will only discuss the choice I made of Sp-4 as a treatment for someone born with a heavenly stem *Jia* with a weakened great movement earth. Let us go back together to that day when this angry boy with a disgruntled face allowed me to diagnose him. The gallbladder *qi* (*Jia*) is fine, he likes sports and

---

11   Ellis, Wiseman and Boss 1989.
12   In Chapters 24, 26, 29, 32, 36, 38 on earthly branches, it is discussed that there are more *qi* than stomach *qi* and spleen *qi* that are qualified as earth.

is good at that. His social skills are poor. Only because of his skills in sports does he feel that he deserves a place in this world. He sees no reason to take care of himself physically (great movement earth). He can train and exercise all day without eating and is completely exhausted afterwards.

My diagnosis focused mainly on the disordered pregnancy in weeks 20–24, in which the spleen and stomach *qi* are activated. Proper development in these weeks is important for the transformational phase of birth, which also induces the proper functioning of *chong mai* (*jing*).

The principle of treatment first focused on strengthening the *jing* along with the *qi* of the earth in general. Then I treated him with Sp-4 to open the bridge between pre- and post-natal *qi* and directed the *qi* of the pre-natal pattern to Ki-5, *Shui Quan*, water spring, which regulates the *ren mai*[13] and *chong mai*. During the next treatments I continued to work on strengthening the *jing* and earth. After five treatments (once a week) the boy shared that he only rarely suffered from abdominal pains now, that he felt tense but otherwise okay. For the first time in months, he had been at school all week. He looked more vibrant and ate better too and gave me a smile. His pulse however was still tight and restless.

Unfortunately, I lost touch with him. All sorts of dreadful things happened to him and his family and circumstances forced us to stop the treatment.

Still, I took his case as an example to show the possibilities of Sp-4. It can be of help to someone born with a well-developed heavenly stem *Jia* in a poorly developed great movement earth. Sp-4 is not used to support the great movement–heavenly stem relationship when the origin of the problem is rooted in post-natal *qi* only.

THE CONSEQUENCES OF *'JIA*, GALLBLADDER IN EARTH' IN THE *WUXING*

The active great movement earth that dynamizes the vital strength of the heavenly stem *Jia* easily subdues the great movement water which can be observed in the qualities and quantities of all the energies that belong to the phase water such as the *qi* of the bladder and kidney, *wei qi, jin yé, zhi* (willpower), *jing, san jiao* and gallbladder.[14]

In years with '*Jia*, Gb in earth', there is a higher chance that the potentially weaker great movement water will become too weak in winter or that the *qi* of

---

13   Which supports yin and nourishment in general.
14   See the chapters on earthly branches for the relationship between the *san jiao* and gallbladder and water. *Wei qi* is mainly produced in the kidneys (*Nan Jing*).

water, *wei qi* and *jing qi* are insufficient. Reduced resistance can cause diseases to develop deeper or more superficially, depending on the rest of the constitution.

In years when, due to the natural rhythm of *qi*, the great movement water tends to be insufficient for everyone,[15] people with innate weaker great movement water must be prepared.

In general, symptoms and diseases can manifest in the active as well as subdued passive great movement. Practice has proven to me that it is generally more pleasant and easier for the patient to nourish the passive great movement first – in the case of '*Jia*, Gb in earth' the great movement water – before the symptoms and imbalance of the active great movement and the heavenly stem *Jia* are treated.

In the past I was taught to choose to balance the (over)active great movement earth first. It usually resulted in a slow recovery of the insufficient great movement water. It worked well, but it gradually became clear to me that people were quickly reverting to their old habits and short-term solutions. The challenge of addressing the underactivity of a great movement water in a healthy way had only been temporarily postponed. Importantly, I also noticed that their learning challenge to feed the underactive great movement water was less clear. Features of a strong great movement earth and heavenly stem *Jia* (vitality, positive input, taking initiative and the ability to effect change) can easily boost willpower and propel people to exceed their limits. The difficult task of fine-tuning their will was taken away by treatments that work on the balance of the great movement earth only, with the result that they soon exceeded their limits again.

I then started combining the treatments: During the same treatment I worked on balancing the overactive great movement earth along with promoting the insufficient great movement water. The outcomes of this approach didn't satisfy me either.

Later, I started to give advice first, along with acupuncture treatments, to support the underactive passive great movement water and found the results more satisfactory because they proved more durable. By nurturing the underactive passive great movement, people suddenly started to show responsibility for their own health and felt the inner impulse to change. They were more open to advice and conversations. Only when the first symptoms of recovery, along with the first signs of facing the challenges of the great movement water, were visible was the active great movement earth treated. This treatment was, in contrast to previous attempts, nearly always experienced by patients as the 'icing on the

---

15   Years ending with a 4 and 1 such as 2024 and 2021.

cake'. It soon became apparent that this approach was just as positive for the other active great movements.

People born with 'Jia, Gb in the earth' generally show a positive sense of identity that allows them to achieve much without becoming intrusive or boastful. They can work hard with vitality and a positive presence, without getting tired quickly, and are happy to do it with dedication, patience, service and responsibility. The earthly qualities make it possible to carry this out with empathy and sympathy. They generally show interest in change processes and developments such as guiding people and groups in reorganizations of companies or guiding the transformation of individuals' consciousness. There is interest as long as there is the opportunity for change. However, there is a pitfall. The properties of great movement earth can be negatively affected by the wood qualities of *Jia*, gallbladder. This leads to exhaustion of the great movement earth. In those cases, direct treatment and advice regarding the great movement earth is the only sensible approach. Unfortunately, besides exhaustion, there is often a lack of certainty and firm footing in life or a build-up of resentment and competitiveness with the tendency to criticize others. It is wise for practitioners to take this into account, because these patients then tend to jump from one therapist to the next.

CHAPTER 13

DYNAMICS OF THE HEAVENLY STEM *YI* 乙¹

YI 乙, THE SECOND HEAVENLY STEM

The quality of *Yi* is shown in the yin of wood, the liver.

Like *Jia*, the heavenly stem *Yi* is related to the East, descending from the emanation *yuan* and the green azure dragon heaven. It expresses the growing spring season with the incredible variety of green colours that shape the fullness and beauty of the promise of new life. The heavenly stem *Yi* continues the creative, vitalizing principle of *Jia*, giving birth to the new strength, growth and flexibility that characterize spring.

Jia links the subtle world of oneness with the world of phenomena and division. The world of cooperating and conflicting phenomena is fragile, so transformation and guidance from the impulse of heaven is offered by the character of *Yi*: vital, flexible, gentle, compassionate and always with strength and alertness to enable support and defence of the evolving life.

To build, *Yi* gathers and guides the impulse from heaven towards qualities known as temperament, inspiration and insight. To sustain, a healthy *Yi* provides people with strong, rapid, flexible *qi* to benefit growth at all levels of existence. It represents the power of gathering and delivering unconscious movements of *wei qi* and *xuè* whenever and wherever they are needed.

The Chinese character *Yi* depicts a shoot that leaves the bud. The joined energy of fast-growing bamboo plants is a fine example of its strength and ability to support rapid growth. Some sources describe *Yi* as a picture of a twisted twig. A flexible, twisted branch shows strength and is harder to break than a straight one. It will find its way into nature more easily, being able to adapt to the dangers and challenges of life.

---

1   Born in years ending with a 5 such as 2005 and 1975, after the Chinese New Year.

In the body, *Yi* is expressed in smooth and firm movements of the hands and fingers, a smoothly working immune system (through strong *xuè*, *jin yé* and *wei qi*), flexible muscles and tendons, an ability to go with the flow and provide the body with necessary improvements. Uncontrolled rapid growth, including the development of diseases that thereby become uncontrollable (such as in cancer), can be caused by an overly vital *Yi* where vitality and adaptation have become an end in themselves. This imbalance is often accompanied by outbursts of anger that serve to release tension.

THE GREAT MOVEMENT METAL AND THE HEAVENLY STEM *YI*

The great movement metal and the wood aspect of *Yi* are in a *ke*-cycle relationship. This cycle is usually understood as the controlling cycle in which one phase is in control of the other. However, the *ke*-cycle has a broader function than only control. It too is in service of wholeness and balance, guides, monitors, purifies and limits overactive components to keep the wholeness healthy. When the *wei qi* travels more internally in the body at night, it purifies the organs in a *ke*-cycle sequence before emerging and travelling externally again in the morning through the *tai yang* channels near the eyes. It nourishes the physical form, and promotes and guides the expression of life.[2]

The great movement metal has its archetypal background in the white tiger heaven and the emanation *li*, the symbols of beneficial gathering, centripetal movements, harvesting, nourishing, prevention and protection from the cold of winter. These properties are accompanied by a clear understanding of the relationship between the internal and external world and the ability to exclude what is disagreeable and harmful. The great movement metal provides the proper *qi* and direction for self-knowledge and inner cultivation.

The passive great movement metal is yin in character, as demonstrated by its responding, receiving, following, gentle, submissive, guiding, providing and nourishing abilities. Its yin aspect is opposite to the wood aspect of the heavenly stem *Yi*, being based on the emanation *yuan*, the *qi* of the beginning of all things and beings, the initial cause, the yang, creative principle and origin of movement, growth, guidance and inspiration. The combination of wood and metal spans the conscious horizontal field, the space between the East and the West, between sunrise and sunset, when people are awake and active. And it

---

2   The *ke*-cycle relationship plays an important role in the treatment of the constitutional nature of a person. It is discussed in Chapter 17 on five methods of treatment.

spans the unconscious horizontal field, the space between the West and the East, between sunset and sunrise, when people sleep and purify their minds and bodies. The cooperation between the yin and yang forces is necessary in both realms. Outward presence requires prudence and self-knowledge; purification requires internal focus in addition to the power of discernment, cleansing and refinement, and so on.

People born with '*Yi*, Liv in metal' feel the need to interpret and understand experiences and explore their learning so as to develop goals for future growth. They might have a hard time talking about emotions – they want to process emotions themselves first – but they appreciate clear interpretations by others on issues they face. It supports them to collect data to process so that life can become more manageable.

The 'horizontal field' of wood and metal is a practically realistic field, which must yield tangible benefits. Mental, spiritual and creative impulses that mainly originate from the active great movement fire are always placed by these individuals along the bar of practical value and interpretation. Since spirituality encompasses infinity and invisibility, there may also be interest and fascination with the afterlife, but it can also lead to anxiety, especially among those who feel possessed by the influences of others that leave them little power over their own lives. It is important for them to get enough sleep to process and incorporate their feelings.

When the combination of the great movement metal and the heavenly stem *Yi* is strong, people born with it come across as very present and inspirational, but their demand for attention may absorb the energy of those around them, who can be left empty and tired when they leave. Complaints appear when this combination is too weak. The lack of metal results in too much fluid, liver blood stagnation, fluid retention leading to digestive problems, oedema, nausea, vomiting, back pain and menstrual cramps, shortness of breath and bladder problems.

Other signs and symptoms are related to imbalanced wood channels: headaches, migraines, muscle and ligament injuries, sexual dysfunction, gallbladder and liver disease, insomnia and so on. Interestingly, these people can summon compassion from others to increase their own resilience. However, the help offered may disappear into an insatiable space. Whatever is done, it will always prove insufficient until the power and balance of this combination is restored.

ACUPUNCTURE POINTS THAT INFLUENCE THE PASSIVE GREAT MOVEMENT METAL AND THE HEAVENLY STEM *YI*

The following acupuncture points support yin and bridge the outside world with the inner world.

St-25, *Tian Shu*, heavenly pivot. *Tian* means celestial, heaven and sky; *Shu* means pivot, hinge and axis. The name refers to one of the stars of the Big Dipper, Dubhe (*alpha ursae majoris*), a bright star in the ursa major constellation that points the way to the North Pole star, the seat of the heavenly emperor. St-25 bridges the relationship of yang-heaven with yin-humans. On the stomach channel it is the last opportunity to connect yang-heaven-outside-environment with yin-human-inside. The location in the centre of the body marks the horizontal plane of humanity, with the sky above and the earth below.

St-25 brings yang into the body and tonifies, warms and moves yin in general. It harmonizes the centre and the stomach and regulates the spleen and meets the liver. Being a meeting point for *shao yang*, it hinges between heaven and humanity.

St-25 is used with yang fullness (above and outside) and yin insufficiency (down and inside) in people with symptoms such as hypersensitivity, talking nonsense (delirious), overexcitement, anxiety and irritability with chronic abdominal yin symptoms.

Sp-15, *Da Heng*, great horizontal, strengthens the spleen and promotes transformation and transportation. It influences the large intestine and promotes smooth flow of liver *qi* in the abdomen. As a point of the *yin wei mai*[3] it connects between yin and yang, as do the great movement metal and the heavenly stem *Yi*.

Sp-15 is used during the peri-menopause period, when the *yin wei mai*, spleen and stomach *qi* diminish. This gradual transition from the creative yang period of life to a created yin period of life can be accompanied by symptoms such as sadness, crying and sighing and self-pity.

Sp-21, *Da Bao*, great embracement, along with Sp-8, *Di Ji*, earth pivot. Sp-21 is the great *luo* acupuncture point of the spleen. It regulates the relationship with the outside world that people seek through movement, thus using muscles and joints, and it focuses on the movements in the inner world of emotional and sensory perceptions. It is the great regulator to balance the bottom–top, left–right,

---

3   'Yang wei mai connects together various yang while the *yin wei mai* connects together various yin; When the *yang wei mai* and *yin wei mai* fail to connect together, it will give rise to a loss of willpower and weakening of physical strength, as powerless as soft water.' *Nan Jing* Question 29.

inside–out. As the *Ode to Elucidate Mysteries* says: 'Man consists of top, middle and bottom. The major points for these three areas are great embracement (Sp-21), celestial pivot (St-25) and earth pivot (Sp-8).'[4] Top, middle and bottom are parallel with the concepts of heaven, earth and human.

Sp-8 is an essential point for treatment of diseases of the central earth part of the body. It is an important point in the treatment of spleen and stomach (earth) disorders, such as lack of appetite and thin stools. Sp-21, St-25 and Sp-8 together maintain the balance of the whole body.

Liv-4, *Zhong Feng*, mound centre or middle seal.[5] This is called the stem point for its connection to the liver and the phase metal. It is mainly known as an acupuncture point to treat ankle injuries with pain. On the other hand it is used for stagnant liver *qi* in the lower burner. These indications seem very different, but they have something in common: *san jiao*. Free flow of *qi* in the ankle and lower burner indicates a healthy free exchange between a person and the environment. According to J.D. van Buren, the *qi* of the ankle on the lateral side is controlled by the gallbladder and on the medial side by *san jiao*. The ankle as a unit is controlled by *san jiao*. The function of *san jiao* in the lower burner has been discussed above.

San jiao is the hinge between the subtle world of heaven and the denser world of our three dimensional existence. The ability of Liv-4 to treat ankle injuries and lower burner stagnation relates to more than relieving pain and discomfort. A free-moving ankle and a free flow of *qi* in the lower burner provide and facilitate the natural exchange people have with the environment.

In addition, Liv-4 balances the three *hun* and seven *po*, the balance between immaterial and material, between intentional and instinctive, especially when accompanied by signs of a weak great movement metal and weak heavenly stem *Yi*, characterized by a flaccid, passive body and constitution.

Tonification of Liv-4[6] restores the liver *qi* and releases the contraction in the lung.

> Treating Liv-4 is used when people are overwhelmed by stimuli from society. For example, they work a lot of overtime, are too busy with social media, travel too much or do something else that drains them. The liver *qi* becomes too tight and constricted by stress and excessive use of the will. The free flow of *qi* becomes blocked, causing stagnation, heat and insufficiency of other organs. It is often enough to sedate Liv-4 and restore the free flow of *qi* by

4   Bertschinger 1991, p. 31.
5   J.D. van Buren advised not to treat people's essential *qi* directly. In rare cases, the stem point may be sedated. One has to be careful with sedation as it reduces the innate essential *qi*.
6   Usually accompanied by Liv-5 and Gb-40.

using Liv-3. The symptoms that present with imbalance vary from hay fever and herpes simplex to heartburn and arrhythmia of the heart.

Because of the differences between people's tolerance and our often mentally overheated, demanding society, great tension may arise in the relationship between the passive great movement metal and the heavenly stem *Yi*. This is manifested in stagnation and constriction of the liver *qi*. Of course, it is not always easy to change this pattern but treatment should go hand in hand with good behavioural advice and hints that spur and stimulate the patient's own responsibility to get healthy.

THE CONSEQUENCES OF '*YI*, LIVER IN METAL' IN THE *WUXING*

People with '*Yi*, Liv in metal' should be able to deal with the stimuli of the outside world and respond appropriately. When, for whatever reason, the great movement metal malfunctions, these people have a hard time. They feel quickly influenced and overwhelmed by the world, creating an inner urge to set up a defence system, especially when introspection is adversely influenced by external stress. Their defence is nearly always observable in the quality and quantity of the pulses of *tai yang* (bladder and small intestine) and heart constrictor, which can be powerful, more superficial and tight.[7] Symptoms can be expressed physically, emotionally or mentally, but all these conditions illustrate the weakness of the great movement metal. The more physically oriented person tends to compensate for the weakness of the defensive *qi* through pride and untouchability. The emotional defence manifests itself in 'I'll take care of it myself'. These people are ready to help others, but find it difficult to ask for and receive help. The mental defence often consists of hiding behind philosophical lines of thought. It is then difficult to truly get personal contact, because the vulnerable individual hides behind the dogmatic principles of philosophical concepts. Uncertainty is then compensated for by fixed habits, which can develop into compulsive rituals: for example, only feeling good when the laundry is done, or leaving the house only when the kitchen is neatly organized in a very personal way. This can even develop into a pathological fear of infection and germs.

Someone born with a passive great movement will generally be challenged to maintain strength in that passive great movement. However, gradually over the years it has become clear to me that the challenges usually appear more in

---

7   Because of *tai yang*'s external position in the six divisions and the heart constrictor that can be overwhelmed by emotions and passions if it doesn't follow the heart.

the resulting active great movement. With the passive great movement metal, diseases, signs and symptoms refer more clearly to excessive fire, rather than insufficient metal. The active great movement fire symptoms can be found in the heart, small intestine, *san jiao* and heart constrictor and in all *qi* that is influenced by fire, such as spleen *qi*,[8] rising *qi*, heat, increase of physiological processes, behaviour, memory, relationships and so on. People born with a passive great movement metal are therefore faced with the challenge to calm down their fire on all aspects.

To relax, and to calm the speed of life, is in general the main challenge for people affected by an active great movement fire. Calming applies in the first place to thinking, which never seems to stop. Past experiences, future expectations and ongoing sensory perceptions lead to yet more thinking rather than focusing on what is happening in the present. Thinking seems to be aimed at assessing how things can be adjusted and how satisfaction can be achieved and seems to distract people from the experiences of the present. A characteristic consequence of overactive great movement fire is a repeated feeling of frustration from the constant, active demanding mind and an inability to be in the moment.

This might be the reason why people with active great movement fire issues like to be distracted by events and hobbies that do not require them to think so much, like binge-watching Netflix, watching sports or using alcohol, cocaine or MDMA/ecstasy. Distraction that involves strong sensory input helps them to experience the often illusionary present. Short-term solutions can range from sports to sex, from alcohol consumption to lavish parties and an extreme focus on study or teaching. A special escape route from the reality of the present is obsessive-compulsive behaviour, where a ritual expression of wanting to control life is acted out physically, as opposed to through thoughts. For these people, ending control by thoughts seems to be the only option for gaining a calm mind, but that usually does not prove easy. Although the exercises in themselves are not complicated, the regular training required is a challenge because it requires perseverance and patience. In addition, such a practice can evoke sorrow and suffering from which people like to flee. However, there is no durable solution to be found in escape routes.

It helps in these cases to practise awareness exercises, body scan meditations, and to be more open to the power of intuition from the heart that goes beyond the distortions of the rational mind. Creativity and free dancing are other options that may lead to calmness. These refer the person to experiences, inventiveness and originality, in which thinking often plays a subordinate role. With creativity and dancing there is less room for the restless mind and more room for intuition and the awareness of the present moment.

---

8   See the chapters on earthly branches.

In my practice something remarkable happened: As with the previous great movement, I first applied the methods of balancing the passive great movement, as I had learned. And, while I wasn't expecting it, I saw that the strengthening and balance of the passive great movement metal reduced the dominance of the great movement fire. Further study of the controlling *ke*-cycle and insulting *wu*-cycle was needed.

In the *ke*-cycle the grandmother subdues the grandson, as fire controls metal and metal controls wood, to inhibit and control unlimited growth. If the controller becomes too strong, the strength of the controller should be reduced; in practical terms, if the fire is too strong and the metal is subdued, the responsible fire channel should be calmed down by sedation, *luo*-source treatment or otherwise. However, the grandson is *conditional* for the grandmother to function properly. It has a strong effect on the grandmother if the grandson becomes insufficient or is out of balance. This could be another reason why the insulting cycle (*wu*) in some traditions is called the cycle of friendship.

The functions of the *ke*- and *wu*-cycles can be described as follows:

The metal axe cuts the tree but metal needs wood: Some minerals and stones of organic origin arise from vital elements of plants or animals. The roots of a tree (wood) break up the earth, but the trees need earth for growth (water and minerals) and stability. Earth controls water through dykes, but earth needs water and moisture to be compact. Without moisture, the earth is too light and will be blown away in the wind. Running water can control the fire, but water needs fire or heat to have the correct temperature and prevent it from turning into ice. Fire melts metal but fire needs a solid form (metal) to cling to. When there are not enough solid forms or the solid forms are already in a state of fullness to which the fire cannot attach itself, it will look for other ways to express itself by, for example, rising *qi* and spreading heat. The better the grandson, the less tension with the grandmother.

To be honest, I have been teaching for a number of years that reducing the reaction in the active great movements first is better than strengthening the insufficient great movement. This made sense since most of the signs and symptoms are in the active great movement fire. However, in most cases it turned out to be sufficient to treat and balance just the passive great movement metal. Nevertheless, it is prudent to advise people to reduce the active fire behaviour to prevent future failure of the great movement metal. Treating the 'grandson great movement metal' offers the form, structure and more physicality. It usually restores the normal function of the 'grandmother great movement fire', but it will not change people's habits.

The outcome of my study and observations made it clear to me that it is more applicable to deal with the balance of passive great movement first. It reminded me of a statement by Lavier, one of J.D. van Buren's first teachers in the field of acupuncture: 'It never hurts, it can't go wrong and it is safer to treat the insufficient *qi* first.'

A FINAL NOTE

It can be challenging to really find the correct personal balance between the ego and the environment. A long-lasting process towards an integrated life with a long-lasting imbalance can still lead to illness. People born with '*Yi*, Liv in metal' regularly seem to seek balance by meeting other people or being active outwardly rather than cultivating their inner selves. In addition to treating the great movement metal and the heavenly stem *Yi*, liver, a number of other acupuncture points have a positive effect in supporting a healthy interaction between the ego and its environment:

Lu-3, *Tian Fu*, heavenly palace, calms the *po* and is used with situations of sadness, depression, weeping, disorientation, forgetfulness and somnolence and/or insomnia caused by lung *qi* imbalance. Lu-3 enlivens and allows a free communication with cosmic *qi* when people are locked in themselves.

This also concerns complaints caused by instability of the neck as a result of whiplash.

Pc-6, *Nei Guan*, inner pass/gate, enables an appropriate communication in general.

The first combination of great movement and heavenly stem ('*Jia*, Gb in earth') promotes the quality of the centre that we may call the identity, the second combination ('*Yi*, Liv in metal') organizes the nature of the relationship between the identity and environment, while the third combination ('*Bing*, S.i. in water') promotes the integration of identity and influence of the environment into the roots of everyone's personal authentic source.

Perhaps you are sitting at your desk or in your armchair reading this text: you and the sentences I once entrusted to these pages. Only when you have internalized and integrated the meaning of the text with your own knowledge and being do you say goodbye to the first two combinations and open the door to the great movement water and the heavenly stem *Bing*.

CHAPTER 14

DYNAMICS OF THE HEAVENLY STEM *BING* 丙[1]

This chapter on the combination of the great movement water and heavenly stem *Bing*, S.i. is essential. Each combination operates to a greater or lesser extent in everyone, but the water–fire axis is essential for integrated social and personal health.

The heavenly stem *Bing* is fire in its yang phase, visible in nature in the lush bloom of flowers during the summer. In the human body it is represented by the fire of the *qi* of the small intestine. The active great movement water that dynamizes the heavenly stem *Bing*, small intestine, simultaneously subdues the great movement fire, which the small intestine is part of.

For people born with '*Bing*, S.i. in water', the strength of the small intestine can, and often does, compensate for the possible insufficiency of fire factors. This however can turn out to be a pitfall, because overcharging of the small intestine *qi* can lead to insufficiency elsewhere. It is like a see-saw, for when yang rises, yin falls. The small intestine guides and protects the outward development of the *qi* of the heart, but when the practical outward-facing reinforced ego is too focused on confirmation from the outside world, this can be an obstacle to the weakened heart *qi* that focuses on inner alignment, self-knowledge, but above all on the health of the 'empire', the body. The practitioner must be alert to this and prevent the *qi* of the heart from weakening.

When the *qi* of the small intestine prevails, the heart yin tends to become insufficient with symptoms of empty heat and heart yang that overflows. The first symptoms that appear are excessive purposefulness and strength along with hidden sadness and loss of self-esteem.

Water and fire are opposite and, in conjunction, they can be each other's

---

1   People born in years ending with a 6, such as 1966, 2006, after the Chinese New Year.

resistance and can also merge with each other. They unite in sexual life, will and wisdom (*zhi*). The combination of water–fire energies gives strength and charisma, purpose and perseverance. When desires and expectations are paramount, these forces work outwardly in the fulfilment of ideas. When they turn inward, they increase authenticity and self-awareness.

'S.i. in water' is a special combination in which people have both a lot to gain and to lose. I have often seen people with problems with '*Bing*, S.i. in water' achieving great things, while at the same time deep fears and insecurities put a strain on their lives. The combination of authenticity, competence, willpower, drive and purpose motivates people to the limit, so that adventurousness prevails but exhaustion and depression lurk. It is remarkable that people are often aware of this pattern and yet seem unable to change; to truly examine themselves and to acknowledge discovered fears and insecurities.

BING 丙, THE THIRD HEAVENLY STEM

Bing is represented in the small intestine, the yang of the emperor fire. The Chinese character shows a yang line entering a space from above. It illustrates the broadening of the observability of seemingly infinite forces of the life-giving source within the limits of a three-dimensional space. The perception of vital fire produces sensations and feelings of pleasure that are transformed into vitality, excitement and original vibrancy of the heart-*shen*.

The heavenly stem *Bing* provides the limitation through form necessary for life and is symbolized as an enclosed space that houses the concentration of the power of fire. The other symbol for this stem is the flame of a wooden torch, which reveals that fire and light only become visible and functional when they are limited and attached to a form principle. Without forms the fire and light are not 'caught' by a fixed shape and are not perceptible. The light reflected on the moon at night is not visible in the empty space between the sun and the moon, even though it is present there. A passing satellite that captures the sun's light can be visible as a moving bright little light in the sky.

FORM PRINCIPLES CATCH AND LIMIT THE POSSIBILITIES OF LIFE PRINCIPLES

The fulfilment and expansion of the life forces of seeds that can be seen in the splendour of flowers in summer is inherently limited in further growth, but fortunately emerging fruits with new seeds ensure the further course of the cycle. The lush shapes of flowers express *and* limit life, just as the *shen* needs a body to express itself but at the same time limits itself in its possibilities. There are no other options for life to express itself once the choice of attachment is made.[2]

LIMITATION AND SEPARATION VERSUS COMPLETE COMPLETION

The first manifestation of visible form principles is represented by the first heavenly stem *Jia*. The second heavenly stem *Yi* focuses on the growth, defence and support of these manifested phenomena. The third heavenly stem *Bing* provides understanding and maintenance for the further development of the vital spark of life in physical form. *Bing* provides insight into life's expression in the body and in particular in digestion – in the broadest sense of the word – through limitation and separation.

The fire quality of the heavenly stem *Bing* is based on the red vermilion bird heaven, the source of all transformation and transcendence and the emanation *heng*, the ever-penetrating consciousness which expresses completion as a natural consequence of what has been started in the emanation *yuan*. In other words, *Bing* completes what has been initiated by *Jia*.

In our language, completion means partial completion, that is something that has been completed and that has ended. A book, a football match, the implementation of a plan, even the growth of a plant can come to a finishing point, making it a closed finite unit. Partial completion always has a beginning and an end. The restrictions on both sides inherently result in inclusion of what the phenomenon contains and exclusion of everything else. This is the source of separation and duality, the opposite of complete (true) completion. It is about (for example) this special book which excludes another book, it includes this specific content and no other content and so on. Complete completion means that everything is present and no further development is required. Complete completion is the end of evolution.

The process of partial completion describes the development that takes place over time until someone or something decides that it has come to a final end. Complete completion does not exist in time, has neither end nor beginning and yet subtly but profoundly affects humans. Before we elaborate on this subject, the phenomenon of distinctive thinking will be discussed.

---

2   Acupuncturists use the subtle realm of the channels of *qi* to direct the life principle for the benefit of the body. The quality of *Bing* and the health of the *qi* of the small intestine converge and align the realm of physical forms with the realm of subtle life principles, determining the outcome of acupuncture treatments.

THOUGHT IS DIVISION IN TIME

Thought is perhaps our most important asset, our best talent. Without thoughts and memories, what would we be, how would we remember each other's stories? Thinking in general, and about ourselves in particular, characterizes human beings, but thinking can also be our biggest pitfall.

Thought is bound and limited by time and space. Thoughts about emotions you anticipate experiencing, thoughts on a specific topic, thoughts about your friends and the party you had together and so forth. Thought is capable of keeping the past vital in the present while distracting from the actual present. In doing this, it diverts the human perception of connection, presence and involvement in the now. Thought is omnipresent, but is limited by its focus in time and space, including and excluding, making it part of partial completion.

The thinking conceptual mind is an expression of duality and separation. Its task is to be distinctive, to separate everything that it perceives into dualities: yin and yang, black and white, good and bad, down and up, me and you, here and there and so on. The ego uses this: Thought distinguishes the ego from the world by the fact that the mind and thought search for contradictions, comparisons and similarities. The heavenly stem *Bing* facilitates this kind of thinking and therefore contributes to the skills of thought, including having a memory.[3]

The difference between complete and partial completion is demonstrated in the distinction between the unity of the pre-natal *yuan-shen* and the acquired, divided, post-natal *wu-shen*. Thought belongs to the acquired *wu-shen*, in which the ego, that uses thought, is in the grip of time, duality, change, challenges, desires and passions. Thought divides and speaks of my and your (or our) consciousness/mind/body/feelings and these differences shape and frame who we are. Distinction and separateness make everyone an 'I' that is most necessary for our self-image, self-evaluation and self-development, which gives us a place in this world! It is just as necessary for growth and evolution; human beings will eventually learn to transform their identification with instinctual material desires into abilities that relate to spiritual principles.

Thought seems unable to fulfil completion. It fails to experience the unity of the *yuan-shen*. Only when people die does the *yuan-shen* seem to be within reach, but at this time the ego may profoundly fear what is perceived as the deep abyss of nothingness. Death seems to be able to hint at the possibility of

---

3   Maybe J.D. van Buren therefore taught that the *qi* of the small intestine governs the function of the circle of Willis, a circle of arteries at the base of the brain, which forms a network of connections that ensure preservation of blood supply to the brain.

an experience of complete completion through the perception of unity and togetherness, but even that may often be avoided by the idea of reincarnation.

So do we not experience 'complete completion' at all? We actually do.

Maybe you once tried to unravel or discuss a complicated problem and finally, after weighing, talking and understanding everything, you came to the conclusion that thoughts and words were not enough to get to the point. Just after giving up and allowing yourself to not know, the essence of the issue was suddenly felt and then easily expressed. The reflection of complete completion has to do with that specific kind of perception when thought ends, but you still are connected fully and present. Just as this complicated piece of text can be nothing more than words, at a certain moment, when thought stops and you still feel its resonance, its essence can inspire, precisely because the ego and thought are no longer actively involved.

DIGESTION

The mind that stops thinking is similar to the functioning of the digestive system, which like thought is based on impressions from the past and on the ability to distinguish, separate and unite, but this happens without the intervention of the ego. The digestive system functions in line with the origin (*yuan*) of the being instead of the desires of the ego, thought and other expressions of the mind. The uniqueness of everyone's essence determines what and how the digestive system separates, uses or rejects. The purer the *jing*-essence, the better the body can discern the good and the bad, the pure and impure, the useful and the useless. The body makes an undisturbed coordination between the great movement water and the heavenly stem *Bing*, small intestine, the heart-*shen* and the *jing*, a coordination that is indispensable for proper digestion – in the broadest sense of the word.

EGO AND LANGUAGE

The ego creates a central point in the being, precisely through the use of the properties of *Bing*, small intestine – such as distinguishing, separating and integrating the input of the senses. It is – certainly as a child – the experience of the ego that the world revolves around it, and it is the ego that secures us a place in the world. Through all these qualities and through personal growth[4]

---

4   The great movement metal and the heavenly stem *Yi*.

and understanding,[5] humans gradually integrate and process what the ego has differentiated through perception so that the ego learns to think and speak.

As an example: Listening[6] is an important condition for the ego to learn to express its identity[7] through the use of language. A few weeks after birth, a baby begins to make movements[8] with the tongue and mouth,[9] resulting in first sounds, yet without a clear directed interaction with the environment. Integration of movements of the tongue, mouth and sounds is only made possible by the interaction between the baby and the immediate environment.[10] Sounds then begin to gain meaning and become a first attempt at language; however, at this stage the sounds are still mostly undifferentiated. All intimate people are probably called mummy or daddy. By further interaction and especially by listening to language and development of improved processing, integration, understanding and co-regulation, the child's words acquire more focused meaning. Children understand many more words in the first phase of life than they can actually speak.

One of the effects of this development in speech is that small children begin to understand that mum and dad are different people and that parents are different to and separate from themselves. The distinction between their environment and themselves creates the first impressions of a 'me' and a 'not me'.

A specific feature of the heavenly stem *Bing* and the small intestine in adults is the art of eloquence and the development of safety rooted in self-esteem. People with prominent features of the heavenly stem *Bing* accurately describe the 'not me', as well as deriving certainty and confidence from self-awareness, although this may sometimes lead to self-centredness and self-glorification.

INTERACTION AND INTEGRATION

The quality of the heart-*shen* and its influence on the health of the body is determined by the degree to which the different inner parts of the human energetic field[11] and the physical body are integrated with each other and adjusted to the environment. Integration, and thus health, depend on the health of *Bing*,

---

5   The great movement water and the heavenly stem *Bing*.
6   Kidney *qi*.
7   Great movement earth.
8   Great movement wood.
9   Great movement fire, the heart and spleen *qi*.
10   The great movement metal and the heavenly stem *Yi*.
11   *Shen, hun, po, yi, zhi, qi, xuè, jin yé* and *jing*.

small intestine, which always seeks integration by limitation and separation.[12] Illnesses can arise when the balanced integration of the *shen* is disorganized, which shows as stagnation or confusion. Circumstances of no or little integration always involve to some extent disorganized *qi* of the small intestine. Integration and thus the healing and self-regulating abilities of the heart-*shen* depend on the health of and collaboration between the great movements metal and water and heavenly stems *Yi*, liver, and *Bing*, small intestine.

The basic conditions for integration that the great movement metal provides are extremely important. Not only does the great movement metal provide the necessary material, it is the prerequisite for the essential integrative interdependence of various internal and external *qi*. Health of the great movement metal and the heavenly stem *Yi* allows the various *qi* to interact and collaborate. This is how integration functions. Interaction precedes integration, which implies that an integrated heart-*shen* can only function well by means of a healthy great movement metal and heavenly stem *Yi*, liver. As a result, when the great movement metal and the heavenly stem *Yi*, liver, function well, direct treatment of the *qi* of the heavenly stem *Bing*, small intestine, may no longer be needed, even when there are signs of fire symptoms such as mania due to stagnation of *qi* and food, insomnia and mental confusion. When healthy interaction is secured, integration and health may return on their own.

The ego ascertains its place in the world through its awareness of and cooperation with the inner and outer perceived worlds. Awareness of the separated worlds is a precondition for conscious interaction and integration. Only through separation can interaction and integration exist.[13]

'*Bing*, S.i. in water' determines the sensitivity of the discernment and helps to distinguish, integrate and understand the nature of the exchange between the self and others.

---

12 'The small intestine receives the food from the stomach, it further digests the food, divides it into essence and the dregs, then absorbs the essence and sends the dregs to the large intestine.' *Huang Di Nei Jing Su Wen* Chapter 8. The impure dregs in the small intestine are sent to the large intestine, and the impure fluids to the bladder. The impure *qi* is sent to the kidney yang to transform it into *wei qi*. The essential pure fluids are sent to kidney yin where they are transformed into two kinds of fluids: impure body fluids as mucus, saliva, sweat and the like, and pure fluids to become *jin yé* that eventually becomes *xuè, ying qi* and *wei qi*. Disorders caused by disrupted *qi* of the small intestine such as abdominal pain, intestinal problems, urinary tract disorders and disorders in the fluids *xuè, ying* and *wei qi* are all due to improper separation *and* integration of the pure and impure substances.

13 Interaction and integration are respectively related to the great movement metal and water.

THE GREAT MOVEMENT WATER AND THE HEAVENLY STEM *BING*

The dark warrior heaven and the emanation *zhen* are the archetypal background of the great movement water. The heavenly stem *Bing* is based on the red vermilion bird heaven and the emanation *heng*. These omnipresent aspects of *qi* are in a *ke*-cycle relationship which, as mentioned in Chapter 13, is in service of the health of the wholeness. This combination of forces guides the heart to set goals, the essence of the kidneys to nourish the heart, and sets the direction. Finding your passion or making an authentic choice is guided and initiated by a healthy '*Bing*, S.i. in water'.

The dynamics of water and fire operate via the vertical creative axis of heaven–earth–humanity, perpendicular to the dynamics of metal and wood that focus on the horizontal field of created forms and physical reality, together with interpretations of and practical responses to life and circumstances. '*Bing*, S.i. in water' and '*Yi*, Liv in metal' are perpendicular to each other, just like yin and yang, creativity and creation, life-giving and life-receiving forces, horizon and meridian, practicality and theory, but they are all inextricably linked and influence each other, even in treatments.

HENG AND *ZHEN* AND THE GREAT MOVEMENT WATER

The emanation *zhen* means perfection. It is the invariable, determining, unchangeable emanation. It means natural and perfect development by being upright, sincere and pure and is the impersonal infinite source of creation that results in people's personal authenticity. *Zhen* in nature and in humans manifests in the great movement water and generates the state of 'being', meaning the overall open, present condition of the physical-emotional-mental body. In this state there are no expectations or assumptions. Everything can arise from and disappear into the potential creative source of the North. Water adapts to circumstances, but always flows back to the deepest point where it strengthens the source. Nothing is constant and immutable.

The emanation *heng* inspires the world of shapes, giving it content and meaning. Consciousness (*heng*) builds and relies on the infinite possibilities of the limitless source of *zhen*, but is in a state of 'becoming' instead of 'being'.

The state of 'being' of the great movement water is the dynamic source behind the fiery heavenly stem *Bing*. It is characterized by being non-conceptual and open to what IS, rather than having expectations, making concepts and personal ambitions of thought. In reality, in many people, the opposite is more often the case: Instead of authenticity determining one's direction, the direction is determined by desires of thought and the demanding *wu-shen*. This is partly because the path to finding one's own authenticity is usually accompanied by encounters with traumas and fears that we would rather not face. In this situation, fire takes the lead and likes to draw on the infinite source to achieve its goals. 'Becoming' then precedes 'being', instead of 'being' as the foundation and source of 'becoming'.

When 'becoming' precedes 'being', this may overstretch limited human resources. It might ultimately lead to physical, emotional and/or mental exhaustion. When the *qi* of the great movement water fails to dynamize the heavenly stem *Bing* sufficiently, there is too much 'becoming'. The meaning of 'being' should be explained to a patient: It is a state realized by quiet obedience rather than imposing the will to achieve goals. This message will only come across if the practitioner conveys it with understanding and presence.

People born with this combination of water and fire are often noticed for their strength and capabilities. They long for and often have the natural power to become authentic, despite present (un)conscious feelings of insecurity. They are guided by their strong willpower to achieve set goals and usually navigate their way through life by thoughtful planning. They seem rooted and centralized, and their dedication and purposefulness may give hope. However, their strengths and single-mindedness can also backfire. Their authenticity, vitality and mental capacity may evoke feelings of inaccessibility, distance and fear in those around them. As a result, they tend to prove their strength but yearn for confirmation and attract people who give them confidence. They endeavour to make other people dependent on them and demand fidelity to their stated goals. This leads people to look up to them, worship them or fight them. Both (worship and struggle) seem to strengthen the ego of these '*Bing* in water' people. Over time, the inflated ego usually becomes frustrated and resentful due to less recognition or insatiability. It's like the story of the very hungry caterpillar. Not infrequently, this behaviour is visible in political and spiritual leaders and CEOs, who are not all born with this combination, but who manage their positions with it. This kind of conduct may be due to neglect and attachment disorders during parenting; the ego struggles to conquer and establish a place in the world.[14]

With '*Bing*, S.i. in water', the ego is challenged to surrender to the naturally flowing path of circumstances and to the originality of human nature that can be found through fidelity to the inner truth. This applies to everyone, but in people born with this combination of forces it is very present.

---

14 In the case of health issues, trauma therapy may offer the prospect of recovery but it is not easy for them to make that choice.

ACUPUNCTURE POINTS THAT INFLUENCE THE ACTIVE GREAT MOVEMENT WATER AND THE HEAVENLY STEM *BING*

The stem point S.i.-2, *Qian Gu*, anterior valley, receives relatively little attention in TCM. It is used to increase urination and reduce sweating and for clearing heat in the regions of the head, eyes, nose, throat, cheeks, neck, as well as in the breasts and bladder. It can be used in people who feel frustrated because they cannot accept that something unforeseen and unwanted but inevitable is happening. S.i.-2 strengthens the state of 'being' and helps people to calm their strong drive to succeed.

> A woman born in 1971 suffered with gynaecological problems and low back pain, based on heat and dryness in the lower burner. When she visited for the first time, she gave the impression of being authentic, saying that fear and insecurity didn't allow her to really be herself, especially in social settings.
>
> S.i.-2, the water point on a fire channel, strengthens the state of 'being'. To also treat her physical and other emotional complaints, the heat and dryness present in the lower burner as well as the fear and lack of determination, I used Cv-4, *Guan Yuan*, gate of *yuan qi*, along with Bl-66, *Tong Gu*, passing valley. Much can be said about these points, but in this context it is essential to know that the water points of *tai yang* division were treated: the most superficial division, the first layer of interaction with and protection against the surrounding world. These two water points are used to support people with low self-esteem who question themselves or are looking for self-worth.

Sp-12, *Chong Men*, rushing gate. This point tonifies all yin in general and has a strong effect on the *yuan qi*. It opens yin to the outside world and is used with cases of urine retention, constipation, fullness of yin in the abdomen, problems with breastfeeding, mastitis and so on. It can be used when a person is stuck in their mind, is ready to move on but feels unable to do so, who is much worried or deceives themselves.

In most cases where I have used Sp-12, patients had exceeded their limits and were in dire need of relaxation. Despite the exhaustion, they felt the need to keep going. They almost always shared that circumstances forced them, such as the emotion surrounding a parent's death or the stress of an upcoming surgery, the confusion of a traumatic experience or the pressure of a training schedule. These people suffered from severe pains and exhaustion, had little contact with their own degree of fatigue and could not feel at ease in any way. They were guided by the circumstances and their own (often unconscious) overdrive, in which their minds and souls were working overtime.

THE CONSEQUENCES OF '*BING*, SMALL INTESTINE IN WATER' IN THE *WUXING*

Activity of the great movement water affects the *qi* of water in general and might be reflected in the condition of the bladder, kidney, *san jiao* and gallbladder,[15] *jing qi*, sexual drive, willpower, strength of *wei qi* and so on.

The active great movement water tends to subdue the great movement fire, which might result in deficiencies of any *qi* related to fire, but especially of the *qi* of the heart. Practice showed me that the heart needs attentive care with people born with '*Bing*, S.i. in water'. Whether this is really the case is diagnosed on the pulse at Ht-7, *Shen Men*, spirit gate.

In people born with the heavenly stem *Bing*, the *qi* of the small intestine should be powerful. The active great movement water that dynamizes the heavenly stem *Bing* may exert pressure on the *qi* of the heart with symptoms such as insomnia, lethargic behaviour, stuttering, lack of stamina or manic behaviour and hyperactivity, sadness and loss of self-esteem and so on. And in more severe cases it causes circulatory problems, stroke, heart problems and panic attacks, as well as compensation mechanisms such as drinking too much coffee and alcohol, a sweet tooth, the need for excessive confirming social contact or confirmation through sexual satisfaction.

The main challenge for these patients and the practitioner is to protect and support a healthy heart-*shen*, both in terms of cognitive mind and perception of a person's true nature. Unfortunately, the latter happens less often. People seem to listen more to the drive of having a task in this world and consider that as their true self. This can be reinforced by the fear of facing the self and the depth of the great nothingness of complete completion. People with weaker heart *qi* tend to seek safety in using their mental abilities and strong skills to distinguish, wanting to explore and understand everything down to the smallest detail. On an emotional level, they feel vulnerable and are difficult to access.

The drive for research and gathering information requires a lot of the great movement metal. It can go well for a long time, but in the long run it takes its toll. Physical complaints such as high blood pressure, eczema and tendon problems arise, mainly due to the dryness and constriction of the great movement metal. It often is accompanied by a disturbed social life and loneliness.

---

15   See the chapters on earthly branches.

The following well-known quote from Chapter 8 of the *Huang Di Nei Jing Su Wen* is about the central role of the heart, but the text shows also the enormous trap: The felt leadership of the heart can also lead to self-overestimation.

> The heart is the supreme commander, sovereign, or the monarch, master, of the human body, it dominates the spirit, ideology and thought of man.

Downgrading others and upgrading the self may compensate for insufficiency of the *qi* of the heart, but eventually leads to long-lasting, often irreversible, complaints that are the result of exhaustion of the *qi* of the heart.

The way to discover true heart nature is through self-knowledge, sensitivity and living wisdom. Self-knowledge arises through openness and tolerance for what is, without the desire to change anything, neither for the benefit of the self nor for others. It is hard work internally to calm all impulses of the desire for action and explore the self in it. Sensitivity does not use the mind and aspirations. It opens the eyes to the now and thus to the omnipresent expression of life.

Living wisdom surpasses fear and pain by focusing on the infinite and not on the temporal nature of the mind. Living wisdom scrapes and polishes the self and makes it a clear transparent crystal through which the light from the original source shines gently. Then the ego and the heart-*shen* can become interpersonal (earth) and impersonal (heaven), formed through interaction, collaboration and integration. This occurs without the efforts of personal will, because the true nature cannot be found, but appears when the real obstacle, the ego, calms down. Freeing the path to authenticity with the housing of fire of '*Bing*, S.i. in water' is the key to open the lock to integration and love.

A FINAL NOTE

As discussed above it is important to focus on the subdued great movement first, especially on the *qi* of the heart. Then it becomes easier to balance the active great movement water, if still needed, also because the heart itself is the underlying basis of the will (*zhi*).

When the active great movement water becomes too dominant, people are too focused on achieving goals. Maybe they are fanatical, but with patience and perseverance, in the search for the cause of a problem. As a result they lose touch with reality and connection with those around them. Sexual issues can be prominent and people can be supercritical and very difficult to approach.

We adults often say that 'where there is a will, there is a way'. But maybe it should be 'where there is a way, there is no will'.

TRINITY *JIA-YI-BING*

The heavenly stem *Jia* is the initiating, future-oriented beginning of the cycle of the ten heavenly stems. The first three heavenly stems *Jia-Yi-Bing* function in a dependent and creative coherence: identity–interaction–integration. The next heavenly stems *Ding-Wu-Ji* give shape to the creative impulse of the first trinity.

The last heavenly stem in the trinity always elevates the qualities into a coherent collaboration. Therefore the balance and collaboration between the three are important to the health of the whole. For example, if the third heavenly stem *Bing* is out of balance, one must take into account the collaboration and balance of the other two heavenly stems in the same trinity. The three heavenly stems operate as a unity. This rule applies to the two following trinities in the cycle of heavenly stems: *Ding-Wu-Ji* and *Geng-Xin-Ren*. The heavenly stem *Gui* is the apotheosis[16] and conclusion of the spiritual incarnation of human beings and has similar dynamics of water and fire as '*Bing*, S.i. in water'.

---

16   The quintessence, the apex, the culmination.

CHAPTER 15

DYNAMICS OF THE HEAVENLY STEM *DING* 丁[1]

'If we don't even know life,
how can we know death?'

Confucius

Humanness arises from the heavenly stem *Ding* and the heart. The state of identity, interaction and integration of the previous three great movements and heavenly stems determines the degree of expression of the basically unlimited possibilities of humanness. Unfortunately, society seems to be more often characterized by conflict, terror and inhuman behaviour. We do not seem to realize that the nature of society is determined by the nature of our relationships, including the relationship we have with our own nature, which makes each and every person fundamentally responsible for the kind of society that is desired. This leads to the justifiable question of how we might respond and initiate positive change. Every human being carries the seed of love and compassion and is approachable for it. It can be awakened by simply noticing it.

DING 丁, THE FOURTH HEAVENLY STEM
The quality of the heavenly stem *Ding* is shown in the yin of fire, the heart.

Ding stems from the red vermilion bird heaven of the South and the emanation *heng*. Together with the heavenly stem *Bing*, it fulfils the desire for inspiring, passionate, warm, friendly, benevolent and vibrant experiences. Everyone possesses these human qualities and is able to use them, although the circumstances

---

1   Years ending with a 7 such as 1957 or 2007, after the Chinese New Year.

of life can make this very complicated. Nevertheless, there are many examples of people in bad conditions who were able to find and share love. They are examples of the positive development of humanity.

There are three ways to illustrate the character *Ding*: a nail, the flame of an oil lamp and the natural character of vegetation in a warm season.

The Chinese character *Ding* depicts a nail.[2] The material from which the nail is made, for example iron, is melted by fire to mould it into a nail. It symbolically indicates that something takes on meaning when it is completed by the active intervention of fire. For the development of humans, this applies to fire, awareness and consciousness[3] (*heng*/fire), by which *Ding*, heart, connects and gives meaning to life, both in relationship with others and with the self.

The flame of an oil lamp is different to the flame of a wooden torch of the heavenly stem *Bing*. Unlike the torch's dry wood which comes straight from nature and is readily available, oil is created by pressure and can only be used in the oil lamp through active human intervention. Oil is earth's gift to humanity and can provide spiritual and physical well-being. Metaphorically, it may kindle the inner light of human consciousness. The wooden torch illuminates people from the outside, whereas the oil lamp is the luminous conscious human body itself.

The process of extracting olive oil, in which hard fruits turn into liquid oil, is similar to the transformation process in which the stubborn ego learns to align itself with the subtle realm. Before ripe olives are pressed, they are first mashed and kneaded. The juices that emerge are still very bitter and unappealing. A centrifuge separates water from the oil and leaves oil behind. In life, personal fears, desires and goals (water) often lose their importance in extreme circumstances of intense pressure, which gives the possibility of steering life in a new direction. Suddenly the essential light of the essence of being can be rekindled. It barely diminishes the sadness, pain and fear, but warms the frozen scars of the ego and bridges connection to the light that supports us all.

The heavenly stem *Ding* manifests in an awake and alert consciousness of the heart-*shen* inspired and infused with love and compassion.

After the vital *qi* of spring and summer and the floral splendour during the time of *Bing*, moisture released by heat evaporates during the time of *Ding*. It generates movement of the more deeply located fluids to regenerate life in the form. This is part of the cycle of life: Regeneration starts with releasing the superficial so as to make the deeper move.

---

2   Some sources say the pain of a bee sting.
3   Consciousness is awareness of the self in its broadest sense along with the interactions between the self and its environment; self-awareness is the confirmation that consciousness belongs to a thinking and feeling being that realizes it can think and feel about it.

Trauma, illness and bypassing of the path of self-knowledge create stagnation and freeze the conditions needed for regeneration. The heart *qi* suffers. This is evidenced by abnormal perspiration, problems with the tongue and mouth, the blood and blood vessels and, on a deeper level, personal imbalance and emotional dependence due to difficulties with emotional processing.

A young girl of 12 with the heavenly stem *Ding* in her birth chart enters my clinic room. Her parents ask me if I can help her with her fear of failure at school. She tells me that she is tired and often has a headache with a heavy feeling in the head. She suffers a lot from wet hands and feet (hyperhidrosis) and she sleeps restlessly and wakes up in the night. Her father shares that she feels ashamed of her wet hands and that she finds it difficult to become more independent, for example she finds it difficult to cycle to school on her own.

Pulse diagnosis confirms that her symptoms are related to insufficiency of the *qi* of the heart, resulting in an insufficient nourishment of the *qi* of the spleen.

She is quite tall for her age. Upon inquiry, it appears that she has grown very quickly in recent years. Bone growth in childhood is mainly governed by *Ding*, heart.[4] Despite the fact that the heavenly stem *Ding* is a stronger aspect in her birth chart, the rapid growth and the demands that school places on her are an overload. These conditions put her under so much pressure that even the potentially strong heart *qi* is affected and this causes symptoms. Being ill in her 'own' *qi* is quite serious because the disease manifests itself in a potentially stronger *qi*. Usually, it takes more treatments to balance and treat the potentially stronger 'own' *qi* compared to the potentially weaker 'absent' *qi* of the birth chart.

In this case in particular, explaining to her that growing in itself is a very tiring period of life and advice to her parents to ensure more rest and regularity – they really encouraged her to do her homework well – were important contributions to the success of the therapy. She was and still is a radiant being and an example to many. The positive approach and support of the parents was probably more important than the acupuncture treatments that merely opened the door to cure.[5] All complaints disappeared in about two months and have never returned since. She is happily married, has a part-time job and is a caring mother of two beautiful children.

---

4   In older children growth is generated from the *qi* of the heart constrictor and spleen. Bone tissue is protected by the *qi* of the kidneys.

5   The treatment of 'own' *qi* focuses on five phases, like and unlike *qi* and the four possibilities. See Chapters 17 and 22.

THE GREAT MOVEMENT WOOD AND THE HEAVENLY STEM *DING*

The development of the cycle of great movements and heavenly stems is valid on many levels: It can be applied to (for example) the evolution of the human race, new paths of development and the developmental stages of babies, children, young adolescents and so on.

During childhood the first great movement and heavenly stem are needed to feel trust and safety. The second pair supports interaction and the drive to communicate. Feeling safe and encouraged activates the sense of authenticity that comes with the third great movement and heavenly stem. The early absence of safety and encouragement may complicate the development of authentic individuality and the process of individuation at an older age. Many illnesses and complaints are caused by injuries to the *qi* of the heart as a result of personal and collective traumatic experiences during the first years of life, which are dominated by the first three great movements and heavenly stems. Before anything else is treated, the balance of the first three pairs must be addressed first.

'*Ding*, Ht in wood' leads people to the meaning and experience of their true purpose in life. People start to wonder who they are, what the meaning/purpose of their life is and whether future perspectives should be reassessed. Under the guidance of '*Ding*, Ht in wood', people make important decisions that change their lives and make them feel more autonomous but, on the other hand, people find it difficult to change when this *qi* has stagnated or is confused.

The bigger picture

The bigger picture describes the energetic origin and development of human consciousness and of humanity as a whole. The first three combinations of great movements and heavenly stems embody the stages of development of potential form and truth through interaction and integration into an authentic wholeness. For humanity this wholeness means consciousness. At that point, the creation process stops briefly, takes a short pause, as if the breath was being held. The further development of the first impulse is about to reveal the inspired physical incarnation. The fourth great movement and heavenly stem represent the birth of humans and humanity, enriched with a loving and compassionate consciousness.

In practice, this means that when people or humanity are severely confronted with the right to exist, it is advisable to cease the intense struggle for survival and not to discuss or fight, but to wait for the moment when it is possible to exhale and inhale again. When people do not take the time, it is not uncommon that diseases force them to take the necessary rest. In those cases, it is wise to take time and to pause. Time is then an ally in the healing process.

During the Covid-19 crisis, this interruption of life was experienced individually and collectively as traumatic and transformative. There were people who were positively surprised by the benefits of a reclusive life and there were opposing forces who considered change to be dangerous and illegal. The confronting of deep-seated inner scars has led to campaigns and aggression. In 2019 and beyond, the balance of the great movement wood and the heavenly stem *Ding* was greatly challenged.[6] I suspect that during this time the development of humanity as a whole was encouraged to evolve by forces driven by the great movement wood and the heavenly stem *Ding*, bearing in mind that people are individually influenced by all the great movements and heavenly stems. The inspiration and creativity gained during the Covid-19 crisis may lead to further evolution of humanity in the direction of the great movement fire and the heavenly stem *Wu*.

THE *SHENG*-CYCLE

The *wuxing* relationship between the great movement wood and the fire of *Ding* is called *sheng*. The *sheng*-cycle is the generating cycle in which every phase generates another phase, for example wood generates fire. During waking consciousness, the physical body is nourished by the *sheng*-cycle that operates more during the day. During the night at the stage of sleep and dream awareness, the body regenerates via *ke*-cycle principles. In addition to the purification of *qi* at night, experiences are processed and organized, all of which happens outside people's conscious will or thought.

Treatments with *ke*-cycle interactions during the day are beneficial for conscious processing. This is especially true for people who are mainly concerned with the past and the material world. In the evening and at night it is better to concentrate treatments on the *sheng*-cycle, especially when people are physically affected and exhausted.

Practicality and visible reality are most appreciated by people born with a *sheng*-cycle relationship between great movement and heavenly stem. Ideas and expectations are fun, but they need to be implemented, they need to take shape, whatever it takes. Only philosophizing is not appreciated. The combination of wood generating fire makes people tend to look ahead and enthusiastically set

---

6   This book was written during the Covid-19 pandemic and I had no idea when the crisis would be over.

a goal, with the danger that continuous progress and purpose might distract from what life means to people in the 'now'.

HAPPINESS AND THE RAT RACE OF LIFE

Western society seems to be primarily concerned with what can be and has been achieved, rather than what people experience in the present. For people born with this combination it is difficult to slow down. In addition to acupuncture treatments they need help and support from, for example, yoga, running and meditation. Not infrequently they turn to alcohol and drugs to give their brains and bodies peace.

The passive, yielding quality of great movement wood can assist in finding a break. Rest is needed for self-reflection and understanding the motives behind the active behaviour of 'Ding, Ht in wood'.

This rest is actually indispensable for good health and happiness. After 'applying a little pressure', people with 'Ding, Ht in wood' understand their own responsibility fairly quickly but still often fall prey to the expectations that society and they themselves set.

A happy life is about the path of happiness, not about achieving happiness. Focusing on a goal only inhibits the potential of the self. For people who are too preoccupied with the demands of their hard-working lives and feel no way out, I read them the following text by Joseph Campbell:

> If you follow your bliss, you put yourself on a kind of track that has been there all the while, waiting for you, and the life that you ought to be living is the one you are living. Wherever you are – if you are following your bliss, you are enjoying that refreshment, that life within you, all the time.
>
> A sacred space is an absolute necessity for anybody today. You must have a room, or a certain hour or so a day, where you don't know what was in the newspapers that morning, you don't know who your friends are, you don't know what you owe anybody, you don't know what anybody owes to you. This is a place where you can simply experience and bring forth what you are and what you might be. This is the place of creative incubation. At first you may find that nothing happens there. But if you have a sacred place and use it, something eventually will happen.[7]

People born with 'Ding, Ht in wood' often experience emotional events or

---

7   Campbell and Moyers 2011.

illnesses that prompt them to learn to hold back and relax in order to find their way to happiness. This is a beautiful but often confronting mystery in which people are challenged by life and are enabled by this process to gain more insight into the self.

DOING NOTHING

Treatments and advice should be practical, clear and feasible, but two things are paramount. First, the practitioner must be persistent and, second, time and space to do nothing are essential to regain strength. People with '*Ding*, Ht in wood' tend to participate fully in everything. The question 'Are you able to do nothing?' is often not even understood at first.

Signs and symptoms are usually yang and fiery. There are only two options: Either the fire becomes too excessive and uninhibited and people may suffer from headaches, pains (due to heat) in the throat, mouth and face, anxiety, anorexia or numbness of the toes; or they suffer from insufficiencies and exhaustion, often from water-related channels with symptoms such as Achilles tendon problems, restlessness or more severe illnesses due to insufficient *jing qi*. Remarkably, these patients often only come to the clinic at an advanced stage of disease.

ACUPUNCTURE POINTS THAT INFLUENCE THE PASSIVE GREAT MOVEMENT WOOD AND THE HEAVENLY STEM *DING*

Sp-4, *Gong Sun*,[8] grandfather grandson, bridges between the pre- and post-natal *jing qi*. It connects personal and social interactions and aligns the influence of society and ancestral *qi* with the personal *qi*. It is especially indicated when people are chronically unable to cope with life, when they feel that everything is too much. This is accompanied by physical complaints due to general underactivity of wood. Coping exhausts people because they constantly feel compelled to take initiative and be active.

It is advisable to first treat Sp-4 in combination with other points that treat the great movement wood and at a later stage strengthen the deep function of the *san jiao* with points like Cv-4, *Guan Yuan*, Sj-2, *Ye Men*, Sj-3, *Zhong Zhu*, Sj-4, *Yang Qi*. To ground, these acupuncture points can be combined with the *yuan source* points such as Ki-3, *Tai Xi*, Sp-3, *Tai Bai*, Liv-3, *Tai Chong*, Lu-9, *Tai Yuan* and Ht-7, *Shen Men*.

---

8   *Gong Sun* is a family name of the Yellow Emperor.

Stem point Ht-9, *Shao Chong*, little rushing or lesser surge. *Chong* indicates that something essential moves, rushes, surges or thrusts through it.[9] It is similar to *chong mai* which moves and mobilizes *jing* from the pre-natal design level to the post-natal level. Ht-9 awakens the awareness and moves the aptitude of the heart-*shen* to the channels to fulfil the personal human destiny that arose at birth.

Like other *jing-well* points, it restores consciousness in the event of unconsciousness. Ht-9 helps to increase alertness and presence when people suddenly become withdrawn.

A PATIENT BORN WITH THE HEAVENLY STEM *REN*, BLADDER

In Chapters 17 and 22 we discuss the topic 'unlike *qi*'. People born with the active great movement wood and the heavenly stem *Ren* tend to have overactive or stagnated *qi* of the bladder with symptoms such as neck pain, back pain and headache, frontal sinusitis and so on. It often goes together with insufficiency of the *qi* of the heart (heavenly stem *Ding*) with symptoms such as exhaustion due to hard work, mental fatigue, emotional vulnerability and the like.

This male patient is quite satisfied with his life and work. He works more than forty hours a week and regularly flies within Europe. During the initial consultation he shares that he has been sad for a number of years because he has long-term relationship problems, which make him feel emotionally and mentally exhausted. He has insomnia but, when he sleeps, he suffers from nightmares: 'I still feel physically good, although I regularly have headaches with neck and upper back pain.' Upon inquiry it appears that he uses paracetamol and nonsteroidal anti-inflammatory drugs (NSAIDs) on a daily basis. It is tempting to treat the pain with points on the bladder channel, but constitutional acupuncture does not directly treat the 'birth *qi*'.

The most important characteristics of his pulse diagnosis:

- generally dull pulse – meaning that it lacks vitality, which is a sign of insufficiency of wood in general. This is an indication for great movement wood issues
- a deep spreading pulse in the heart position – meaning *qi* and *xuè* insufficiency of the heart

---

9   Just as other points do with the name *chong* as Liv-3, St-30, Sj-1, Gb-9.

- a deep and soft pulse in the kidney and liver position – meaning deficiency of kidney yang and insufficient kidney and liver *qi* and *xuè*
- a push pulse in the bladder position – meaning exhaustion and pushing himself into activity
- all post-natal *qi* feel tight and thin – in combination with the rest of the pulse this means being overworked.

Treatment principle: First nourish post-natal *qi*, balance the great movement wood (with *Ding*/heart and *Ren*/bladder) using heart channel points; build kidney *qi*.

Treatment: Sp-4, *Gong Sun*, and Sp-1, *Yin Bai*, Ht-9, *Shao Chong*.

In addition to what has already been said, Sp-4 strengthens and regulates spleen *qi* and calms the *shen*. This point supports the processing and digesting of experiences along with the emotions and thoughts that come with them.

Sp-1 roots the *qi* of the *chong mai* and brings fluids and blood to the phase earth and the post-natal *qi*. It is indicated for agitation of the heart *qi* with propensity to sadness and works well in cases of insomnia with excess dreaming and nightmares. It provides clarity of thoughts where there is congestion or mental agitation, especially when combined with Ht-9.

Sp-4 with Sp-1 supports kidney *qi*.

Ht-9 tonifies heart *qi* and *xuè* and balances the great movement wood in people born with the heavenly stem *Ren*[10] and therefore calms the bladder *qi*.

The combination of these three points supports the phase earth and the stomach *qi* and therefore nourishes the post-natal *qi*.

At the next meeting, after four weeks, I treated Sp-4 and Cv-4, after which most of his physical and emotional problems were resolved, despite the ongoing relational problems.

THE CONSEQUENCES OF '*DING*, HEART IN WOOD' IN THE *WUXING*

Due to the passive great movement wood, the previous great movement in the *ke*-cycle (metal) is more active. The great movement metal influences all *qi* of

---

10 See Chapters 17 and 22.

metal: the large intestine, lungs, bladder, kidneys,[11] along with all conditions related to a tendency to become too dry such as dry skin, tight tendons, tight arteries, brittle bones and so on.

Flexibility and adaptability decrease and people adopt rigid and hardened behaviour and gain stiffer muscles when passive great movement wood is under increasing pressure from great movement metal. Too much metal can lead to behaviour driven by money, systems and structures, a need for justification and justice and dogmatic thinking. Stiffness is interpreted as realistic and practical: Self-reflection is absent.

People born with 'Ding, Ht in wood' are more willing to engage in introspection when they feel the intensity of a joyful, free and unthreatened life. It can help if they are reminded of their playful and pliable time as children.

More structure, introspection, physical orientation and boundary setting (associated with the great movement metal) are needed when the passive great movement wood and heavenly stem Ding lead to excessive yang, fiery behaviour in which the person assumes that the boundless is a virtue, even if it exhausts them physically and emotionally. There is a danger, however, that the great movement metal becomes too powerful and itself causes complaints.

People born with 'Ding, Ht in wood' can go beyond their own limits very easily for a long period of time. Often they need the attentiveness of others to protect them from themselves. I have often heard the justification for self-imposed servitude: 'You do that for each other, right?' or 'Everyone does that anyway.' Advice to take better care of themselves is heard, but often has to be repeated. And even then, it remains difficult for 'Ding, Ht in wood' people to sense their own limits. It is difficult, in part because of our fast-demanding society, for these people to limit their yang, fiery nature, their desire to expand, to care for others, to have goals, to feel actions and to take initiatives.

For the practitioner, the challenge is to transform creativity and rich imagination into perseverance through softness and flexibility. I usually give patients the example of long marram grass that moves softly and flexibly with the wind and resists the force of the wind due to its soft resilience and strong texture.

A FINAL NOTE

The heavenly stem Jia, which has the gallbladder qi as an exponent, is dynamized by the great movement earth. What are the consequences of earth that is

---

11   See Chapters 24, 33, 34, 38 on earthly branches.

affecting the gallbladder *qi*? And what about the great movement metal influencing the liver and the great movement water influencing the small intestine?

The phase earth is in contact with all directions so that it can harmonize the totality of different forces and enable the necessary transformations. But earth can also have a dominant and stagnant effect due to too much damp. The heavenly stem *Jia*, gallbladder, responds to the inhibitory force of earth with a certain forcefulness against the limitation of its form. It causes initiating dynamic vitality by strength and sprouting. The normal pulse of the gallbladder is therefore slightly superficial, a little short and slightly elastic. It is especially sensitive to too much damp.

The phase metal tends to introversion, dryness and constriction. The heavenly stem *Yi* and the liver despise these dry and tight qualities and respond with rapid growth and free flow of *qi*.

The normal pulse of the liver is, therefore, gentle as a waving hand, as soft as the tip of a long bamboo being lifted up. A healthy liver responds with flexibility and adaptability that opposes the constricting qualities of metal. It is especially sensitive to too much dryness and constriction (tight and wiry pulse).

The phase water internalizes and flows to the depths. It forces the heavenly stem *Bing* and the small intestine to ensure the expression of the phase fire in, for example, upward and expansive movements, warmth, prosperity and vital *qi*. It functions despite and due to the distinctions of the properties of the phase water.

The colour vermilion of the red vermilion bird heaven is found in nature in the mineral cinnabar. This special mineral, known in Chinese alchemy, indicates the process of transformation of one substance into another. When food has passed through the stomach and enters the small intestine, food is no longer a foreign object but has passed beyond recognition into particles in the blood. It has become part of the human system. This kind of irreversible transformation is only possible through the capacity of fire for division and integration of yin and yang. Objective distinctiveness and being able to direct yin and yang, the impure and pure in the body, is possible only by being aware and having an overview.[12] To distinguish between foreign and known/native plays an enormous part in the digestive and mental-emotional functions of the small intestine. The small intestine receives relatively little attention in our profession, but it is not for nothing that it is connected to the heart, so that it is able to discern what is useful. Useful is everything that can be integrated and is intended for

---

12 The bird is the only animal that can overcome gravity and oversee the world.

the rightfulness of the heart which is based on inner judgements. The purer the heart, the purer the judgements.

The normal pulse of the small intestine is a nicely formed and moderately superficial pulse. A small intestine pulse that is too deep or too rough deviates from the expression of the fire and loses its distinctive properties. The small intestine regulates objective thinking and repels the overly subjective wishful thinking that belongs to the water phase.

The manifestations of the phase wood, just like the wind, are difficult to control. Wood is flexible, supple, pliable and moving. In order not to risk the upward expanding force of the fire being pushed up too much, the heavenly stem *Ding* and the heart are forced to rest in solid matter, but even more in the silence of the hidden and peaceful space in the heart itself. The normal pulse of the heart is therefore a steady flow, sliding as a string of pearls and smooth as jade stone. Any form of unrest in this distracts from the quiet presence of awareness. A scattered pulse, especially, shows the overwhelming dynamics of the wood.

The lesson to be learned from this section is that *qi* is composed of collaborative and opposing dynamic forces. In this case, between the dynamic action of the great movement and the receptive response of the heavenly stem and the related organ. The description of the normal pulses indicates the strength and quality of *qi*, as well as the degree of resistance and acceptance of the responses of the heavenly stems to the dynamics of the great movements. The collaboration of the dynamic dualities largely determines the health of the organs and channels.

CHAPTER 16

DYNAMICS OF THE HEAVENLY STEM *WU* 戊[1]

Without leaving home, you may know the world
Without looking out the window,
you may be able to experience the *Dao* of Heaven.
The further you go, the less you know.

So the sage knows without going;
He understands without looking;
He acts without doing.[2]

FIVE, THE BREATH OF LIFE

One of my teachers answered my question about the meaning of numbers as follows: 'If you desire to understand the language of heaven, learn all about music, vowels and numbers.' He continued: 'There are three ancient concepts that manifest themselves only through and in every material form. *Qi*-breath, *Li*, the immutable laws and designs of nature and *Shu*, numbers and rhythm.'

Though numbers may appear to have been invented by humans, they are in fact regarded as the revelation and unfolding of the rhythm of creation. One (一) is considered to be the great monad, the undivided heart of every being. Two (二) is the expression of the undivided heart in the manifested world by two opposite and complementary forces: heaven and earth, yin and yang. Three (三) is the trinity, the three in one, the cosmic foundation of creation. In Chinese philosophy and medicine they appear in the sky as the sun, moon and stars, on earth as

---

1   Born in years ending with an 8, such as 1978, 2008, after the Chinese New Year.
2   *Dao De Jing* Chapter 47.

water, fire, wind, and in humans as *jing, qi, shen*. Four (四) are the four cardinal directions that define the space and time of the manifested world. They are the four pillars that sustain heaven. Five (五) is the breath of life that guides every transformation for which it holds the centre. Six (六) organizes in the form what is created by five. Together with five, six guides the expression of the undivided heart in three-dimensional space. Seven (七) is often considered inauspicious because of the relationship with the seven *po* and the seven emotions. The seven stars of the Big Dipper, the chariot of the heavenly emperor and the seven orifices of the head indicate that seven is the gateway for heavenly inspiration and self-cultivation. Eight (八) organizes the creation by dividing, separating, ordering and collaborating. The eight directions and eight trigrams display and reveal what appeared in seven. Nine (九) is the most heavenly number, the completion of creation and thus the other number of transformation. Standstill means decline, moving forward means progress to the next realm of development. Ten (十) symbolizes the integration and inspired vital energy of all the previous numbers. It is the universal life force in created life elevated to the way of heaven.

Five, then, is known as the number of life and change. Six is known as the one that organizes and distributes life in form. Together, these are the central yin and yang that link the subtle realm to the self and give it its experience of being and consciousness and are the cause of intentions, regardless of whether they are expressed in behaviour or not.

The fifth great movement/heavenly stem combination 'Wu, St in fire' and the sixth combination 'Ji, Sp in earth' together hold the centre of the ten great movements and heavenly stems and determine the state of the whole. They are the terrestrial representatives of the undivided heart, the heavenly emperor and the North Pole Star; they are the axis of the spinning cosmic wheel on earth.

To understand the meaning and role of number five in numerology we need to look at the number two first. The Chinese character two consists of two horizontal lines, one above the other, symbolizing heaven (yang) above and earth (yin) below. The number two creates the condition for interaction by positioning opposing and complementary forces, that communicate in all animated beings by means of the flow of *qi* between yin and yang, heaven and earth. The Chinese character five depicts the movement of *qi* between the two primal forces yin and yang, heaven and earth. The interaction between yin and yang refers to the back-and-forth movements of the flow of *qi* in channels. Five holds the centre between and in connection with heaven and earth, and enables smooth change through neutrality and stability.

Not long before J.D. van Buren died he gave me a bundle of papers with notes he was working on in Portugal during his vacation. On one of the papers he had written a text relating to a well-known painting, known as the Vitruvian Man (Leonardo da Vinci c.1490). The man stands with his arms outstretched and touches the circumference of a circle with his hands and feet displayed in two different positions:

> 5 and 6 are very closely related. This shows diagrammatically MAN standing in a sphere representing the Universe. He touches the sphere at 5 points; 3 above the waistline (Yang) and 2 below (Yin). The Chinese character for 6 is 六, which resembles this stance.

The text speaks of five contact points with the universe (heaven). The human being is the 'six', the breath of form in which the flow of the vital six *qi* arises and falls.

J.D. van Buren's comment about the three points that touch the sphere above the waist is actually not quite correct. The two hands and two feet touch the circumference of the sphere; the fifth point is the centre of the circle in which all the tensions of the sphere of the universe come together, merge and are balanced. This point coincides with the centre of the Vitruvian Man at the umbilicus. Here, Cv-8, *Shen Que*, spirit gate, is where the *shen* rests and is in balance. This point is considered the abode of the source of life. The diagonals of the depicted square (earth) intersect at Cv-2, *Qu Gu*, curved bone, which supports and carries post-natal *qi*, strengthens perseverance and builds self-confidence. Furthermore, it is remarkable that the head does not touch the sphere but the square; the mind and thought are linked with the earthly realm, the centre, the spirit gate of the Vitruvian Man at the umbilicus with the heavenly.

The Vitruvian Man stands with his hands stretched out above the head. Yang channels flow down from the fingers to the head and then on to the feet. Yin channels flow from the feet to the thorax and then rise up to the extended hands above the head. This flow is opposite of what would normally be expected from the nature of yin and yang: Yin is like water that moves to the deepest point; yang rises like fire.

The flow of *qi* in the channels shows the expression of potentiality from pre-natal conditions, in which heaven directs to earth and vice versa. The channel system is the sacrifice of heaven to human. Sacrifice corresponds to the emanation *heng* and the many mythical stories in which the universe is created through a sacrifice of the creator to the created. The universe is usually created by a mythical creature, as told in the Chinese myth of Pangu, the primitive hairy giant with two horns who sacrificed his life for the creation of heaven, earth and humans. This is a principle worth considering. Just as the *shen* sacrifices its ubiquity in order to make a temporary appearance in humans and evolves from it, and form principles sacrifice their infinite possibilities for the limited form expressions of the body and evolve from it, so humans might sacrifice some of their endless choice of opportunities in favour of the development of other beings and thereby further evolve. This mutual exchange is the essence of the heavenly stem *Wu* and of creation in general.

WU 戊, THE FIFTH HEAVENLY STEM

The quality of the heavenly stem *Wu* is shown in the yang of the earth, the stomach. *Wu* refers to the centre that provides harmony, stability and firmness. It represents the post-natal aspects of *Qian*, Heaven, the life-giving source that creates and supports life and all forms.

Wu maintains balance in all possible ways but does not itself participate in the transformation process. Its function follows the natural path, including seasonal cycles that sometimes lead to abundance and prosperity, and sometimes to decay and death. An example is the stomach pulse. In the course of the seasons, the stomach is an energetic compass for the other organs and *qi*: In winter the stomach pulse is small, like a stone, inside and enveloped; in spring it beats like the vibrating sound of the string of a lute; in summer it flourishes and resonates like the beat of a fine hammer; in late summer it turns inward again and is thin, soft and feeble; in autumn small and rough. In general, the stomach holds the centre with a moderately superficial, slightly thick and short pulse.

In nature, *Wu* is revealed in mountains and hills. From the highest point descent is the only possible path. It is the point where decay and letting go embarks. The development of the spark of life in spring has evolved to its peak in the summer and can only decrease to return to its original source in winter.

The Chinese character *Wu* shows a hand holding a cutting instrument used in harvesting. The cutting follows the natural process of letting go of what is no longer necessary or appropriate. It promotes the process of natural withering, but on the other hand it cuts fruits to benefit others.

THE GATEKEEPER

The person using the cutting instrument must be able to distinguish healthy and unhealthy, useful and useless, good and evil, alignment and harmonization versus discord and disharmony.

When food has passed the level of the stomach, it becomes part of the human being. In the small intestine food is broken down into nutrients that are absorbed into the blood and can no longer be distinguished as food. The same applies to other inputs such as opinions, ideas, thoughts, emotions and so on, which are judged, approved or rejected by *Wu*, stomach, whether or not to be part of that person's ideas and feelings. In this sense, the stomach is the gatekeeper. People can swallow food, but also refuse or reject it by vomiting.

Wu, stomach, should only accept what is consistent with the inner order (heaven), allowing people only suitable food in the broadest sense of the word, to enable them to follow the path of their soul's destiny and their own point of truth.

When *Wu*, stomach, is too fragile, people 'swallow' too much. They may be too late to realize that they have fallen into an unpleasant situation. This is one of the most challenging energetic aspects for people born with '*Wu*, St in fire'. Despite an innate aptitude for feeling and supporting others and yet not getting too much involved with them, it often proves too difficult for these individuals to distance themselves. They overempathize when others struggle with emotions and the suffering of others can have a major impact on their health.

A balanced heavenly stem *Wu*, stomach, allows the inner processes to proceed naturally by keeping people focused appropriately inward towards themselves, not being overly distracted by the demanding challenges of others and by their own personal will.

A harmonious focus is possible through the cutting instrument (*Wu*) that allows the self to release unnecessary personal and cultural desires and reveal the person's true spirit and true *qi*. However, suppressing emotions and feelings of concern can lead to complaints: muffled, stagnant, action-seeking *qi* that turns inward, causing frustration, sadness and anger. This stagnation may lead to heat with stagnated *qi* in the abdomen, chest and face, and symptoms such as irritable bowel syndrome (IBS), dyspnoea, asthma, red spots on the neck, sore throat or sinusitis. It is worth noting that the harmonious focus of *Wu*, stomach, is inherently natural and not organized by will, coercion, visualization or imagination.

THE GREAT MOVEMENT FIRE AND THE HEAVENLY STEM *WU*

The great movement fire and the earth-related heavenly stem *Wu* have a *sheng*-cycle relationship. What was discussed in the previous chapter therefore also applies to this combination; however, with this relationship it particularly affects the centre (earth).

The *yuan-shen* is part of a *collective* network that connects all living beings that express themselves in creativity and selflessness. The *wu-shen* and the associated great movements connect people *individually* and socially. They are subtle tools for self-perception. Collective and individual-social sensations of joy can cause people to desire to stay excited. They desire to feel more and more, experience more and more, achieve more and more and so on. A stable, harmonious and firm stomach *qi*, with its associated feeling of positive self-esteem/'I am', keeps people with both feet on the ground. A confused, chaotic or stagnant stomach *qi* is a sign of low self-esteem that is often muted by workload and a full agenda or emotional self-neglect. It shows itself through, for example, fatigue and migraines; when it is directed inward, it is revealed by deeper conditions such as autoimmune diseases.

Being overenthusiastic and setting more goals than is healthy is typical for people born with '*Wu*, St in fire', even if they are already too tired and overloaded. Sometimes taking a break is tolerable, but often not for too long. The underlying cause of this tendency is often a fear of the finiteness of life, which they determine must therefore be fully lived.

EAGERNESS

Throughout my life, I have come to know desires that are difficult to fulfil, not only for myself, but also for friends and family, and for large numbers of patients. Desires for a different kind of relationship, desires for a less stressful life, desires for children, desires for some free time, desires for more work and so on. The abundance of desires determines and directs a large part of our lives. However, persistent eagerness hampers and is uncomfortable in the long run. The powerful and harmonizing properties of the heavenly stem *Wu* become unbalanced, causing people to lose themselves and become truly ill. People get irritated and confused and feel uprooted. This gives rise to symptoms of heat and rising *qi*, usually in the stomach channel, indicating an imbalance of '*Wu*, St in fire'. Treatments can calm this eagerness, but underlying fears and uncertainties often persist. These are usually so existential and extensive that help from a psychologist is indicated.

The ego may attune itself to the spiritual realm by harmonizing its own tensions, while not neglecting the manifested form. *Wu* is about making subtle spiritual concepts practical. '*Wu*, St in fire' motivates and enhances the connection between the higher and the lower. It is therefore up to the ego to allow both to be present equally and in harmonious connection with each other. This is achieved through making the right choices, by refusing without tension that which does not fit and by taking the time to digest what is needed, so that the ego becomes less and less burdened and more transparent and can align with the heart-*shen* and *yuan-shen*.

ACUPUNCTURE POINTS THAT INFLUENCE THE ACTIVE GREAT MOVEMENT FIRE AND THE HEAVENLY STEM *WU*

The stem point St-41, *Jie Xi*, dispersing stream, the *jing* river-fire point on the stomach channel, is a typical heaven–earth–human point. It takes from the fire phase and is energized by the great movement fire, brings the *qi* to the earth and supports the body and post-natal *qi*, especially through the kidney yin. It can be used in stress and emotions due to collective stress such as collective suffering due to climate change, socio-cultural conditions, the Covid-19 pandemic and so on.

People born with '*Wu*, St in fire' who overwork or burn out are helped when they focus on creative pursuits, transforming inspiration into physical forms (heaven–earth–human).

The Chinese character *Jie* is about dividing, undoing, separating and untying. *Xi* means stream, gorge, ravine, torrent or creek. The free flow through St-41 keeps the path of *qi* clear between heaven, earth and human. St-41 facilitates free physical, emotional and mental movement with both feet on the ground. The freedom of movement of the foot bones is first and foremost determined by the unimpeded flow of *qi* through this point. It determines stability as well as freedom of movement.

Though the foot has lost its grip function during evolution, it can still withstand the great forces of body weight and offers humans the opportunity to walk and run upright. This point is indicated when people feel blocked and have lost the zest for life; St-41 makes it easier for people to lift the feet and to take the first steps towards healing.

Stomach *qi* is concentrated at St-41. Despite the fame of St-36, *Zu San Li*, St-41 is considered the original stomach *qi* point. It takes from fire – especially from the small intestine and *san jiao* – and nourishes the rest of the body. Walking easily and easily lifting the feet without stumbling illustrate the health and nourishment this point offers to the rest of the body.

St-41 activates and warms the stomach channel and dissolves blockages in the channel and beyond. It is used to transform damp and stagnation, to prevent mood swings and to treat internal devils.

St-41 sedation is indicated for diseases such as oedema of the eyes, bloodshot eyes and conjunctivitis, facial neuralgia, general infections and high fever. But one needs to be careful with sedation of St-41. It can seriously drain the kidney yin, causing depression, sadness and increasing anxiety. My teachers advised me to tonify kidney yin when sedating St-41, but in practice I have never sedated St-41 in my life.

Sp-20, *Zhou Rong*, encircling glory or complete nourishment, leads the *qi* to thrive and prosper.

Sp-20 is a meeting point of pre-natal and post-natal *qi*, making it good to use with Sp-4. This combination bridges the *qi* that are linked through birth. This point can be used in hereditary chronic lung diseases and whole-body exhaustion.

Sp-20 emphasizes nurturing and compassion, safety and protection. It can be compared to the energy of a mother figure. It gives a powerful sense of both giving and receiving and relaxes the *shen*. The feeling of confidence and physical support helps when people find it difficult to be physically touched. The relaxed posture and full body support with improved function of kidney *jing* invokes in people a feeling of having both feet on the ground with the sensation of being complete, especially in combination with St-41.

Sp-17, *Shi Dou*, food drain or food hole. Sp-17 can be used for post-natal congestion of the chest and abdomen. The essence of food and fluids accumulates in Sp-17 before proceeding to the lung channel. This point regulates *qi* and promotes water circulation.

In 'Wu, St in fire' constitutional emotional issues, Sp-17 can be used when *qi* stagnates in the chest and abdomen. This is typically accompanied by symptoms of chest congestion with shortness of breath and abdominal distension with ascites, along with belching and vomiting right after eating. Waking up at exactly four in the morning is the core symptom. In cases due to guilt and shame, the *qi* should be directed towards the diaphragm; in cases of grief, perpendicular treatment is indicated; and in cases of lung *qi* stagnation, oblique treatment to move *qi* towards Lu-1, *Zhong Fu*, is best. People often feel immediate relief, but further care for the underlying emotions is essential.

> This patient initially came because he suffered from all kinds of symptoms like insomnia, lower back pain, arrythmia due to heart *qi xu*, *jing qi* exhaustion, liver *qi xu*. He then started to share that he had been looking for a happy relationship for years. After he finally succeeded and got married, both he and his partner had been unhappy ever since. He shared that he made up for his grief and dissatisfaction by working very hard. He felt especially guilty about the wrong choices he had made in his life.
>
> After my diagnosis, he was treated with Sp-20, Sp-17 directed towards the diaphragm and Ki-16, *Huang Shu*,[3] vital *shu*. Ki-16 balances the three burners,

---

3   *Huang* is the area below the heart, the area of the diaphragm.

regulates and warms the intestines and harmonizes the stomach. It can be used for symptoms due to lack of warmth and affection.

When he returned after four weeks, he felt fitter than ever. He was preparing for a divorce. However, things turned out differently. As he felt stronger, the relationship with his partner changed for the better and he got to know himself better. His long-lasting desire for a happy relationship seemed to have finally been fulfilled. It prompted him to end the divorce process. Nevertheless, they fell into old habits and patterns and after some time the unhappy feelings returned.

He continued to receive treatment once a month in which I treated the great movement fire and the heavenly stem *Wu* in different ways, always in accordance with the innate imbalances. After about a year, he began to explore his deeper located emotions: A complicated relationship with both his parents in his youth made him lonely and deeply anxious. He finally had the courage to listen to the silence within by facing his fears. His busy schedule subsided and he was satisfied with himself and the path he was taking. Both partners chose to continue the marriage. Years later, he wrote me a letter saying that happiness was not something to aspire to. 'The moment it is there, it is there. The awareness of it is not in the present but always afterwards.'

THE CONSEQUENCES OF '*WU*, STOMACH IN FIRE' IN THE *WUXING*

The active great movement fire tends to subdue the great movement metal. The quality and quantity of the passive great movement metal can be diagnosed by the strength of the pulse at Lu-9, *Tai Yuan*, great abyss. Some teachers discuss this point as *the* point of the body because it connects the phase earth with all *qi*. It balances the overall *qi* and sends *qi* to the deeper levels of the body for nourishment and defence via the kidneys. It is called the great meeting of all vessels. The *Mai Jing* 'Classic of the Pulse' states:

> The *chong* and *du mai* combined are the way of the twelve meridians. If the *chong* and *du mai* do not function correctly, the twelve meridians do not return to the great meeting of vessels (*Tai Yuan*, Lu-9).[4]

The word *yuan* in *Tai Yuan* means abyss, a deep bottomless gap. It symbolizes the source of endless flow and supply of *qi* of the origin of existence that flows from

---

4   Matsumoto and Birch 1986, p. 32.

the source toward Lu-9. It is one of the reasons that pulse diagnosis is performed at the level of Lu-9 and why Lu-9 is the *hui* point for the blood vessels.[5]

Lu-9 affects the lungs and all *qi* that belong to metal.[6] It governs the function of the blood vessels and the descending of *qi* and fluids to the kidneys, the root of all yin.

At lavish parties you may see people born with '*Wu*, St in fire' who can easily go wild and get overexcited (great movement fire), even without drugs or alcohol. When exhausted, they develop a sore throat, shortness of breath and possibly an asthma attack. It is not uncommon for them to suffer from urinary tract disorders such as cystitis or low back pain the next day as a result of a constricted, insufficient great movement metal.

People born with '*Wu*, St in fire' need to take good care of the properties of great movement metal, which involves introspection alongside healthy interactions with the surrounding world. They tend to kidney *qi xu*,[7] which in combination with underactive great movement metal easily causes the *jing qi* to be affected.

The level of the *jing* mainly concerns the physical-emotional realm. People trying to strengthen the great movement metal along with the *jing* require structure and effort, which can be achieved by regular physical training and by taking regular care of others where physical endeavour is required.[8] For those born with '*Wu*, St in fire', this can of course easily be overdone and lead to undesired consequences.

The level of *jing* requires clear structures, clear agreements and good planning but also needs to be pleasurable and involve the exchange of shared experiences and good feelings.

INTEGRITY

The human equilibrium needs physical, emotional, mental and spiritual interaction and integration, with integrity being paramount. Whether physiotherapist or accountant, police officer or estate agent, we all need an internal human scale

---

5   It is noteworthy that four of the six *yuan source* points of the yin channels contain the Chinese word *Tai*, big. It indicates the extent and importance of the functions of these points and emphasizes the enormous effect. Lu-9, *Tai Yuan*; Sp-3, *Tai Bai*; Ki-3, *Tai Xi*; Hc-7, *Da* [great] *Ling*; Liv-3, *Tai Chong*.
6   Large intestine, bladder and kidney. See the chapters on earthly branches.
7   See Chapter 17 on unlike *qi*.
8   I regularly met people who travelled long distances to care for sick friends and relatives to strengthen their own *jing* in the short term.

that registers a healthy balance. 'Wu, St in fire' is the centre point and keeps an eye on the balance between self- and other-interest.

The level of the *shen* also includes and expresses integrity. It is based on introspection and acceptance of the temporary nature of existence (which the 'Wu, St in fire' person usually chooses to avoid). Rational thinking is often used by these individuals as a form of self-regulation. It ensures that they have something to do to avoid facing inner emotional problems. The key to avoiding this pitfall is a consistent practice of justice to the self, which is not the same as procedural justice, but is aimed at maintaining integrity and selflessness.

CHAPTER 17

FIVE METHODS OF CONSTITUTIONAL TREATMENT[1]

Heaven	① 1 Jia Gb +	□ 2 Yi Liv –	③ 3 Bing S.i. +	□ 4 Ding Ht –	⑤ 5 Wu St +
Human	**Earth**	**Metal**	**Water**	**Wood**	**Fire**
Earth	Ji Sp – □ 6	Geng L.i. + ⑦ 7	Xin Lu – □ 8	Jen Bl + ⑨ 9	Gui Ki – □ 10

Figure 17.1 Great movements and unlike qi of the heavenly stems

We are halfway through the series of ten great movements and ten heavenly stems. The second series of five great movements follows the same order as the first: earth, metal, water, wood and fire, with two main differences:

1. The great movements that share the same phase are opposite in their activity. For example, the first great movement (earth) is active, the sixth great movement (earth) is passive, the second is passive, the seventh active and so on.
2. The heavenly stem and its corresponding organ in each great movement are different. The relationship of the two different organs within one great movement is called 'unlike qi' because the qi that are housed by

---

1 These are the most commonly used methods. Other methods are discussed throughout the book.

the same nature of great movement are not alike. So for great movement earth we have: Gb and Sp; for great movement metal: Liv-L.i.; great movement water: S.i.-Lu; great movement wood: Ht-Bl; great movement fire: St-Ki. The relationship between the organs of unlike *qi* is always in a *ke* or reverse *ke*-cycle relationship, that accentuates the life side of the energetic model. It activates vitality, brightness and authenticity, the dynamic qualities that are independent of and complementary to the physical material world. In contrast to the *sheng*-cycle relationship, that supports and nourishes form, the *ke*-cycle relationship supports the spark of life of the eternal that binds to all forms.

Five methods of constitutional acupuncture are discussed in this chapter.

A. Five phases
B. Unlike *qi* of the heavenly stem
C. The three treatment options
D. Like *qi* of the heavenly stem
E. Great movement mother point

A. FIVE PHASES
Treatment according to the five phases is part of constitutional acupuncture. I assume that the reader is aware of this treatment method. The five phase relationship between *great movements*, however, differs somewhat from the well-known five phase theory.

An example:

1. Determine the great movement and heavenly stem of the year of birth.
   Let us assume that someone is born with '*Yi*, Liv in metal'. The innate *qi* of the great movement (metal) and heavenly stem (*Yi*, liver) are considered strong aspects of the person involved.[2]
2. Determine the relationship between active and passive great movements in five phases.
   The effect of the passive great movement in '*Yi*, Liv in metal' is that there is a reasonable chance that the active great movement fire will become too active. The temptation to excess is considered a weaker

---

2   A constitutional passive character of a great movement is also a stronger aspect, as long as it does not lead to excesses or insufficiencies elsewhere that are too disturbing.

aspect of the birth chart. In general, passive great movements can also be considered as a weaker aspect in relation to the active great movements, especially when an active great movement predominates. If 'Wu, St in fire' is indeed too active – to be diagnosed through pulse diagnosis and qualifying behaviour and symptomatology[3] – the great movement metal is further subdued[4] and the great movement fire and stomach *qi* might be treated.[5]

Treatment of an overactive great movement is preferably not done by sedation, as this also sedates essential *qi*. Other options are 'unlike *qi* treatments' (where in the above example, with overactive 'Wu, St in fire', we work instead on the opposite *qi* in great movement fire, i.e. kidneys) or one of the methods of the 'three treatment options' (see below).

B.1 UNLIKE *QI*
Treatment of the *innate* heavenly stem and associated organ

Unlike *qi* treatments are widely used in constitutional acupuncture because they are used to balance and cure the life dynamics of great movements. These treatments are called 'unlike *qi*' because two great movements of the same nature, although one is active and the other passive, are linked to different – unlike – heavenly stems and associated organs. The unlike *qi* of 'Yi, Liv in metal' is 'Geng, L.i. in metal'. Liver and large intestine share the same great movement metal. The unlike *qi* of 'Wu, St in fire' is 'Gui, Ki in fire'. Stomach and kidney share the same great movement fire.

Unlike *qi* treatment restores the balance of great movements.

An analogy for this is to imagine the two bowls of a weighing scale. For example, there is 'Yi, Liv in metal' in one bowl; in the other bowl is 'Geng, L.i. in metal'. Assume that the dynamics between the passive great movement metal and 'Yi, Liv in metal' is disturbed.[6] This may result in a liver *qi* that becomes too tight/metallic causing pain in the flanks or muscle cramps. The tightness changes the weight of 'Yi, Liv in metal' which also influences 'Geng, L.i. in metal' in the other bowl.

---

3   For example, dry mouth, longing for cold drinks, halitosis, red tongue body with yellow coating.
4   For example, weak voice, shortness of breath, loose stools, weakness of the lumbar region, hearing issues and so on.
5   However, practice has shown that, in many cases, treatment of 'Yi, Liv in metal' by unlike *qi* 'Geng, L.i. in metal' is to reduce the activity of the great movement fire, especially when the four possibilities appear, such as wood too metallic; see Chapters 22 and 45. Nevertheless, advice should be given to quieten the great movement fire.
6   For instance, the great movement metal makes *Yi*, liver too metallic, too dry and tight.

The treatment is not approached from the bowl of 'Yi, Liv in metal', but from the other bowl of the weighing scale.

After the disturbance in the liver *qi* and large intestine *qi* has been first examined and confirmed by diagnosis, an acupuncture point is chosen on the large intestine channel, which treats the tight liver *qi* as well, *because the great movement metal* – the weighing scale – *is then balanced*. When the two organs in the same great movement are disturbed, an unlike *qi* treatment balances the related great movement, which in this case treats the unhealthy influence of the great movement metal on the liver *qi*.

We have not yet covered the second part of the cycle of great movements and heavenly stems, but I hope the rationale is clear. The active great movement and heavenly stem is treated via the passive equivalent and vice versa. Unlike *qi* treatments balance the great movement and, with it, the natural reciprocal influence between great movement and heavenly stem. This means that liver problems can be treated with the large intestine and vice versa just as the stomach can be treated with the kidneys and vice versa.[7]

In constitutional acupuncture, these seemingly strange combinations are as normal as the relationships between the gallbladder and liver and between the stomach and spleen in the five phases.

Summary
- The innate great movement and heavenly stem are considered strong aspects, the unlike *qi* of the innate heavenly stem is considered a weaker aspect.
- The consequence of an unlike *qi* treatment is the healing of the dynamics of the related couple of great movement and heavenly stem/organ. Simply put, an imbalance between the dynamic great movement and the corresponding heavenly stem is restored by treatment of its counterpart.
- See the discussion in Chapter 22 to treat the so-called four possibilities with unlike *qi*.

B.2 UNLIKE *QI*
Treatment of the heavenly stem and *diseased* associated organ
The previous discussion relates to the innate *qi* (that is an expression of a person's date of birth). Unlike *qi* principles, however, can also be used to treat diseased organs and channels that are not constitutionally related for a person.

---

7   See also Chapter 22 on the 'four possibilities'.

For example, liver organ diseases in general respond well to treatments of the unlike *qi Geng*, large intestine and vice versa.[8]

CASE EXAMPLE

One hospitalized patient had an enlarged, diseased liver (organ), ear and balance disorders due to toxicity of the body from eating and drinking habits and medicines, and an extensive demanding social life, all of which drain the (yang) liver *qi*. This was accompanied by insufficient *qi* of kidneys and heart, as well as of *san jiao*.

Although in constitutional acupuncture it is not customary to use the same points over and over again, I decided to give the following treatment twice a week for two weeks:

L.i.-6, *Pian Li,* along with S.i.-7, *Zhi Zheng,*[9] that together nourish the kidney yin and *san jiao*, along with L.i.-15, *Jian Yu*. Together these points calm people's excessive behaviour, partly because L.i.-15 tonifies and strengthens the heart. In addition, L.i.-6 affects the ear and balance via the longitudinal *luo* channel of the large intestine and restores the sense of balance. S.i.-7 nourishes the heart.

Because large intestine (*Geng*) is the unlike *qi* of the liver (*Yi*), it balances the great movement metal and restores the *qi* in the liver. Good progress was made after four treatments and his hospital doctor could not understand the rapid improvement of his liver enzyme levels. The patient was discharged from hospital and I started to give constitutional treatments in my clinic, once a week at first, then once a month. It took another month for him to return to work. After six months he was back to good health and had adopted a healthy lifestyle.

There are other alternatives to treat an imbalance in an organ/channel:

C. THE THREE TREATMENT OPTIONS

1. Using the *ke*-cycle relationship within the (diseased) channel
2. The dynamic approach
3. Sedation

---

8   It should be obvious that the (im)balance of *qi* in the birth chart and (pulse) diagnosis are always to be taken into account first.
9   See the discussion in chapters on earthly branches about the unlike *qi* relationship between S.i. and Liv.

1. Using the *ke*-cycle relationship within the (diseased) channel

A too active 'Wu, St in fire' causes fiery stomach *qi* with symptoms such as thirst, dry mouth, conjunctivitis, red tongue with yellow coating, having a constant appetite, rapid fiery pulse and so on.

Using the *ke*-cycle within the stomach channel means to control the fire by water: St-44, *Nei Ting*, the water point, controls and clears heat in the stomach channel.

2. The dynamic approach

The acupuncture points that are used in the dynamic approach do not necessarily have to be related to the five phase theory, or reside on the channel that is imbalanced. In this case, points have to energetically oppose the heat and rising *qi* in the stomach channel in some way.

St-12, *Que Pen*, for example, descends stomach *qi* and clears heat; alternatively, Sp-6, *San Yin Jiao*, nourishes the fluids and calms the mind; St-36, *Zu San Li*, regulates the *qi* in the stomach channel, strengthens kidney yin and clears heat in case of insufficient fluids; Cv-12, *Zhong Wan*, clears stomach heat. The choice of points depends on the (pulse) diagnosis.

3. Sedation

The third option is not preferred, as discussed above: St-41, *Jia Xi*, the fire point, sedation.

Another example:

- Determine the great movement and heavenly stem of birth, and its balance/quality, e.g. 'Bing, S.i. in water' is too active.
- Determine the relationships between active and passive great movements.

Due to 'Bing, S.i. in water', there is a reasonable chance that the great movement fire will become passive, which in most cases mainly affects/diminishes the *qi* of the heart.[10] It is safer to start a course of treatment with nourishing rather than sedation. Therefore, nourishing the heart *qi* in this case is usually best and sufficient to restore balance.

Furthermore, when the small intestine is also affected by water and cold with

---

10 Palpitations, tiredness, pale complexion and tongue, spontaneous sweating, especially under the arms, and so on.

symptoms such as abdominal pain, diarrhoea and frequent urination, treatment can be extended with one of the three treatment options:

1. Using the *ke*-cycle relationship within the (diseased) channel
Treat S.i.-8, *Xiao Hai*, the earth point, to counteract the coldness/excess water in the small intestine. This is not the healthiest choice, though, as dampness and coldness together may cause other problems. Moreover, we want to avoid treating innate *qi* directly because it can lead to imbalances in the constitutional *qi*.

2. The dynamic approach
Bring warmth to the small intestine to oppose coldness. Moxa on Cv-4, *Guan Yuan*, Cv-6, *Qi Hai*, and Bl-27, *Xiao Chang Shu*. The alternative approach (to tonify S.i.-5, *Yang Gu*, the fire point that reduces dampness and coldness in the small intestine channel) is avoided because we want to avoid treating the innate *qi* directly.

3. Sedation
Sedation of S.i.-2, *Qian Gu*. Sedation of the stem point would be possible, but only with serious imbalance and is only recommended once in a lifetime.[11] Preferably this approach would be combined with a point that also nourishes the sedated channel.

Coldness in the small intestine is a manifestation of the 'four possibilities', as will be discussed in Chapter 22, and for which the unlike *qi* treatments are the best choice.

> A female patient born with '*Yi*, Liv in metal' has a bitter taste in the mouth, abdominal pain, constipation, poor appetite, irregular menstruation, mood swings, difficulty with swallowing and suppressed anger. The expected insufficient and stagnant liver *qi* was confirmed by pulse diagnosis. The disruption of free flow of *qi* caused all pulses to show some degree of tightness. Treating Liv-3 was not an option.[12]
>
> Three treatment options:

---

11 J.D. van Buren was quite clear about this. Too much sedation of a stem point could lead to a reduction of essential innate *qi*, which could certainly lead to long-term insufficiencies that might only show up much later.

12 It has already been discussed that innate constitutional *qi* will only be treated indirectly.

1. Using the *ke*-cycle relationship within the (diseased) channel

Since I did not want to treat the liver channel, Liv-2 was not an option. In addition, using the fire point is dangerous for the innate dryness of metal and more stagnation would likely then lead to more heat.

2. The dynamic approach

I could have chosen acupuncture points like Ki-21, Bl-18, both of which act on the liver.

3. Sedation

Liv-4 sedation is not advisable, not just because it is innate *qi* but also, specifically, the stem point (the metal point on the liver channel). Sedation may lead to long-term insufficiencies afterwards and for this reason J.D. van Buren advised practitioners not to sedate birth stem points and, if so, not to do so more than once in a lifetime.

Treatment of the unlike *qi*

For those born with '*Yi*, Liv in the *passive* great movement metal', the unlike *qi* is '*Geng*, L.i. in the seventh *active* great movement metal'.

Any (!) point on the large intestine channel will affect the relationship between the liver and the great movement metal as well as the stagnation of the liver *qi* seen here. In addition, the acupuncture point chosen should ideally improve the flow of *qi* and wood. In nearly all cases, pulse diagnosis provides a definite answer about the point(s) to be chosen. Diagnosis guides the practitioner who knows the rules.

I chose L.i.-3, *San Jian*, the wood point on the large intestine channel. L.i.-3 balances between the metal and the wood without the intervention of water and removes stagnation from the wood; it is known for its good effect on suppressed anger. After three weeks, the patient reported that most complaints had disappeared after a short cold.

In the chapters on earthly branches, it will be discussed that the large intestine channel has inherent wood quality as well as metal. For now, I would like to remind the reader that the large intestine in the Chinese hourly clock occupies the period of 3 to 5 a.m., the time of the rising sun, the direction of the East and the wood.

Symptoms due to the tendency of '*Wu*, St in fire' to become overactive may be caused by increased innate passivity of the great movement metal or can be triggered through behaviour and diet. Treating the passive great movement here (metal) is the first choice of treatment. As an additional treatment, calming the overactive great movement at some point may be useful but certainly advice regarding lifestyle change to minimize this over-activity is advisable.

D. LIKE *QI* OF THE HEAVENLY STEM

Like *qi* treatments are also called guest–host treatments, probably because they are similar to the guest–host relationships between the yin and yang couples in five phases theory. Born '*Yi*, Liv in metal', the like *qi* is '*Jia*, Gb in earth' and vice versa.

Like *qi* treatments are mainly used to support, nourish and prevent innate *qi* from becoming unbalanced. They accentuate the form, material side of the energetic model. For instance, every point on the gallbladder channel supports the physical aspect of the innate *qi* of '*Yi*, Liv in metal'. The precise choice of points on the 'like *qi* channel' should preferably support the actions of like *qi* treatment. For example, to treat '*Geng*, L.i. in metal' to support the innate '*Xin*, Lu in water' is more directed when, for example, L.i.-8, *Xia Lian*, is used, because that point in itself strengthens the lung *qi*.

This method of treatment can also be used in diseases of the organs, regardless of innate *qi*. It is less powerful and effective than treatments that utilize the unlike *qi*.

E. GREAT MOVEMENT MOTHER POINT

The great movement mother point is a method that can be added to the like *qi* treatments. It has not been described in the classics, nor taught by my teachers. It has proved useful for me over my years of practice. The method is only used in patients with major weakness or in the elderly when the *jing* decreases. It happens regularly with these patients that their 'own' innate *qi* is weakened.

An example: When the liver *qi* of someone born with '*Yi*, Liv in metal' becomes increasingly weakened due to chronic disease or ageing, the practitioner is tempted to treat the liver *qi* directly. Until now it has always been said that it is inadvisable to treat the innate *qi* directly, but preferable to work indirectly, for example by using like and unlike *qi*. This method semi-directly strengthens the weakened innate *qi*.

An example of a great movement mother point treatment:

Liv-4, *Zhong Fen*, is a stem point. It is the metal point on the liver channel. The mother of metal is earth. Liv-3, *Tai Chong*, the earth point, has been named the 'great movement mother point', because earth nourishes metal. It strengthens the relationship of the dynamic great movement metal and the heavenly stem *Yi*, liver. This treatment is very supportive and tonifying. It is wise to repeat this treatment only after three months because the great movement earth may become exhausted if this great movement mother point is treated too often.

The great movement mother points are:

Table 17.1 The great movement mother points

'*Jia*, Gb in earth'	Gb-38	'*Ji*, Sp in earth'	Sp-2
'*Yi*, Liv in metal'	Liv-3	'*Geng*, L.i. in metal'	L.i.-11
'*Bing*, S.i. in water'	S.i.-1	'*Xin*, Lu in water'	Lu-8
'*Ding*, Ht in wood'	Ht-3[13]	'*Ren*, Bl in wood'	Bl-66
'*Wu*, St in fire'	St-43	'*Gui*, Ki in fire'	Ki-1[14]

---

13 Needle no longer than ten minutes because Ht-3 tonifies the yin of the heart, which can quickly result in coldness of the heart.

14 It is preferred to use the sinew channel point Ki-1 on the kidney sinew channel, that is opposite Bl-67 on the medial side of the nail, because that is where the wood quality executes best.

CHAPTER 18

DYNAMICS OF THE HEAVENLY STEM *JI* 己 [1]

THE CENTRE

What has happened so far? '*Jia*, Gb in earth' established the foundation. The initiating power of the heavenly stem *Jia* created and animated the new life to come. It can be compared to the first breath that opens the lungs for the cosmic *qi* to serve the body in its meeting with the nourishing *qi* of food. Life is not possible without inspiration.

The second combination '*Yi*, Liv in metal' combines wood of the East and metal of the West. It establishes the horizontal field of human existence with earth, the identity, in the centre. The horizontal field is the level of incarnation where people meet. Inner growth takes place in everyone's personal vertical axis of water–fire. The vertical axis symbolizes human development and conscious recognition of what is being learned, as we live between heaven above and earth below.

The third combination '*Bing*, S.i. in water' combines water and fire. The water of the North and fire of the South represent the inner human vertical alignment with the subtle forces of heaven and the more material forces of earth, which attune us to the natural course of events. A healthy balance of these energies allows people to meet others on the horizontal plane with humaneness and righteousness and act in accordance with the forces of the vertical, that is with love and wisdom. The basic principle of underlying humaneness and righteousness is that all people are equal, which is symbolized by the horizontal plane. Activities and movements in this plane are aligned with inner virtues such as uprightness and consistency of awareness.

The power of the inspired identity in the centre expands both horizontally

---

[1] Born in years that end with a 9 such as 1969 and 2009, after the Chinese New Year.

and vertically, whereupon the wheel of life becomes operational. The circumference of the circle with the cross within is set in motion. The wheel of life is put into practice in '*Ding*, Ht in wood'.

In '*Wu*, St in fire' the *qi* flows from the fire of the South back to the centre again. This is the area where the influx from heaven is received, transformed and passed on to the next stage of development, represented by '*Ji*, Sp in earth'. The integrative power of '*Ji*, Sp in earth' in the centre contributes to the processes of individualization and individuation, the awareness of the distinction between the specific and universal self, between the ego and its environment and the process of emancipation and self-realization.

The heavenly stems *Wu* and *Ji*, stomach and spleen, jointly hold the centre from where the entire network of the five *zang* and six *fu* and the entire network of ten great movements and ten heavenly stems emanate. This reminds me of an oft-repeated statement of my teacher: 'The *qi* of heaven is received by the water of the earth, the stomach. The fire of the earth, the spleen, transforms and transports the *qi* further to the realm of human, the kidneys.'

The heavenly stems *Wu* and *Ji* are the central gateway for the influx from heaven that pervades the being with consciousness. With (or better, without) will, people may accept and surrender to what life presents. It is often hard work. My beloved mother compared this process to polishing a crystal. Friction smooths the surface, makes it clear and translucent, but the rough surface cannot become smooth without heat and the detachment of small but important elements. Therefore, it is understandable that during this self-purifying process, we experience emotions. As she said not long before she passed away: 'Studying the self is forgetting the self, forgetting the self is being one, enlightened by all things.' We have to surrender to the polishing process of life before clarity and inner peace can be found.

Self-knowledge starts with a balanced interaction between '*Wu*, St in fire' and '*Ji*, Sp in earth'. Together, they bring stability throughout the organism that is needed for focus on and intent towards the path of self-knowledge. Intense experiences that evoke strong physical-emotional-mental reactions disrupt the balance between *Wu* and *Ji*, potentially making the path to self-development and emancipation bumpier.

Complaints of the vertebral column and related muscles are among the main symptoms that indicate imbalance and tension of these great movements and heavenly stems. Complaints especially in the area of the neck (the transition from heaven to human) show that the person in question is trying to keep too much control over the process of transformation. It could also be that persistent complaints in these areas show that important personal changes are needed first and that too much outside intervention makes this process difficult.

A young woman, born with 'Geng, L.i. in metal', is going through a troubled relationship, her husband cheats on her. She can't think about anything else and is neglecting her children. She sleeps poorly and is exhausted, has stiff, aching muscles in the neck, head and shoulders, with headaches, cold feet and frequent diarrhoea. Blood tests show marginal abnormalities,[2] but too few for the doctor to respond to them. Her first comment upon entering the clinic is 'I am no longer myself, can you please help me to become myself again?'

The main aspects of her pulse diagnosis: Large intestine pulse is tight (Jin Mai) but hidden (Fu Mai), liver pulse is deficient (Xu Mai), stomach pulse is tight (Jin Mai), spleen pulse is not rooted, too soft, stagnant and flooding deficient, also called push pulse,[3] dai mai pulse has signs of stagnation, yin qiao mai pulse is thin and insufficient (Xi Mai).

Without going into the symptoms and underlying syndromes, I would like to highlight the pulses and the related treatment.

Tight but hidden pulse (Jin Mai and Fu Mai) of the large intestine: While we haven't covered the seventh great movement and heavenly stem yet, you probably understand that this may be due to 'Geng, L.i. in metal'; her metal becomes too metallic. A hidden pulse is an indication of severe stagnation. Not uncommonly this pulse is diagnosed as thin and insufficient, Xi Mai. However, by treating the metallic constriction, the pulse recovers in strength and width very quickly.

Any point on the liver channel balances the great movement metal because 'Yi, Liv in metal' is the unlike qi of 'Geng, L.i. in metal'.

Liv-3 ensures free flow of qi, regulates the liver and relieves muscle spasms and, in this case, it also balances the innate great movement metal and regenerates the relationship between the great movement metal and Geng, the large intestine, for which relaxation is extremely beneficial.

The stomach and spleen pulses represent a number of symptoms that are expressed at the blood level. Visible abnormalities in the blood, even very marginal ones, mean that the disease has manifested itself in the physical body, indicating that a disease has or will take root and may develop further in due time. This is a reason to treat the underlying great movement and heavenly stem.

---

2   Such as red blood cell count, thyroid-stimulating hormone, haemoglobin and haematocrit.
3   Feels like excess but does not come up as high as an excess pulse. It means exhaustion and pushing oneself into activity.

The unlike *qi* of the heavenly stems '*Wu*, St in fire' and '*Ji*, Sp in earth' are successively '*Gui*, Ki in fire' and '*Jia*, Gb in earth'. The treatment of the stomach and spleen in this case is undertaken to take care of serious acquired imbalances and not about treating innate *qi*.

Jia: Gb-41 opens *dai mai*, allowing stagnant *qi* in the upper half of the body to descend. Furthermore it is the wood point on the gallbladder channel that generally spreads *qi*.

Gui: Ki-6 on the right with Lu-7 on the left side treat *yin qiao mai*, rooting her in herself.

Gallbladder is unlike *qi* of the spleen, kidney the unlike *qi* of the stomach and the lungs are like *qi* of the large intestine.

The moment the treatment Gb-41, Liv-3, Ki-6 (right) and Lu-7 on the left side[4] started, she closed her eyes, began to cry softly for a few minutes, took a deep breath and said, 'Thank you.'

THE DYNAMICS OF THE NUMBERS FIVE AND SIX

Five is the symbol of change and the breath of life which is received and organized by the number six, the vehicle for life. The number five shows in the five *zang* that produce and store the five fundamental substances.[5] The number six is represented in the six original *qi*[6] and the six *fu* that ingest, propel, digest, absorb nutrients and secrete the impure residues. The merging of the *qi* of the five *zang* and six *fu* is responsible for all life activities.

The yin number six represents the space in which the subtle *qi* organizes the human microcosm in the image of the heavenly macrocosm. Six portrays the movement of heaven within humans and is the 'house of channels' that organizes the yang-life within yin-form and is revealed in the twelve channels and the six divisions.[7]

Life develops at the bridging place between the opposing forces of numbers five and six. For example, in the treatment of infertility, hormonal dysregulation,

---

4 In constitutional acupuncture we generally treat women on the right side and men on the left.
5 *Jing, qi, shen, jin yé* and *xuè*.
6 The archetypes of the six divisions: growing *qi*, expanding *qi*, full grown *qi*, changing *qi*, gathered *qi*, hidden *qi* leading to *jué yin*-wind-wood, *shao yin*-fire-emperor fire, *shao yang*-summer heat-minister fire, *tai yin*-dampness-earth, *yang ming*-dryness-metal, *tai yang*-coldness-water.
7 Six pairs of related *qi*: *tai yang*, Bl-S.i.; *shao yang*, Gb-Sj; *yang ming*, St-L.i.; *tai yin*, Sp-Lu; *jué yin*, Liv-Hc; *shao yin*, Ki-Ht; and six pairs of opposite *qi*: Gb-Ht, Liv-S.i., Lu-Bl, L.i.-Ki, St-Hc, Sp-Sj.

shortened menstrual cycle, low sperm count and low libido (all representing deficient 'life'), it is advisable to first treat 'Wu, St in fire' and 'Ji, Sp in the earth' before other organs such as kidneys or san jiao are treated. Five and six create the framework on which all life can manifest itself in form.

JI 己, THE SIXTH HEAVENLY STEM

The quality of the sixth heavenly stem, Ji, is shown in the yin of the earth: the spleen. It marks the beginning of the yin/second half of the cycle of heavenly stems. 'Ji, Sp in earth' is the fulfilment of the promise of the first expression of life at the time of 'Jia, Gb in earth'. Bloom, prosperity and vitality, that were previously still hidden and hardly expressed, are now evolved to support and vitalize the body, making it a perfect vehicle for qi. Ji carries out the mandate of the emanation qian, Heaven, the life-giving source that produces and supports all life forms to mature.

Ji enables people to master and embody the values of integrity and reliability. These begin with accepting one's own body and being and, by doing so, fulfilling the heavenly mandate that every human being receives.

Ji is naturally expressed at the time of late summer, the break in the seasons between the yang of spring and summer and the yin of autumn and winter. It brings gentle, harmonious and yielding movements that are firm and stable when challenged. These movements can be observed in the soft and stable breathing of the body when it moves without any coercion. Nothing needs to be achieved, nothing but incessant movement. My qigong teacher advised me to be aware of my centre and observe the breathing of the whole body rather than just the lungs. 'That is the true power of the heavenly stem Ji,' he said.

After the mountaintop of the heavenly stem Wu comes a valley. Ji is expressed in plains with panoramic views up to the horizon, so it has views of the whole area. It symbolizes overview and insight into the future. The body can anticipate the coming winter and precautions can be taken to use the abundance of late summer as a source of nourishment for later hibernation.

The Chinese character Ji 己 shows the threads when weaving on a loom. The warp threads are the longitudinal threads, that are barely visible in the woven fabric and can be compared to the vertical connection to heaven. The woof (or weft) threads are the horizontal threads that go over and under the longitudinal threads. These are more visible and represent the temporal realm. The reciprocating movements of warp and woof reflect the cycles of blossom and decline, of life and death. The woven fabric symbolizes the temporary fundamental structure of any organism that is animated by universal qi. Ji is the ground of existence that supports the body and yet knows that it will decline and die.

Ji, spleen, possesses the yang of heaven needed to cultivate the mind and body. It is called the root of post-natal *qi* because it personalizes the yang essence through transformation, transportation and absorption of beneficial nutrients and *qi*. It possesses the yin of the earth that leads the digestive system, houses the *yi*, remembers life events, helps in the production of *qi* and *xuè* and is involved in generating ideas and opinions. *Ji*, spleen, is the portal of life that supports, maintains and animates the temporary form.

Over the years, I have guided patients with pancreatic cancer,[8] many of whom showed great activity of the yang of the spleen, so much that it extinguished the warmth of the heart *qi* via the reverse *sheng*-cycle. It caused cold, leaving the heart unable to nourish the spleen yin, causing the whole body to suffer. Due to the excessive yang of the spleen these patients are active, vital and lose weight. They have poor digestion and diarrhoea due to spleen yin insufficiency. They seem emotionally involved due to the active yang of the spleen, but have difficulty making real emotional connection due to the coldness of the heart *qi*.

The treatment principle to guide these people is to reduce the coldness of the heart, and especially to calm the fire of the spleen. This is incredibly complicated because life for those involved feels dynamic and energetic, inspiring and full of challenges. Calming the fire should be accompanied by supporting spleen yin.

Treatments in these cases are as difficult as a balancing act on a high wire. For instance, some points on the gallbladder channel[9] subdue the spleen *qi* too much and are not eligible – such as Gb-38, *Yang Fu*, yang support – for treating the great movement earth. Notable are Gb-12, *Wan Gu*, that calms the spleen, Gb-21, *Jian Jing*, on the left, which affects spleen yang and might be sedated, and Gb-21 on the right that affects spleen yin and might be tonified. There is a danger that recovery of the warmth of the heart might lead to strong emotions that generate the spleen yang and bring apparent vitality, but in the long term subdue the spleen yin again. Guiding these people can contribute to emotional and spiritual peace, but early diagnosis and preventing the derailment of spleen yang is just as important.

THE GREAT MOVEMENT EARTH AND THE HEAVENLY STEM *JI*

The earth nature of both the great movement and heavenly stem in this combination emphasizes the focus on the centre. As the landing site of and the

---

8 The pancreas is part of the spleen *qi*.
9 Unlike *qi*.

response to the heavenly mandate, '*Ji*, Sp in earth' is in charge of the perception and understanding of the heavenly influx and for the exchange between the individual identity and society.

In doing so, *Ji* influences the balance between moral integrity and inner integrity/being true to oneself. In our modern world, moral integrity is determined by the powers of legislation and regulation, intellect and science. In spiritual development, however, moral integrity ideally becomes a reflection of inner integrity and the nature of the self.

The yin nature of this great movement and heavenly stem contribute to receptivity to inner truths and values. They are the true foundation upon which loyalty, faithfulness, reliability, service and care rest. These energies may teach us not to fight others who seem to display disloyalty, unfaithfulness, untrustworthiness, disservice and neglect, but to feel care and responsibility for everyone, including those who appear to be different. Love awakens love, also and even among the indifferent.

The first two great movements and heavenly stems laid the foundation; the following combinations activated the human alignment to the cosmic field; the sixth combination is the reflection of the supreme being in humans themselves. The nature of '*Jia*, Gb in earth' is to vitalize, to begin, to emerge. Its evolved powers are received in '*Ji*, Sp in earth', by manifesting the initiated life in the material world and realizing ideas.

THE COLLECTIVE FIELD

'*Ji*, Sp in earth' contributes to the ability to transcend differences. It may allow people to transcend the ego and feel part of a collective whole.

For people born with '*Ji*, Sp in earth' the observable collective field is important. This is seen in the teacher who takes care of the school children, the dancer and their audience, the politician and the electorate group and the human being who makes other people happy through their presence. Sensitivity to the signals of the unobservable collective field, the collective energetic field of the family, fellow believers, nationality and so on, can lead these people to both uncertainty and strength. Opening up and recognizing sensitivity to the unobservable collective field can encourage confidence and contributes to health. However, it may also lead to the encountering of collective traumas.

In particular, a strong reliance on intellect and science indicates that these people do not focus as much on these underlying forces, but on the other hand it is important that sensitivity and an opening up to the invisible and the inexplicable must have practical value and serve observable reality.

When the great movement earth and spleen dominate, people may become inert, heavy in nature, obsessive in their thinking and emotionally immobilized. They may feel unsafe and, through fear of losing themselves, go along with the opinions and views of others, but appearances can deceive. Beneath the vulnerability lies a great perseverance and a strong presence. It may take a while for that to move, but once it gathers momentum, it keeps moving until the goal is reached.

RAISON D'ÊTRE

In general, people born with equal energetic combinations such as this are challenged to choose between their desires for peace and excitement. Both are necessary for them to find life meaning. However, the equality of the earth easily leads to stagnation, causing boredom. Relaxing into boredom can be very useful. Deeply hidden in boredom lie the vitality and power of the *qi* of water that can contribute to self-knowledge and inner growth, but above all to authenticity.

> One thing that comes out in myths is that at the bottom of the abyss comes the voice of salvation. The black moment is the moment when the real message of transformation is going to come. At the darkest moment comes the light.[10]

The great movement earth and the heavenly stem *Ji* nearly always participate in existential issues, ranging from identity crises to financial problems, from existential questions about human suffering and death to the meaning of life in general. The first appearing physical symptoms can be mild: heartburn, mild shortness of breath, headache, nervousness, eczema or a tendency to faint. These, however, can develop into severe depression if they are not noticed and treated in time. Fighting for the right to exist at times seems to be the only solution, but so also does inner peace and boredom; both ways cannot prevent the fear of apparent loss of ego.

ACUPUNCTURE POINTS THAT INFLUENCE THE PASSIVE GREAT MOVEMENT EARTH AND THE HEAVENLY STEM *JI*

Cv-17 especially and the other points discussed in Chapter 12 in the section 'Heaven meets earth meets human' are applicable.

---

10   Campbell and Moyers 2011.

Cv-17, *Dan Zhong*, chest centre. After being circulated externally, the *ying qi* returns to the interior of the body and descends along the route of the *san jiao* through Cv-17. When Cv-17 is obstructed, the periphery of the body becomes empty, resulting in tiredness, little movement and pain in the chest. The heart-*shen* becomes dull and *qi* does not circulate. The stagnation may develop into serious problems with grief, sadness, anxiety, fatigue and depression with inability to move. In addition the stagnated *ying qi* attacks the *qi* of the stomach with associated symptoms. Chapter 39 of the *Huang Di Nei Jing Su Wen* discusses the pattern in which obstruction occurs as a result of excessive anxiety or pensiveness. Moxa treatment on Cv-17 is advised.

Sp-3, *Tai Bai*, supreme white. *Tai Bai* is the name of the planet Venus, the white evening star of the West, or the white morning star of the East. In the West Venus refers to conditions of decay and internalization, Venus in the East represents the beginning of life and external prosperity. Sp-3 keeps the balance between these two expressions by holding the centre.

Sp-3 strengthens the centre, the spine and spinal muscles and tonifies all joints and bones. It promotes transformation and provides rooting of the self through solidity and security. It regulates the rhythm of the heart and vitalizes the brain. It is used for memory processing problems.

Sp-3 safeguards the body by increasing the amount of white blood cells and by organizing the field of the spleen and the pancreas.

St-42, *Chong Yang*, rushing yang. This may be the best *yuan source* point to restore insufficiency of stomach and spleen, especially when it has led to chronic restlessness of the mind and body. Perpendicular treatment harmonizes the stomach and nourishes the spleen. Oblique needling, with the flow of *qi* in the direction of Sp-1, while gently turning the needle clockwise, moves the *qi* to the spleen and clears stomach heat.

Sp-21, *Da Bao*, great wrapping, great *luo* point of the spleen. Although Sp-21 is mentioned in treating the great movement metal, it is a great acupuncture point for '*Ji*, Sp in earth', especially when the *shenming* is weak.

Sp-21 is used in cases of insufficiency with flaccidity and pain of all joints. It makes people feel enveloped in warmth, calmness and strength.[11]

---

11 See Chapter 12 about Gb-34 for external issues.

THE CONSEQUENCES OF '*JI*, SPLEEN IN EARTH' IN THE *WUXING*

The passive great movement earth results in an active great movement wood that influences all *qi* of wood such as gallbladder, liver, large intestine, lung[12] and all other expressions of wood such as agility of *wei qi* and purposeful behaviour. For people born with '*Ji*, Sp in earth' it is important to relax by moving and to have a clear purpose in life. This natural emphasis on the wood seems beneficial, because the gallbladder is unlike *qi*, but it may lead to unexpected problems.

Looking at all passive great movements we see the following:

'*Yi*, Liv in metal' leads to active great movement '*Wu*, St in fire' and can influence the strength of the unlike *qi* '*Geng*, L.i in metal'.

'*Ding*, Ht in wood' leads to active great movement '*Geng*, L.i. in metal' and can influence the strength of the unlike *qi* '*Ren*, Bl in wood'.

'*Ji*, Sp in earth' leads to active great movement '*Ren*, Bl in wood' and can influence the strength of the unlike *qi* '*Jia*, Gb in earth'.

'*Xin*, Lu in water' leads to active great movement '*Jia*, Gb in earth' and can influence the strength of the unlike *qi* '*Bing*, S.i in water'.

'*Gui*, Ki in fire' leads to active great movement '*Bing*, S.i. in water' and can influence the strength of the unlike *qi* '*Wu*, St in fire'.

With '*Ji*, Sp in earth' the active great movement and unlike *qi* both belong to the wood phase. But the action of '*Ren*, Bl in wood' works out very differently from the action of '*Jia*, Gb in earth'. As we will see in Chapter 21, '*Ren*, Bl in wood' carries the burden of life instead of the inspiring, innovative *qi* of '*Jia*, Gb in earth' that generates ambitions. This does not necessarily have to be negative. Burdens can be incentives for a courageous life and enhanced self-knowledge, but the pressures of existence can be overwhelming and people can feel fearful, rejected and devastated.

The healthy pulse of the gallbladder should be slightly superficial, a little short and slightly elastic. If the great movement wood is too dominant, the gallbladder pulse will be affected too. It may become too active, fiery and superficial, but often the opposite happens: The pulse becomes too constricted, loses flexibility and becomes insufficient in response to the overdominance of wood.

As a result of the subdued spleen *qi* by significant activity of the great movement wood, symptoms of spleen *qi* insufficiency occur: digestive problems, fatigue, pale complexion, easily full after a meal, weakness in muscles and so on.

---

12 See chapters on earthly branches.

Depending on the pulse diagnosis, the severity and duration of this imbalance, the following treatments are possible:

At an early stage, balancing the wood is sufficient. Over the years I have found that the combination of the two *luo* points, Gb-37, *Guang Ming*, and Liv-5, *Li Gou*, balances the wood and calms the stress of the emotions.

When '*Ren*, Bl in wood' is too dominant or has persisted for an extended period of time, it causes hypoglycaemia, restlessness and nervousness, shortness of breath, oedema in the feet and existential problems.

Not only is the spleen subdued but, more remarkably, the increased activity of '*Ren*, Bl in wood' subdues its own unlike *qi*: '*Ding*, Ht in wood'. Life is experienced as complicated, difficult and uninspiring. To calm the overactivity of '*Ren*, Bl in wood' '*Ding*, Ht in wood' may be used – of course depending on the pulse diagnosis: Ht-9, *Shao Chong*, or Ht-6, *Yin Xi*, or Ht-3, *Shao Hai*. Especially when people feel too vulnerable, Hc-7, *Da Ling*, the *yuan source* point of the heart channel,[13] is beneficial.

Serious complaints of hypoglycaemia associated with existential issues – due to the insufficient '*Ji*, Sp in earth' – require nuanced guidance that usually starts with calming the great movement wood by using Cv-14, *Ju Que*, and/or Cv-15, *Jiu Wei*, and possibly sedation of Bl-65, *Shu Gu*.

TRINITY *DING-WU-JI*

The heavenly stems *Ding-Wu-Ji* give shape to the creative impulses of the first trinity *Jia-Yi-Bing*. *Ding* shows in intuition and supports intentions that energize life to become mature. *Wu* provides inspiration and intelligence that nourishes the powers that are bound to the form. *Ji* stands for integrity and intellect that radiates as reliability. These characteristics are respectively empowered and guided by love and compassion, creativity and the capacity for individuation. This trinity generates harmony in the growth and freedom of the spirit and centralization of the self.

Disturbances between *Ding* and *Wu* usually go hand in hand with problems between the heart-*shen* and *yi*, where intentions in particular are influenced more by the opinions of others rather than being carried by what people themselves have in their hearts. In other words, when the heart is overpowered by thought, when intellect and cognition prevail over intuition and intelligence,

---

13   In Chapter 1 of the *Ling Shu* the importance of Hc-7 is emphasized as the *yuan source* point of the heart channel.

the reverse *sheng* movement may quench the warmth of the heart. This misalignment impedes the development towards individuation. Physically it may result in digestive problems based on a disarranged production of *qi* and *xuè* or chronic fatigue syndrome. These kinds of complaints that at first glance seem to be caused by impaired spleen *qi* should first be treated by restoring the nourishing *sheng*-cycle between '*Ding*, Ht in wood' and '*Wu*, St in fire'.

What is special about this illness is that the severity of the illness and the fatigue, pain and changed expectations for the future it brings may give people the necessary space to make such an inner turn so that the voice of the heart can be followed, allowing *Ding* to nourish *Wu*. It cannot be forced and is never an excuse, but suddenly there can be emancipation and individuation and loyalty to the self. This process can be very intense and is not simply over and done with. Treating the great movements and the associated heavenly stems and organs offers people a gentle method and opportunity to open this door to the heart. When this path is confirmed and recognized, healing has begun.

CHAPTER 19

DYNAMICS OF THE HEAVENLY STEM *GENG* 庚[1]

The more understanding of the heavenly stems I gained, the more questions arose. How can we view the upcoming sequence of heavenly stems after *qi* has returned to the centre with the heavenly stem *Ji*? The impulse of life has now returned to the source, hasn't it? What is the significance of four more combinations of great movements and heavenly stems for the development of nature and development of humans and humanity? These are questions that have puzzled me for years.

They were answered as expected by my teacher: 'Study the questions carefully first. The answer is hidden in the question.' Well, it wasn't until much later that I got confirmation and the comment: 'Keep up the good work.'

The first trinity is creative. *Qi* evolves from the stage of being into becoming. The second trinity transforms the life of becoming into that of interactive psycho-social beings. These two developmental phases of trinities may be understood as heaven creating earth and earth receiving heaven. It is time for humans and humanity to develop further through internalization and interest in the inner way of heaven. It is this way that transcends thoughts and the self, to return to 'being' again. The essence of the true self has no other purpose than being. This is the eternal condition of heaven. The focus is attuned to what IS, connected, peaceful and intuitive.

The phase of introversion begins with '*Geng*, L.i. in metal'. It is the start of a new trinity: the heavenly stems *Geng, Xin, Ren* make humans humane. Unfortunately, everyday experience only seems to show the external protective side of metal, namely the tough, defensive and confrontational. It manifests itself in rigidity and the use of power through money and intimidation, violence and

---

1   Born in years ending with a 0 such as 1960, 2000, after the Chinese New Year.

the use of weapons. Relentless instinctual forces are usually in the foreground: Powers of victory and coercion that often lead to death and destruction usually win over inner values like compassion and righteousness.

What do Chinese medicine and philosophy have to offer here? Can the horrific reality created by humanity up until now itself be changed?

The third trinity starts in the West, the direction of metal and autumn that represent decline and decay. The forces of the West are also represented by the seven *po*, which are usually seen as annoying entities with no other purpose than to make life difficult.[2] The *po* are said to 'go out and come in, in association with the essences'. To follow the essences means that they appear at conception and birth and disappear with death. The seven *po* are animal instincts that guide and protect people during life through reflex impulses, driven by unconscious feelings and sensations.

The Chinese characters for *po* 魄 and *hun* 魂 contain the character *gui* 鬼. The name *gui*, ghost, calls for caution – people are afraid of ghosts – but they are an expression of the same original energetic source as everything else. Ghosts seem to have personal powers, especially those who fear them. Yet the seven *po* are indispensable for pleasure, pain sensations, awareness, self-development, communication, physical strength and flexibility, sexuality, expression of emotions and purification. The 'human' faces of the *po* and *gui* that cause pain and suffering are in my opinion the compelling forces of the ego to which the seven *po* are sensitive. The demands of traumas, desires and fear force the ego and make the *po* hard and inflexible, relentless and almost uncontrollable.

When people are emotionally distressed or depressed, the seven *po* are usually described as if they have a life of their own that affects people negatively. They seem not to care about human life at all. The power of the ego is usually not perceived as playing a role in this, but it is precisely the ego that determines the direction of the *po* and the power of metal as a compelling source that seeks a goal.

However, despite the fact that the seven *po* are animal instinctive powers, they can be transformed from demanding to supportive capabilities that elevate humans above animal instincts. Processing trauma and transforming fears is not possible without the intervention of the seven *po*. Along with the great movement metal they are at service to humans and humanity.

Physicality, clarity, surrender and acceptance support the essence of the being rather than the desires of the ego. Desires to satisfy the ego's own goals can awaken the seven *po*, making them the annoying entities that make life difficult.

---

2   The seven *po* represent the seven emotions of joy, anger, worry, pensiveness, grief, fright and fear that occupy people and the seven openings in the head through which sensory information can enter and agitate.

The **earth** stagnates when the *po* influence it too much. This causes obsession, regret, worry and feelings of insecurity about identity and fear of doom scenarios. The pulses become taut and tense, sometimes hidden. A deep, forceful and tight pulse is an indication of pain due to stagnation.

The *po* lead the *qi* of earth. They are the earthly souls that correspond to autonomic systems that sustain life and are stimulated by touch. This is one of the reasons why it is so difficult to live without being touched. Cuddling, a hand on the shoulder, massage, sex, belong to the life-supporting qualities of the *po* that relate to earth.

The quality of the earth–*po* connection manifests in the strength of the muscles and the nature of a person's physical impression: the strength of hand-shaking, an open or closed posture, the strength of eye contact, and so on. In addition the *po* assist the earth to purify and cleanse the body and strengthen the concentration, making consciousness active. Targeted focus depends on the strength of the metal and the *po*.

The **metal** that is upset by the *po* gives rise to grief, sadness and shame. The *qi* stagnates at the level of the diaphragm and the pulses become taut. A tight pulse means that people are threatened for their safety.

The *po* regulate breath and the awareness of smells that in turn affect the five aspects of the *shen*: the scent of burning affects the fire, aromatic scents affect the earth, a fishy smell affects the metal, a rotten smell affects the water and the smell of sweat affects the wood. In addition, smells can generally arouse greed that reduces the power of the *jing*.

Unlike the heart-*shen* that can travel where it desires and infuses the whole body, the *po* are limited to the space of the lungs. The breath, the rhythm of the *po* that directs all *qi*, animates the whole body. It makes the *po* indispensable for the functioning of the body and the *shen*.

The metal–*po* connection transmits information into the level of the *jing*. Introspection that supports awareness and focus (earth) is possible due to the interconnection between the *po*, skin, lungs and kidneys. These properties are indispensable for the process of self-cultivation.

The **water** that is disturbed by the *po* gives rise to fear, insecurity and loneliness. The *qi* sinks to the lower burner where it often encounters stagnated *qi* caused by feelings of guilt. The pulses feel sunken and become jumpy with fright.

The water/*jing*–*po* connection determines a person's physiological and physical resilience. The *po*, in addition to the extra channels, are the vehicles through which the *jing* communicates with the body. White structures such as bones and teeth express the close relationship between the *jing*-essence and the seven *po*.

During the first months, even possibly the first years of life, babies are mainly *jing-po*. This combination allows babies to grow and develop. The body is adequately maintained and fed; enough waste is removed so that assimilation processes can function properly. This process continues throughout life, but in the early years of life it is the most important source of good physical development. As people grow up the same characteristics apply, but more focused on emotional, mental and spiritual development. Nourishing the useful and releasing the unnecessary are important qualities that support the resilience of the soul. A weak connection between water/*jing* and *po* causes weakness and reduced mobility on all possible levels of development. Physical weakness makes people fall more frequently, emotional weakness makes people become more nervous, mental weakness makes people more insecure, spiritual weakness makes people more fearful.

Physicality[3] is the basis for the development of the more subtle realms of feeling, thinking and spirit-mind. The development of those areas becomes discernible as they reveal themselves by moving the physical. Touching the physical body, in whatever state, supports growth on any of these levels. The water/*jing–po* connection keeps people alert and is the basis of physical awareness. Physicality and the accompanying capacity to feel are the foundation of health and cure on all levels. Consciousness and inner orientation connect the earth with *qi*. This supports health through nutrition, safety and love through water/*jing* and *po*.

The **wood** that is adversely affected by the *po* gives rise to irritability, frustration, resentment and anger. The pulses become agitated. A leather pulse (*Ge Mai*) indicates that agitation is (partly) caused by lack of fluids, *xuè*, yin or *jing*. This is often due to too much dryness emerging from firm metal resulting in judgemental and disdainful behaviour. The three *hun* are no longer nourished by virtues, meaning that the *hun* can no longer follow the *shen* – 'What follows the *shen* in its coming and going is the *hun*'. As a result of the overwhelming dryness of metal *qi*, the *qi* of the body can no longer be a proper vehicle for the *shen*. This causes the *hun* to travel downward, making the *qi* slower. The focus of awareness is more directed on matter and the physical world. As the strength of the *hun* diminishes, people become apathetic, anxious and find it difficult to make decisions. The five senses become harsher and more rough, less flexible and resist change. This makes people light-sensitive during the day and restless at night because of a more active dream consciousness.[4] As the *hun* affect the *shen*, it is no longer possible to properly coordinate perception and

---

3   Physicality refers to the physically perceivable world, not the perfection of the body.
4   The *hun* houses in the eyes during the day and in the liver at night.

intuition, cognition and intelligence, differentiation and integration, leaving people confused and isolated.

The *hun* cannot function without the seven *po*. Human development, sexual relationships, social communication and the relationship with the more subtle realms of the spirit are based on physical experiences and memories that are stored in the water/*jing–po* connection. Sensual passions, conquering the heart of a loved one, conditional love, biological drives, sexuality, lust and desire, and assertiveness are all expressions of a healthy wood-*po*.

The *hun* and *po* together create the world of experiences and perceptions, which ultimately serves to nourish the *shen* so that the self can find its place in harmony with the virtues of heaven. Finding this place is about the balance between seeming opposites: fixed structures/habits and freedom of the spirit, introspection and creativity, letting go and all-embracing, exclusivity and inclusivity. The balance is healthy as long as the *shen* interacts with integration rather than stagnation and chaos. In the latter cases, treatment should start with healing the *hun–po* balance.

The **fire** confused by the *po* gives rise to nervousness, tension and restlessness, possibly trauma. The pulses become scattered, larger and faster.

The seven *po* control the seven openings of the head that process sensory information received by the heart. Fire–*po* imbalance can lead to sensory problems such as skin hypersensitivity, reduced skin perception with paraesthesia, pain and itching along with hypersensitivity to light, sound, smells and taste. Mental problems such as depression and even psychoses can arise when the *po* overwhelm fire. Due to the restriction of metal, the fire struggles to break out to inspire the channels, leaving the *shen* empty.

The fire and the *shen* both need the physicality of the *po* and the *jing*, because the fire can only express itself when it is bound to the physical.

The **yin** affected by the *po* causes an emotion that is difficult to control: jealousy. The more you want to resolve it, the worse it seems to get. In this situation the pulse of the lung is deep, yielding and insufficient, making the wood overactive and agitated. In the depths of jealousy lies an incredible source of creativity and vitality. Jealousy should not be combated, but rather deeply felt and explored, despite existing fears and despairs. Then forgiveness might open a source of seemingly unlimited energy.

At night, at yin times, the *yin-po* really comes into its own. The *qi* returns to the inside, cleanses and purifies the being on all levels. Sleep is essential for that.

The **yang** affected by the *po* causes restless sleep and nightmares. The pulse of the heart is deep, yielding and insufficient. People feel victimized, have mood swings and may even have delusions. This *po* directs sexual energy, not just sexual arousal, but a ubiquitous life energy that penetrates the body and vitalizes interaction.

GENG 庚, THE SEVENTH HEAVENLY STEM

The quality of the heavenly stem *Geng* is shown in the yang of metal, the large intestine. *Geng*, large intestine, belongs to the West and autumn.

As the days get shorter the amount of sunlight decreases; there are autumn storms that alternate with calm sunny autumn days. It is a time for long walks to enjoy beautiful bright colours in the forest, hot chocolate and a cosy fireplace. As it gets colder outside, nature withers faster and life returns to its source; the flow of fluids decreases in trees and plants. The leaf green retracts into the trunk and a cork layer forms at the base of the leaf, preventing nutrients and green dyes from reaching the leaf. The plants and trees organize protection against cold and central dehydration. The dried leaves fall to the moist soil and the tree directs its forces inward.

Geng refers to gathering and harvesting, depicted as two hands that move a basket to thresh rice. It is the time of the emanation *li*, the beneficial power and the white tiger heaven. The power to protect and gather the fluids in a healthy way presupposes a clear sharp mind and the power of instinctive abilities. By the actions of the heavenly stem *Geng*, the large intestine, which is represented by weapons such as swords and axes, the inauspicious is rejected, attacked and excreted, and the auspicious is accepted and integrated. There are no half measures for survival. Metal swords or axes are unshakeable deadly powers that can be used to separate good from bad. They are used to protect and preserve life, property and belongings.

The human fight mechanism is intended to defend itself against dangerous forces such as pathogenic attackers, whether internal or external, or circumstances of insufficient nutrition. The necessary must be preserved and protected, the unnecessary can be released and eliminated. The process is similar to the leaves of the tree that fall to the ground. The flow of fluids recedes into the roots, the unnecessary is given up and eliminated.

The large intestine is mainly seen as the organ that keeps the body healthy through excretion, but reaping the benefits is just as important.[5]

In an emotional, spiritual sense, weapons are the ability to let go. Letting go of something that is no longer really necessary is often difficult because it

---

5   There is recent scientific evidence about the large intestine's central role in immunity and brain function.

continues to attract attention. Strength and clarity are needed to turn away from something that demands attention. Yet the necessity of turning away may give the feeling of being punished. Letting go of the ego's desires is not easy, especially since it should not be done half-heartedly, but irrefutably. It requires a clear and honest view of one's situation, with good self-judgement. A blurred image of one's own psyche can easily lead to delusions and overestimation as well as depression, melancholy and hatred for oneself or others.

An unhealthily functioning heavenly stem *Geng*, large intestine, pollutes and disturbs the clarity of the body, soul and spirit.

GENG: SELF-KNOWLEDGE

In the depth of our being resides a life-giving source. You may call it pre-natal *jing*, *yuan-shen*, or the Universal Spark. Essentially, the life-giving source doesn't actually have a location or name. The primal source and understanding of it does not derive from rational thinking and what the ego knows. The ego operates independently of this source in its search for feelings, sensations, thoughts, consciousness, growth and development. Due to past traumas that cause inse-curity, denial, sadness and other intense emotions, the internal trajectory to the essence and its connection with the primordial source seems dangerous, paved with fear and pitfalls. Usually, we prefer projection of our inner emotional storms. The outside world seems more familiar, more fun and more controllable and we often seek the source of life in the outside world with its overwhelming number of impressions and forms.

The question arises whether we have forgotten the essence in the inner world or deny it – consciously or unconsciously. We are often increasingly anchored in the world of shapes and desires (which we seem to understand better), in which we feel more at home and definitely seem to enjoy more. How-ever, our alienation from the essential experiences of the inner world results in conflicts of power and hardens the human external behaviour that is desperate for satisfaction. It is precisely through the connection with the life-giving source that the integration of health and disease contributes to the development of individual and collective existence.

Geng, large intestine, is perhaps the most powerful energy that serves us to consciously deal with traumas. I am not saying anything about the speed of this process, only that the process of self-knowledge can make use of *Geng*, large intestine. In the *Geng*-process of anthropogenesis, people can find the right balance between outward behaviour, along with protection, and the inner path of self-knowledge.

This is the drama of the heavenly stem *Geng*, large intestine: Potentially *Geng* is the bright and clear energy that opens and illuminates the path to the core of the being. The ego, however, uses the qualities of *Geng* to strengthen the desire for life through hardening and enforced authority.

Yet there is hope. Years ago a change began that is becoming more and more common. Yoga, meditation, awareness exercises and the like are gaining ground and fortunately there are more and more people and groups who care about the importance of life, in themselves, but also the importance of the living earth and the communities in which they feel involved.

GENG: ANGER AND SELF-CULTIVATION

Geng can explore and resolve inner personal conflicts. However, the endangered ego prefers to defend itself and tends to wage war. While understandable, anger is often used inappropriately to fight and protect rather than explore the underlying feelings of disappointment, defeat, frustration and so on.

Geng, large intestine, is about making the world a better place. But it is a misunderstanding that fighting for a better life can be enforced on others. *Geng*'s weapons and combats do not target others, they are metaphors for an inner process of self-development. The sharp weapons are used to distinguish and separate the non-beneficial and the beneficial. The brightness of the metal sword and axe is the mirror in which one may see the self. As a result of this process, a source of truth and love for life can unfold that contributes to the health of the self and the communities to which the individual belongs.

I elaborate on this subject because humanity has been at this crossroads for many years. People suffer from the inner struggle that accompanies discomforts of the *qi* of the large intestine. Introspection and a clear self might actually be the most useful contribution to the healing process of society in general.

Large intestine problems and diseases, including those in children, are existential. Consciously or unconsciously, large intestine issues are almost always related to underlying questions of being. What does this life mean to me? What am I doing here in this world? What is the meaning of my difficult childhood? Where do my tensions come from and how can I function with this handicap? How do I face and digest these problems?

Introspection, which so often comes with storms of emotion, is challenging. There is often fear, fighting or avoidance. Yet, for healing to occur, there is an inevitable task of taking time to process underlying trauma. I strongly believe that healing personal trauma contributes to the healing of existential issues for humanity as a whole.

THE GREAT MOVEMENT METAL AND THE HEAVENLY STEM *GENG*

After the centralizing *qi* with '*Ji*, Sp in earth' we again see equal qualities in the great movement and heavenly stem, this time concentrated in metal. People born with '*Geng*, L.i. in metal' adhere to fixed habits, structures and patterns and tend towards introspection and inner development. They fight for justice and they often take responsibility or claim it. They can work hard and with great concentration and focus and, not infrequently, they face questions of guilt.

Domination of the great movement metal causes physical stiffness and rigidity along with headstrong behaviour. Too hard, tight skin, muscle cramps, reduced mobility with complaints such as back and neck pain, high blood pressure, agitated, suppressed emotions, abuse of authority and all kinds of other complaints are due to reduced flexibility, which in turn is caused by a decrease in the amount of fluids. The normal decrease in the amount of fluids as people age can be amplified by *Geng*. People born with '*Geng*, L.i. in metal' should therefore pay much more attention to flexibility as they age than others. This applies to both the physical and the mental-emotional body. The keys to this are self-development and a good soothing, moisturizing diet.

In general, sour food supports the process of contraction in autumn. Excessive use of sour causes the connective tissue to contract, making it stiff, tough and inflexible. It makes the lips dry. Therefore, normal use of sour food can be beneficial in autumn, especially when summer was very hot – which usually means that the pores were open with a lot of sweating, and the activity was mainly directed outward. For people born with '*Geng*, L.i. in metal' sour is inadvisable; it is more beneficial to have a slightly pungent diet that lubricates the body, unless there is outward-directed anger and/or defensive behaviour; in that case, slightly sour food can be advised. The astringent quality of sour flavours contracts the externally directed behaviour.

ACUPUNCTURE POINTS THAT INFLUENCE THE ACTIVE GREAT MOVEMENT METAL AND THE HEAVENLY STEM *GENG*

L.i.-1, *Shang Yang*, merchant yang or metal yang, is discussed in more detail along with Lu-11, *Shao Shang*, lesser merchant/metal, in Chapter 27.

L.i.-1 is a stem point well known for treating heat, pain and stagnation such as sore throat, toothache, deafness, vertigo, tinnitus, eye inflammation. It pulls *qi* down from the head very quickly.

I like to use L.i.-1 when the majority of the seven openings in the head are attacked by pathogenic *qi, po* or *gui* and when the senses are hypersensitive to light, sound, smells and tastes. In these cases, it can be tonified or sedated depending on the pulse diagnosis.

Tonification is indicated in cases of a weak pulse with signs and symptoms of weak *wei qi*; sedation is used in cases of a tight pulse that goes along with signs and symptoms of dryness such as constipation, pain and emotional stagnation.

During supervision I have often seen the large intestine pulse diagnosed as weak, insufficient and thin when the pulse was actually very thin and tight: so tight that it was no longer noticed. A thin pulse can be pushed away; a constricted pulse, even if it appears as very narrow, keeps its intrinsic strength. In this case the stem point can be sedated. The relaxing effect is immediate, provided that not too many other acupuncture points are used at the same time.

The other acupuncture points influencing the great movement metal (St-25, *Tian Shu*, Sp-15, *Da Heng*, and Sp-21, *Da Bao*) have already been discussed in Chapter 13.

THE CONSEQUENCES OF '*GENG,* LARGE INTESTINE IN METAL' IN THE *WUXING*

'*Geng,* L.i. in metal' tends to constriction. Together with the tendency for insufficiency of the unlike *qi* '*Yi*, Liv in metal', this easily leads to constriction and a lack of flexibility and adaptability.

Introspection – the inward movement and interaction with the self – of the great movement metal goes together with the desire for movement and exchange with others of the passive great movement wood and '*Yi*, Liv in metal'. The quality of these is determined by the degree of integrity, commitment and general understanding of the transience of life. This in turn is influenced by the stability and trust that is based on the health of the great movement earth. This is a trust that comes from stability and harmony of the heavenly stem *Ji* through its direct connection with heaven.

Integrity is often defined as being honest and trustworthy or as a concern for generally accepted social and ethical norms. However, there is a different kind of integrity, based on understanding and acceptance of the transience of life. A person who consciously integrates the idea of death confirms as a consequence the essential values such as trust, harmony, involvement, intimacy, integrity, friendship, love, the beauty of nature and value of music and so on.

Fear of death makes people want to hold tight to fixed social patterns or seek confirmation by breaking agreed rules and living as though there were no consequences. Seriously ill people, confronted with the finiteness of existence, face the task of overcoming this fear and, if achieved, they can then be more aware of essential values. When we are healthy, we tend to look away from death. And yet the realization of death causes the essence of life to be felt and given meaning. Inner integrity is free from outside norms and values, yet acknowledges the inner essential similarities with those outer norms and values. Life experience, attunement with an inner sense of justice, an inner balanced trust of the great movement earth and an awareness of the insurmountable finiteness of life preserve the inner norms and values. The compass for inner integrity arises from within.

The acceptance of the transience of existence relates to the great movement water. A well-functioning great movement metal is determined by the collaboration between the three great movements earth, metal and water. Problems with interaction and integrity should first be addressed by restoring stability of the great movement earth and then, if possible, interaction and inner integrity of the great movements metal and water.

Flexible integrity of the great movement metal is an important keynote that supports healing and builds fundamental trust. Attention to the significance of the role of integrity in private and work life is extremely important for healthy interactions with others. Therefore, it is important that practitioners conduct peer review and supervision and examine their own psyche. Flexible integrity is an inner principle that is constantly trying to align with improvement and development. When social norms become too dominant or there is fear of facing something, integrity becomes overly challenged and therefore rigid: 'Geng, L.i. in metal' evokes constriction.

Maintaining healthy flexibility and adaptability in the broadest sense of the word is the main challenge for people born with 'Geng, L.i. in metal'. Stiffness quickly reduces the functions of the senses and the natural motility of body and mind.

In children, however, this lack of flexibility and adaptability is particularly physically noticeable. As people grow up and the more subtle bodies develop, maintaining subtler forms of flexibility will also be a prerequisite for maintaining health.

CHAPTER 20

DYNAMICS OF THE HEAVENLY STEM *XIN* 辛[1]

There is a silence of the tongue,
there is a silence of the whole body,
there is the silence of the soul,
there is the silence of the mind,
and there is the silence of the spirit.

John of Apamea[2]

4 May 1955 was the first time that I had consciously listened to silence. I was a little boy. My parents turned on the radio to listen to two minutes of silence in Dam Square in Amsterdam in memory of the fallen during the Second World War. They told me that everyone in the Netherlands would be quiet for two minutes at eight in the evening. Dam Square is normally a very busy and noisy square. I looked into my parents' sad eyes and heard the eight church bells, which I counted unnoticed. Occasionally there was a buzz, but after the sound of the eighth bell it got really quiet. All I heard was the sound of the pigeons.

For years, silence equated to the sound of cooing pigeons, until I headed to a small island in Norway called the Land of God. My friend told me I was going to hear something incredible. We navigated on a small motor boat across a calm sea to the sea side of an island close to the coast. As we went around the island, I saw a small bay at the base of a fairly large mountain. The boat slowly entered the narrow entrance and we went ashore. Suddenly there was a deafening silence, there was no sound. The entrance to the bay and the mountain blocked the wind and sounds of the sea. I remember being shocked at first. I was so aware

---

1 Born in years ending with a 1, such as 1961, 2001, after the Chinese New Year.
2 A fifth-century Syriac writer.

of all the noises in my head. Thoughts and feelings overwhelmed me. I stood dead quiet, frozen to the ground, and looked and felt and listened in the eyes of nothing. I don't know how long it took, but suddenly I noticed that there was also a void in me. Actually, I can't say I noticed, instead I was emptiness. We looked at each other and tears streamed from our eyes. Suddenly we heard the loud bleating of a sheep. We burst out laughing. There was no sheep to be seen at all. My friend said it was probably somewhere in the mountains. I felt happiness like I had never felt before.

This experience of inner emptiness, awe and silence has been with me all my life. It is the presence of something that is nothing, but means everything.

The *Dao De Jing* in Chapter 45 states 'peace and quiet govern the world'.

This text reminds me of my acceptance of the ever-present silence that I believe everyone has, the place where there is no longer a desire for distraction or a goal that must be achieved. There is no need for control. I recognize and accept this innate inner silence as my foundation, but I know that I still have a long way to go to consciously and fully integrate it into my existence.

XIN 辛, THE EIGHTH HEAVENLY STEM

The quality of the heavenly stem *Xin* is shown in the yin of metal, the lung.

The heavenly stems *Geng* and *Xin* are manifestations of the emanation *li*, the beneficial force and the white tiger heaven. Like *Geng*, *Xin* distinguishes between the useful and useless, generates health, strengthens the interior and protects against external pathogenic factors.

The lungs are seen as the father of breath/*qi*. They control the rise and fall of *qi*, inhalation, exhalation and regulate the circulation and metabolism of fluids. In the lungs, the beneficial cosmic *qi* meets the nourishing *qi* of food from which the flow of *qi* in the channels is dynamized, including *wei qi* stored in the liver, lung and skin. In addition to the lung, the great movement water strengthens the body's resistance and supports the production and transformation of *wei qi*. The lungs excrete unbeneficial substances through exhalation, perspiration and urine through the movement of fluids in the body.

The Chinese character *Xin* depicts serious, arduous attacks and relates to times of difficulty, hardship and suffering. In ancient times it stood for punishment and death penalties. It looks violent and it is. With targeted defensive actions, *Xin*, lung, protects the essence from any disturbance of the natural order.[3] A good example of protecting and strengthening the inner is Lu-4, *Xia Bai*, guarding white. It protects the lung, strengthens *wei qi*, descends lung *qi*, relaxes the upper burner, allowing for an adequate and responsive flow of *qi*.

Xin is associated with behaviour or activity that is punishable by law. Enforcement of order through laws was originally designed to maintain peace and integration of the state and the people. Order was and is intended to protect lives and property. Any form of disintegration in the body such as stagnation, counter-current flow of *qi*, chaos, emotional disruption, mental confusion and so on excites *Xin*'s defensive and inner order-promoting qualities and activates the lung.

In nature, *Xin* protects the crop and synchronizes each *qi* with the natural order. It operates through withdrawal and silence. The goal is to protect the harvest by leaving it undisturbed until the growing season starts again.

Xin is associated with a kettle or cooking pan. During cooking, flavours and food compositions change significantly. This reference indicates that '*Xin*, Lu in water' is not only involved in physical protection, strength and order. *Xin* and the authentic, dynamizing great movement water generate inner transformational and alchemical processes that eventually illumine the *shen*. They contribute to the purification and fine-tuning of the body and mind through the transformation of *jing qi* into *qi* into *shen*.[4]

Participation in *tai chi*, *qigong*, diet, herbs, acupuncture, yoga and so on that cause changes in *qi* by influencing the pure authentic *qi* of the great movement water accelerate the movement of *qi* and raise the temperature of the body. The heat released during this transformative process is observed in, for example, warm hands and feet or tingling in the body. These perceptions usually disappear over time, but in the long run the dynamic force of the great movement water contributes to an inner stable source that has no other purpose than synchronizing with time and circumstance. The passive great movement water offers the experience of timelessness because it moves with the times. Past and future have disappeared. The flow of the great movement water is the invisible source of light, fire, heat and movement. They become visible in time, but come from the timeless. The key to this synchronization is the silence and letting go

---

3   The lung is the father of *qi*. Due to its descending properties the lung provides the rhythm of movement in the body and the maintenance of the five *zang* and six *fu*. It works together with the heart, the mother of the *xuè*. The grasping properties of the kidneys causes lung *qi* to descend to the root of the *qi*. The kidneys keep the lungs rooted when the lungs purify the body by exhaling. A weak kidney *qi* therefore deteriorates and pollutes the body. In the *wuxing*, the mother lung nourishes the son kidney, but in physiological functions they act like sister and brother, yin and yang.

4   On this subject I refer to books and schools in *Nei Dan*, inner alchemy.

of the desire for change or for achieving a goal, that is the gift of the heavenly stem *Xin*.

THE GREAT MOVEMENT WATER AND THE HEAVENLY STEM *XIN*

The dark warrior heaven and the emanation *zhen* and the white tiger heaven and emanation *li* come together in the great movement water and heavenly stem *Xin*. In line with this *lizhen* advises using the benefits (*li*) of divination (*zhen*). Divination refers to the principle of synchronicity, a term invented by Carl Gustav Jung, and described as 'an acausal connecting principle'. Simultaneity might be seen as coincidence, but the principle of synchronicity gives meaning to coincidences and change. Interdependence is assumed between 'accidental' events and the subjective experiences of those observing those coincidences.

The great movement water and heavenly stem *Xin* connect to an area and a source where time and space apparently have a different meaning. Its signature is authenticity (*zhen*).

AUTHENTICITY

The fifteenth verse of the *Dao De Jing* says, 'When muddy water is kept still, it gradually becomes clear. That which is still, is gradually being stirred by movement.'

These lines describe the back-and-forth movement that everyone is subject to. Stillness happens when every physical-emotional-mental movement has withdrawn and the mind is clear. Stillness and clearness are like death, but do not mean death. They are symbols that belong to the power of gathering and letting go and establish a peaceful field from which new movements can arise.

Letting go of the ego's desires for appreciation and affirmation does not automatically mean that people should remain withdrawn. Being nourished by the authentic source of the great movement water evokes an unstoppable amount of energy, known as the source of change and creativity. The source of authentic energy is addressed by psychotherapy and other similar methods, but also through constitutional acupuncture, allowing people to feel liberated and energized.

Silence and clarity manifest themselves eventually in movements like activity after rest, waking consciousness after sleep, and happiness that emerges out of awe. Silence and clarity are the yin revelations of each cycle that generate yang. A primordial eternal source is hidden in silence and clarity, a source with which the still and clear mind knows itself connected. The primordial eternal source of nourishment is equal to authenticity, the personal design, and may be called the primordial mother of *qi*.

> The world has a primal source, which acts as primal mother for the world. Those who acknowledge the primal mother have recognized their own inner child.[5]

The beauty of silence is comparable to the peace of a baby being nourished at the mother's breast. Clarity lies hidden in the baby's relaxation, the stillness of the heart-mind.

A child must develop an ego that can take up a place in the world in which it moves. All existence, and thus also the evolved ego with personal will and desires, comes from the original source. The will (*zhi*) and desires may feel authentic, but the ego, identity and personality are influenced by upbringing, education and society. Still water, unaffected by outside movements, is a metaphor for the stillness of the heart-*shen*, the receptive ego and pure *jing*, allowing a release of the turbulence of the moving and longing ego-will. Everyone has access to stillness of the original source.

A calm and clear mind does not mean sitting back and doing nothing; it means being alert and observing developments, intentionally experiencing and understanding inner restless feelings that focus on changes and adaptations. The inner motives behind intentions are explored and reassured. Desires, needs, fears, frustrations emanating from the conditioned will could have clouded the inner 'waters'.

Perhaps it is up to the very wise person to always have still and clear 'waters', but for most of us it is a life's work, because this process towards self-knowledge breaks the intimate identification of the ego's will with its source, the primal mother. What we are, do, think, feel, have, is directly connected to the will. We are husbands, wives, alone, we have children or not, we feel sad or happy, think scientifically logically or emotionally and so on. All this directly moves the willpower that desires to act accordingly.

As we learn from our automatic, often unconscious, compulsive behaviours, we allow our true nature to emerge. This is not a theoretical concept, but a reality for those who accept that love is not based on answers and expectations, but on openness of *shen*, *qi* and *jing* to others as they are to yourself.

Authenticity is accepting yourself as you are, daring to be yourself, meeting your own needs, listening to what your intuition gives you and presenting

---

5   Personal English translation of the first sentences of verse 52 of Paul Salim Kluwer's Dutch *Dao De Jing* (1995).

yourself freely based on your own experiences and perceptions. You protect and take responsibility for yourself, but leave what belongs to others with those others, even if you don't like their behaviours. Authenticity follows its own ways, based on sincerity and truthfulness and the awareness that it is precisely authenticity that is the channel of expression of the *shen*, *qi* and *jing*. Then authenticity merges with its source, which is love, unbound, undivided and connected with and building on the living source.

Xin synchronizes with the natural sequence of events without the ego playing a leading role.

The most important advice for people born with '*Xin*, Lu in water' is to listen carefully inside, to the voice of 'intuition'.[6] All the more so, because in these people advice received is often ignored, as, however well intentioned, external advice is often seen as deviating from their own idea of what is beneficial. So ignoring advice turns out to be beneficial. Refusal is not based on stubbornness, but is an appropriate means of opening awareness and attunement to 'intuition'.

An additional dilemma for people born '*Xin*, Lu in water' is that expression of the source of authenticity may change from day to day, sometimes even hourly. For themselves, this is natural and feels very invariable – after all, changeability is the constant of life – whereas others who like order and principles sometimes find this extremely uncomfortable.

'*Xin*, Lu in water' can induce people to seclude themselves. This applies to those born with this combination as well as to everyone with lung problems. They need time to themselves on a regular basis. Sitting in a safe bubble gives air and increased sensitivity to the needs of the authentic source of *qi*. Some people are unable or unwilling to seclude themselves regularly. They can unwittingly create distance through strong reactions, offensive comments, oversocializing or catching diseases which may lead to unexpected sadness and despair.

Unconscious needs can be sublimated by continuous animated communication that distracts people from their own inner turmoil and avoids the discomfort of uncertainty and fears, thereby losing contact with their true needs. It is then insufficient to balance the great movement water. The great movement earth and the power of the ego and identity occupy a more crucial position in the healing process than the great movement water and the heavenly stem *Xin*, lung. These energies therefore require the most attention at the start of acupuncture treatments. The option of unlike *qi* treatments is not always the first and best choice.

---

6   Intuition is in quotation marks because it is not the intuition of the heart but the arising authenticity associated with the great movement water.

'BING, S.I. IN WATER' THE UNLIKE QI[7]

For these people separation and integration should be explored. Where *Xin* focuses on the integration between the authentic self and the authentic source of existence, *Bing* mainly focuses on the differences and similarities between the outer world and the inner world which facilitate the ego to find a safe place in this world. The ego-reinforcing effects of '*Bing*, S.i. in water' – although for people with '*Xin*, Lu in water' it often appears to be an issue as well – put pressure on the relationship between the self and its authentic source; a powerful ego and the importance of identity motivate the active great movement earth to subdue the passive great movement water further.

A healthy balance between the ego and its authentic source creates a strong presence and a clear mind with freedom of artistry and intuition. An unbalanced relationship can lead to feelings of (misplaced) trust and certainty about certain beliefs. However, these 'certainties' are accompanied by all kinds of other inner insecurities and fears such as one's choice of a profession or hobby. The passion is followed, but there seems to be fear, uncertainty and doubt in its pursuit.

FIRE, GREAT MOVEMENTS EARTH AND WATER

The path of self-knowledge but also treatments should not be judgemental in any way. It is about recognizing the imbalance in the dynamic operating system of the self. It is about maintaining the natural balance that is given by the birth chart. Elements that are underexposed are likely to need more attention to restore balance and health than overexposed elements.[8]

Imbalance in this operating system of the self causes complaints due to the disturbed communication between fire and the great movements earth and water.[9] The resulting diseases can include heart rhythm problems, lymph vessel and bone issues, breast diseases, digestion and skin issues and so on. It is advisable to first balance the great movement earth through restoring the balance between the heavenly stems *Jia* and *Ji*. Only then may the power of the ego normalize and be nourished sufficiently by the interconnectedness between small intestine, *san jiao*, heart and the heart constrictor. This regulating approach again needs to precede the unlike *qi* treatments.

The careful reader has observed that this process balances the three treasures

---

7   Unlike *qi* treatments are discussed in the chapters on treatments. The word refers to the inequality of *qi* in the same great movement. The unlike *qi* for '*Xin*, Lu in water' is '*Bing*, S.i. in water'.

8   Other struggles that affect the control of the ego are the battle between the mind and the heart, between intellect and intuition and between sense and sensibility.

9   Between heaven, earth and human.

jing-qi-shen, water-earth-fire, human-earth-heaven. A healthy balance between the heart and heart constrictor[10] along with a healthy great movement earth seem the best choice to solve '*Xin*, Lu in water'-related issues.

A 55-year-old male patient, born with '*Xin*, Lu in water', is super social. He combines a strong practical personality with a good intuition to solve problems. He develops heart rhythm problems when he overworks, often in times of personal stress. The small intestine pulse is weak. The *jing* and nearly all water-related *qi* are insufficient, which indicates insufficiency of the great movement water. The *shen* is overactive and the gallbladder insufficient (opposites in the Chinese hourly clock). All aspects of the earth are weak. This indicates insufficiency of the great movement earth.[11]

The first treatment Ht-5, *Tong Li*, Gb-34, *Yang Ling Quan*, Sp-3, *Tai Bai*, and Ki-4, *Da Zhong*, reduced the heart rhythm problems by 80 per cent. The second treatment S.i.-4, *Wang Gu*, and S.i.-5, *Yang Gu*, cured it. In order to further balance him and prevent future problems, I treated him a little longer.

Ht-5 connects to the inside. It is the *luo* point of the heart channel and sends an internal channel to S.i.-4. It brings yang back to its origins, calms the *shen* and regulates the heart rhythm and connects people with themselves.

Gb-34 and Sp-3 balance the great movement earth. This is the keystone of the first treatment.

Ki-4 is the *luo* point of the kidney channel and sends an internal channel to Bl-64, *Jing Gu*. It strengthens the will, but also softens the too driven will. It benefits the *jing qi* of the kidneys and regulates the *ren* and *chong mai* that are rooted in the kidneys: It regulates *qi* and moves *xuè*.

This treatment operates on the level of *jing-qi-shen* via heart-*shen*, great movement earth and *jing qi*.

S.i.-4 is the *yuan source* point of the small intestine. It brings peace and stability to taking decisions and gives confidence. It opens the chest and mobilizes *qi*.

S.i.-5 is the fire point of the small intestine channel. It calms the *shen* and clears the mind and gives mental clarity. It often balances fire better than heart points.

Small intestine points balance the great movement water in people born with '*Xin*, Lu in water'.

---

10 See chapters on the earthly branches and specifically Chapter 36. The heart belongs to fire, the heart constrictor influences fire, earth and water.

11 See chapters on the earthly branches.

THE CONSEQUENCES OF '*XIN,* LUNG IN WATER' IN THE *WUXING*

Water that affects metal is a reverse *sheng* movement. Although it is inverted, it is still a *sheng*-cycle relationship. Nourishment in this case is not the result of support, but of gradual resistance. There is a headwind. It is like cycling against the wind, and despite the fact that it takes more effort, the muscles become stronger and the condition improves. Reverse *sheng* resistance may create conditions that are obstructive and troublesome, but it evokes strength. It can generate heat, causing the temperature to rise, perspiration to increase, emotions and intense feelings to become overwhelming and the mind to become confused. Too much resistance can lead to extreme fatigue syndromes and emotional and mental disorder. Understandably, people become stronger through resistance and setbacks than through luck and windfalls. People born with '*Xin,* Lu in water' seem to know this implicitly, although I understand their desire for an easier life. Seeking silence and clarity, especially when there is none, is the recurring lesson.

For '*Xin,* Lu in water' the passive nature of the great movement water may cause the great movement earth to become overactive. This puts even more emphasis on the ego and identity. The extent to which this becomes unbearable for the great movement water depends on other input, which can be personal, social, cultural and/or national in nature. For example, an ego can be challenged to perform in sports in such a way that, partly due to exhaustion, water/authenticity comes under great pressure. This can initially express itself through incomprehensible back pain, but eventually in depression and despair.

ACUPUNCTURE POINTS THAT INFLUENCE THE PASSIVE GREAT MOVEMENT WATER AND THE HEAVENLY STEM *XIN*

Treatments of lung complaints that originate from a disturbed relationship between the great movement water and the heavenly stem *Xin* should first of all focus on balancing the great movement earth, in which the spleen has an important function. In addition to the stem point Sp-3, *Tai Bai,* Sp-19, *Xiong Xiang,* and Sp-20, *Zhou Rong,* are very useful acupuncture points that contribute to a good balance of the great movement earth. Moreover, these points restore the relationship between the spleen and lung. Gb-34, *Yang Ling Quan,* the stem point, is as important as Gb-40, *Qiu Xu.* They nourish and balance the spleen–lung relationship and affect the chest area to a great extent.

Lu-5, *Chi Ze*, cubit marsh, the stem point. This is the water point on the lung channel that regulates the water passage in the body. It descends and disperses body fluids for urination and lubrication of the intestines to facilitate bowel movements. Descending the fluids increases perseverance by strengthening both will and authenticity. People's true nature might be expressed through Lu-5. It is the gate on the lung channel where *qi* opens to the more external aspects of the body.

The fluidity of peaceful water reduces rigidity: It benefits the flow of *jing*, *qi* and *shen*. Physical-emotional-mental rigidity may lead to protest or avoidance, a compulsive mind, unconscious restlessness and complaints due to an impaired digestion and pains based on excessive control. Lu-5 facilitates and eases the flow of water, especially in agitation and stubbornness due to yin insufficiency.

Sp-12, *Chong Men*, rushing gate, was discussed in Chapter 14. Sp-12 connects with the *yuan qi* and facilitates its expression in the outside world. People feel stuck but are ready to move on.

S.i.-1, *Shao Ze*, little marsh, along with S.i.-4, *Wang Gu*, wrist bone, opens the chest and the lungs and mobilizes *qi* in general. Like Lu-5, the name of S.i.-1 refers to a marsh. Marshes function like sponges, they release stored liquids in periods of drought and store fluids in periods of excessive humidity. Moreover, fluids in marshes are purified from pollution. S.i.-1 with S.i.-4 support the lubrication and function of the lungs.

S.i.-7, *Zhi Zheng*, the true branch, works on bodily fluids and *yuan qi* and, along with L.i.-6, *Pian Li*, the side passage, supports *qi* and fluids to descend to the kidneys and strengthen the kidney yin. *Zhi* is the offshoot of the rectifying true-*zheng qi*. *Zheng* refers to protection from external pathogenic factors and therefore reflects the strength of the body's true *qi*. S.i.-7 is treated on the left-hand side (the side of the heart) and L.i.-6 is treated on the right-hand side (the side of the lung). This combination emphasizes the intimate relationship between the lung and heart which are both rooted in the original *qi* of the kidneys. Small intestine and large intestine are unlike and like *qi* of the lung, respectively.

CHAPTER 21

DYNAMICS OF THE HEAVENLY STEMS *REN* 壬 AND *GUI* 癸[1]

The dynamics of the last two heavenly stems are discussed together. They are even more intertwined than the other like *qi* couples. Before approaching the topic of this chapter, the like *qi* couples will be discussed first.

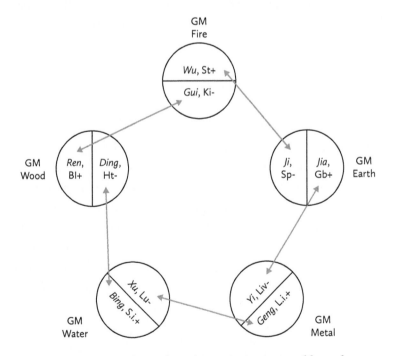

Figure 21.1 Active and passive great movements, like and unlike qi of the heavenly stems and related organs

---

1   People born in years ending with a 2 and 3, such as 1982 and 1983, after the Chinese New Year.

LIKE *QI*

Like *qi* couples: Gb-Liv; S.i.-Ht; St-Sp; L.i.-Lu; Bl-Ki

Like *qi* has not been discussed much yet, but the concept is more important than it may seem at first glance. Normally, for a person born with '*Jia*, Gb in earth', the great movement water will be subdued. However, an *overactivity* has more consequences. First, the passive great movement water becomes more insufficient which makes it less able to nourish the great movement wood. Second, the active great movement fire, which is less under control, becomes overactive.

'*Jia*, Gb in earth' too active → great movement water too passive → '*Wu*, St in fire' too active.

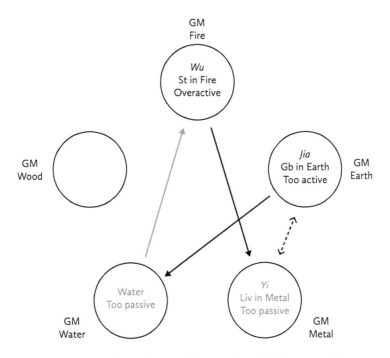

Figure 21.2 'Jia, Gb in earth' too active, 'Yi, Liv in metal'
too passive. Result: 'Wu, St in fire' overactive
The dotted, two-directional arrows depict the like *qi* interrelationship. Black arrows depict the controlling action of an active great movement, grey arrows depict the lack of controlling action due to passivity of the great movement.

Furthermore, the great movement water will become even more insufficient for another reason: when '*Jia*, Gb in earth' is too active, the like *qi* '*Yi*, Liv in metal' has the tendency to become more passive. The great movement metal will be unable to nourish the great movement water sufficiently. The active great movement fire becomes more active than it already was in response to the passivity of the great movement water and of the passive great movement metal.

'*Yi*, Liv in metal' too passive → '*Wu*, St in fire' too active.

Overactivity of '*Jia*, Gb in earth' (ego, identity) eventually results in an overactive great movement fire. This is usually visible by signs and symptoms arising from '*Wu*, St in fire' such as dry mouth, constipation, reduced fluids, unsatisfying hunger, but also heartburn, trigeminal neuralgia, herpes simplex and migraine. Of course, treatment of the unlike *qi* '*Ji*, Sp in earth' is possible, only if the pulse diagnosis indicates it, yet the role of '*Yi*, Liv in metal' should not be missed in this process.[2]

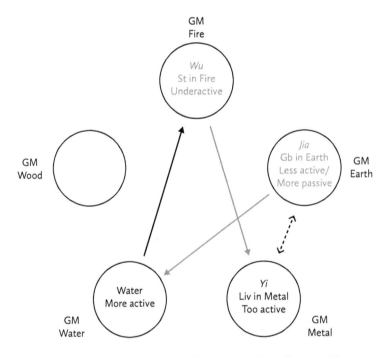

Figure 21.3 'Yi, Liv in metal' too active, 'Jia, Gb in earth'
less active. Result: 'Wu, St in fire' underactive
The dotted, two-directional arrows depict the like *qi* interrelationship. Black arrows depict the controlling action of an active great movement, grey arrows depict the lack of controlling action due to passivity of the great movement.

---

2   With overactivity of '*Jia*, Gb in earth', sedation of the stem point Gb-34 would be possible. However, frequent sedation of essential *qi* is unwise. J.D. van Buren stated that it should only be done once in a lifetime. Sedation of the fire point on the stomach channel, St-41, *Jie Xi*, would be a symptomatic treatment that does not address the underlying cause.

When 'Yi, Liv in metal' becomes too active, the normal activity of 'Wu, St in fire' is reduced. The dynamics of the great movements stagnate and there is a good chance that the liver *qi* will stagnate. An overactive 'Yi, Liv in metal' causes a less active like *qi* 'Jia, Gb in earth'. This causes less suppression of the great movement water, which in turn reduces 'Wu, St in fire'.

This causes issues with excess fluids, digestive disorders, reduced muscle nutrition and abnormalities in the blood.

Thus 'Yi, Liv in metal' too active results in 'Wu, St in fire' too passive.

Treatment of the unlike *qi* of 'Yi, Liv in metal', 'Geng, L.i. in metal' is possible, but in this process the like *qi* of 'Jia, Gb in earth' should not be forgotten.

Unlike *qi* may exacerbate (or balance) disturbances of the dynamic model of the great movements.

> Overactive 'Jia, Gb in earth' → great movement water too passive → 'Wu, St in fire' too active.

> Reduced 'Yi, Liv in metal' → 'Wu, St in fire' too active.

A yin yang imbalance between the heavenly stem *Jia* and *Yi*, Gb and Liv, leads to problems of overactivity of the active great movement fire.

> Overactive 'Bing, S.i. in water' → great movement fire too passive → 'Geng, L.i. in metal' too active.

> Reduced 'Ding, Ht in wood' → 'Geng, L.i. in metal' too active.

A yin yang imbalance between the heavenly stem *Bing* and *Ding*, S.i. and Ht, leads to problems of overactivity of the active great movement metal.

> Overactive 'Wu, St in fire' → great movement metal too passive → 'Ren, Bl in wood' too active.

> Reduced 'Ji, Sp in earth' → 'Ren, Bl in wood' too active.

A yin yang imbalance between the heavenly stem *Wu* and *Ji*, St and Sp, leads to problems of overactivity of the active great movement wood.

Overactive '*Geng*, L.i. in metal' → the great movement wood too passive → '*Jia*, Gb in earth' too active.

Reduced '*Xin*, Lu in water' → '*Jia*, Gb in earth' too active.

A yin yang imbalance between the heavenly stem *Geng* and *Xin*, L.i. and Lu, leads to problems of overactivity of the active great movement earth.

Overactive '*Ren*, Bl in wood' → the great movement earth too passive → '*Bing*, S.i. in water' too active.

Reduced '*Gui*, Ki in fire' → '*Bing*, S.i. in water' too active.

A yin yang imbalance between the heavenly stem *Ren* and *Gui*, Bl and Ki, leads to problems of overactivity of the active great movement water.

'*Ren*, Bl in wood' and '*Gui*, Ki in fire' are the only like *qi* couples in which the effect of mutual imbalance has an effect on their own phase. As a result, initial complaints can quickly worsen. Treating *Ren* or *Gui* as like *qi* prevents this rapid evolution of disease and is therefore essential in any imbalance between bladder and kidneys.

For those born with '*Ren*, Bl in wood' it is best to start with kidney points and vice versa.

REN 壬, THE NINTH HEAVENLY STEM, AND *GUI* 癸 THE TENTH HEAVENLY STEM

The quality of the heavenly stem *Ren* is shown in the yang of water, the bladder. The quality of the heavenly stem *Gui* is shown in the yin of water, the kidneys.

Ren and *Gui* are manifestations of the emanation *zhen* and the northern heaven with the dark warrior, the tortoise and snake. Both heavenly stems are involved in the process of internalization and attunement to the true authentic *qi*, the foundation of existence that is hidden within everyone. The degree of transformation of the self, initiated and guided by the source of existence, is reflected in sexuality, talent and authenticity.

The Chinese character *Ren* shows the burden of someone carrying the weight of a yoke. It indicates a man who is tired of his troubles that he carries with him. At the same time, it shows the time of conception and new beginnings. An old saying is 'seeing in darkness is clarity and renewal'.

In ancient times the Chinese character *Gui* represented hands making sacrifices. There are descriptions that relate *Gui* to grass mats used during ancestral sacrifices. Ancestor worship was and still is an important part of Chinese culture. It is said to be based on the idea that the spirit of the deceased lives on in our world and may influence the fate of the bereaved. Ancestor worship is still practised, usually with the aim of positively influencing personal fate and preventing any negative influence of the deceased. However, sacrificing in a spiritual sense means distancing yourself from personal gain and is intended to contribute to life and humanity.

Both these heavenly stems look back to the past. Standing still and looking back creates a resting place in the unstoppable flow of time. It may lead to a real turning point in consciousness initiated by a moment of peace and quiet, in which distance is taken from the old and an irreversible change can take place.

TRINITY *GENG-XIN-REN*

The heavenly stem *Ren* is the last of the trinity *Geng-Xin-Ren* that focuses on becoming human and humane. The yoke, depicted by *Ren*, bears the influences of the eight previous heavenly stems. The initiated actions of *Jia*, interactions of *Yi*, integration of *Bing*, intuition of *Ding*, inspiration and intelligence of *Wu*, integrity and intellect of *Ji*, introspection of *Geng* and authentic 'intuition' of *Xin* all contribute to the capacity to become human in the heavenly stems *Ren* and *Gui*, including efforts, frustrations, emotions, figments, thoughts and so on.

The road to authenticity is not an easy one; it is a road full of setbacks and soul pain. It can be difficult, especially for people born with '*Ren*, Bl in wood'. Meeting the challenges and integrating what is experienced may lead to the path of authenticity but, irrespective, it definitely provides inner strength and stability. The reverse also happens; avoiding or rebelling against life's challenges exhausts and makes people dissatisfied and insecure. Being authentic means being sensitive and understanding and accepting the expressions of life. One can become a human channel for heavenly *qi* by eschewing personal gain and yielding to the course of things that arise from the inner source of heavenly *qi*.

Diseases and complaints in the field of *Ren*, bladder, and *Gui*, kidneys, are often caused by inner struggle against the natural development of human beings. This is not meant as a normative qualification, but intended as a wake-up call to focus awareness and treatment on possible personal issues that manifest themselves through the bladder and kidney *qi*. Acceptance of fallibility, complaints of ageing, menopause, external gender characteristics and so on frequently provoke feelings of resistance which manifest themselves in bladder and kidney complaints.

A balanced *Ren* is expressed in a soft, nourishing and supple attitude that does not change due to setbacks and resistance. With *Gui* it is somewhat the same, but more internalized. It is characterized by a wise and talented appearance and is attractive to others. Unbalanced *Ren* and *Gui* can cause people to have fears, and become introverted, easily overstimulated and anxious.

THE GREAT MOVEMENT WOOD AND THE HEAVENLY STEM *REN*
THE GREAT MOVEMENT FIRE AND THE HEAVENLY STEM *GUI*

The green azure heaven, the emanation *yuan* and the northern heaven of the dark warrior, tortoise and snake and the emanation *zhen* come together in '*Ren*, Bl in wood'.

The red vermilion bird heaven, the emanation *heng* and the northern heaven of the dark warrior, tortoise and snake and the emanation *zhen* come together in '*Gui*, Ki in fire'.

To better understand *Ren* and *Gui*, two types of development paths are identified separately, but in life the two paths are of course both present and closely so. We discuss the external development path in which people focus their attention on the outside world and the internal development path in which they focus their attention on their inner world.

'*REN*, BL IN WOOD'

On the external path, the encounter of the vitalizing *qi* of the East with the authentic, upright *qi* of the North generates dynamic, purposeful, powerful, artistic, innovative and clever minds. Since genuine existential problems are often suppressed or avoided on this path, one should be vigilant about the effects of underlying anxiety and depression.

On the internal path, the vital *qi* of the eastern heaven enriches the inner being in which communication with oneself and others is characterized by openness and vulnerability. The known world of contradictions touches a world in which contradictions do not challenge but complement each other. Sometimes this state is described as a waiting void; emptiness that is not empty, but is boundless in its possibilities. It is therefore advisable for people to seek silence, both in themselves and in nature, so that their destiny can reveal itself through openness and vulnerability.

'*GUI*, KI IN FIRE'

On the external path, the meeting of the determined *qi* of the South with the authentic, upright *qi* of the North causes a powerful, usually predominant will and devotion. Fulfilling an objective and dedication to a cause is paramount. Urge and activity are so strong that boundaries are not properly observed or are intentionally exceeded. When the urge to be active is hindered by others or is made impossible by circumstances it easily causes frustration, insecurity or anger. One should be vigilant about depression when there are existential problems, but even more so about the possibility of burnout. Limitless behaviour weakens the security and scope of the ego. Instead of finding more inner peace and perpetuating the security of the ego, people are increasingly seeking affirmation through more activities. Usually, I recommend people take a few steps back – I really mean this physically and not as a brain game. After they have taken a few steps back, I ask them to stop and turn and look back. Can they be grateful for the opportunities offered?

On the internal path, the fire of *heng* represents the art of offering. It is the offering of the human being attuned to a deep source of existence and independent of the will to achieve.

When fire comes into contact with water, it stops rising and the heart is no longer full of passions and desires. When the water is approached by fire, steam is created and water stops flowing down. The water–fire axis provides inner vitality and health that is visible and tangible through harmony and balance in all bodily functions.

This way of life cannot be pursued, but can be lived. Health is determined by self-cultivation and the potential of the inextricably linked heavenly stems *Ren* and *Gui*.

You will understand that everyone follows an external and an internal path. Complaints and illnesses can occur if there is an untrue relationship between the two paths, especially if one of the paths is driven by too much will. Understanding one's own contribution to responsibility for health and disease contributes to healing.

THE CONSEQUENCES OF '*REN*, BLADDER IN WOOD, AND '*GUI*, KIDNEY IN FIRE' IN THE *WUXING*

'*Ren*, Bl in wood' has a reverse *sheng* relationship (wood to water). Due to the great movement wood, the appearance of heat develops faster in '*Ren*, Bl in wood' than in '*Xin*, Lu in water'. The reverse *ke*-cycle relationship in '*Gui*, Ki in fire' (fire to water), previously discussed with '*Jia*, Gb in earth', is a state in which life starts to express itself in form. The hidden beginning of the cycle of the heavenly stems starts in the heavenly stem *Ren* and is incorporated into the heavenly stem *Gui*.

Ren and *Gui* are the heavenly stems of winter, when it is cold and the *qi* has turned inward. The creative and guiding influence of the great movement wood on the heavenly stem *Ren* is shown in divine inspiration, spiritual insights, prayers, music and everything else that awakens consciousness to overcome divisions that, unfortunately, characterize humans and humanity. The vital and moving *qi* of the great movement wood keeps the mind and body smooth and supple. It prevents them from getting stiff and hard. Running water keeps everything smoothly connected. That is the essence of (new) life. Standing water gives a hardened mind, which makes adjustment and flexibility difficult. People tend to focus mainly on themselves. Moreover, there is often a lack of vision and future plans.

As water naturally flows downward, the blooming *qi* of the great movement fire naturally rises and spreads. These two forces meet in '*Gui*, Ki in fire'. In nature this happens when the *qi* gathers for the benefit of a new cycle of life. Deep inside human beings lies a similar 'hidden mission' of renewed creation that can elevate humanity into a more subtle realm. The key lies in the conscious descent of the fire that frees the heart from stress, desires and longings, and in the conscious ascent of the water that frees the kidneys from the instinctual will. In this way, the combination of fire and water lays the foundation for future life, movement and maintenance of life. It is a natural process, known as the fire of the *Ming Men*, which is the fire that tunes into the inexhaustible source of water and thus guides the process of evolution. It is precisely human will that easily disrupts the natural process of evolution. We can consciously investigate the encounter of fire with water, for example in sexuality where the merging happens naturally, but in a more spiritual sense, the fire–water encounter is mostly uncharted territory and it is advisable to approach this with patience and caution.

Bearing the burdens of life is not easy. People need time to learn to deal with this. It becomes more difficult when the great movement earth with the ego and identity are subdued too much by the great movement wood. It becomes more bearable when people born with '*Ren*, Bl in wood' walk the inner path and base their trust on an inner source rather than an outer. Setbacks or a hard life cannot be changed, but the way they are carried can be adjusted.

The passive great movement fire causes an active great movement water. The more the will is involved, the more external the '*Gui*, Ki in fire' people are, and the more is required of the kidney *qi* and water phase. The kidney pulse may feel normal in amount, but its tightness betrays the pressure it is under. In the long run, exhaustion arises. The increased drive can cause the passive great movement fire to become (over)active. This puts the great movement metal under pressure and the great movement water is no longer properly nourished and gets further exhausted.

The passive great movement fire remains healthy when people follow the natural course of events instead of being motivated by desires and will. This only works out well if people can face their fears and insecurities. 'Gui, Ki in fire' is the source of the being, the Light bearer, the bearer of pure essence that heals and improves.

Treating patients born with these heavenly stems requires a very hands-on approach. The internal way seems to be the healthy way, but can only be proposed, especially because it makes life tough. Everyone has to find their own way in, in their own time. Trust based on tangible results in particular enables people to find their own way to their own potential.

ACUPUNCTURE POINTS THAT INFLUENCE THE ACTIVE GREAT MOVEMENT WOOD AND THE HEAVENLY STEM *REN*

'Ren, Bl in wood' easily subdues 'Ji, Sp in earth', which is often artificially overstimulated by identity issues. A sweet tooth is the usual short-term solution for spleen *qi* insufficiency. In general, Bl-65, *Shu Gu*, binding bone, the stem point, helps to restore the balance of the spleen *qi* in hypoglycaemia. Sedation or tonification of Bl-65 assists the spleen *qi* in directing sugar metabolism: Sedation is recommended in cases of spleen *qi* insufficiency and tonification in cases of spleen *qi* excess. This treatment is indicated if hypoglycaemia is accompanied by complaints along the bladder channel like neurological problems in the leg, fullness and warmth in the head and neck or bruising pain in the area of the kidneys.

Bl-65 supports bone healing after fractures or operations through the vitality and creative properties of the great movement of wood. It is located opposite Sp-3, *Tai Bai*, great white, the stem point of the passive great movement earth. The balance and health between the two great movements wood and earth and heavenly stems Ren and Ji is evident in the strength and tension of the forefoot support when people are standing.

Bl-65 has additional important connections. I always imagine tension wires running from Sp-3, Sp-4, *Gong Sun*, grandfather grandson, and Ki-2, *Ran Gu*, blazing valley, across the dorsal side of the foot and converging in Bl-65. The tension, strength and flexibility between the acupuncture points Sp-3, Sp-4, Ki-2 with Bl-65 determine the power of the forefoot and midfoot. Flat and spreading feet are related to malfunction of these interconnections.

The tension of the wire Sp-3–Bl-65 shows the strength to stay centred and take good care of the internal organs. The tension of the wire Sp-4–Bl-65 shows the ability of the personal *qi* to socialize without becoming entangled in the pitfalls of the ego or the energetic net of others. The wire Ki-2–Bl-65 shows the weight of desires and goals. Ki-2 is tonified when people have difficulty setting goals due to a lack of needs and desires. It is sedated when people are overwhelmed with desires or when they are overly challenged by themselves or others.

For further information about Sp-20 and Sp-12 refer to Chapters 14 and 16. These acupuncture points are the ultimate expression of the qualities of 'Gui, Ki in fire'. In themselves they express the merging of fire and water, which leads *qi* to thrive and prosper.

A FINAL NOTE

The heavenly stem *Ren* is the last of the human trinity *Geng-Xin-Ren*. It summarizes all previous heavenly stems. 'Ren, Bl in wood' receives the heavenly impulse for the individual human being and develops the personality accordingly. The personality that is bound by knowledge, life lessons, the connection with others and so on is the mirror and response of human beings to the original impulse of existence. It is up to every man and woman to show what this evokes.

The heavenly stem *Gui* gives humans the mandate to exist. Usually this manifests itself through willpower and external activity. The deeper meaning of *Gui,* however, is the other side of *Dao*'s revelation that is not connected with glorification or comparison.

My teachers explained and translated Chapter 67 of the *Dao De Jing* as follows.

I hold three treasures, which I cherish and keep
The first is love
The second is simplicity
The third is modesty

These words reflect my personal understanding of the beauty of *Dao*. These treasures[3] are not ethical, cannot be enforced or taught, they come in freedom and give freedom. They are like water that always finds a natural way; they are like water in which heaven and humanity complement each other and people learn to reconcile with themselves and with others.

---

3   Sometimes called the three treasures of Daoism.

CHAPTER 22

UNLIKE *QI* AND THE DYNAMICS OF THE FOUR POSSIBILITIES[1]

The great movement can impose its *qi* on the related heavenly stem and, conversely, it can happen that the heavenly stem imposes its *qi* on the great movement. This domination can cause new challenges for the person involved and may affect dietary choices, emotional and spiritual preferences and physical behaviour. It may require self-effort, self-responsibility and possibly treatment to balance the great movement and heavenly stem relationship by using so-called 'unlike *qi*' treatment.[2]

Any appearance of the 'four possibilities' in pulse diagnosis indicates an imbalance between great movement and heavenly stem. For example, in someone born with '*Ren*, Bl in wood', the great movement wood may receive too much water from the heavenly stem *Ren*, bladder. In the beginning wood takes advantage of water to support growth. However, too much water stagnates growth, which can cause the liver *qi* to stagnate; this may cause fits of anger, tension headaches, irregular menstruation and so on.

I hope you agree that it makes more sense to treat the cause of symptoms rather than just symptoms; in this case it means a healing of the relationship between the affected great movement and the heavenly stem by using unlike *qi*, '*Ding*, Ht in wood'. Any point on the heart channel restores the relationship

---

1   Some of the 'four possibilities' cannot be explained at this stage of the book, but are described here for the sake of completeness. Please see Chapter 45 for more explanation.
2   See Chapter 17 .

between the great movement wood and *Ren*, bladder. The choice of points is determined by pulse diagnosis.[3]

If you are new to constitutional acupuncture, it may be challenging to find the correct points on the heart channel but, once found, it will prove the benefits of balancing treatments through unlike *qi*.

Four possibilities and unlike *qi* treatments work well in patients, but can also be applied in other situations than acupuncture treatments.

A CEO ASKS ME FOR ADVICE

A small department in his company with seven employees was not functioning properly. He had fired people, hired new people and provided training and education. Nothing helped to change the dysfunction; everyone worked hard but there were often disputes and power conflicts.

He almost gave up because he couldn't figure out what was going on. People got tired quickly and were constantly nitpicking, and with a lot of sick leave it became a huge problem for him. In addition the department did not match the creative, inspiring energy that the company wanted to radiate. The diagnosis of the problems in this story indicated that earth was stagnant and unable to develop.

I asked him about the dates of birth of current employees and new applicants. His employees all had '*Ji*, Sp in earth' as birth *qi* of the year and/or month. One of the applicants was born with '*Jia*, Gb in earth' (unlike *qi* of '*Ji*, Sp in earth') as innate *qi* of the month.[4] I advised him to hire this person.

From the moment this person started working for him the atmosphere in the department changed; disagreements were unexpectedly resolved, requests for improvements in working conditions came and, unexpectedly, the department suddenly became productive. That year there was no department in the company that was so productive with hardly any absenteeism.

The following classification of the 'four possibilities' is far from complete. It is a description of possibilities and cannot be used like a reference book. I especially encourage you to research the underlying energetic concept of the 'four possibilities' and apply it in practice.

---

3   When people become ill in their 'own' innate *qi*, treatment should be done through the unlike *qi*. Treatment of one's 'own *qi*' is possible, but the effect on the essential birth *qi* is uncertain. Treatments that balance the dynamizing great movements with the heavenly stems and related organs are more refined and do justice to the patient's personal constitutional challenges.

4   The innate year *qi* is the essential *qi*, the innate month *qi* relates to social and personal relationships. With work issues the innate month *qi* needs to be considered.

'*JIA*, GB IN EARTH' – '*JI*, SP IN EARTH'

The challenge for people born with '*Jia*, Gb in earth' is to balance their innate qualities to inspire and innovate through confidence with the receptiveness, sensitivity and vulnerability of '*Ji*, Sp in earth'.

The challenge for people born with '*Ji*, Sp in earth' is to master qualities of '*Jia*, Gb in earth'. These people need movement, change and initiatives to prevent stagnation in any form.

'*Jia*, Gb in earth' treat with '*Ji*, Sp in earth'

WOOD TOO EARTHY

The great movement earth influences *Jia* so much that the wood aspect becomes too earthy. This applies to the gallbladder, liver, large intestine and lung.[5]

Too much earth in wood may lead to too much dampness in wood-related tissues such as ligaments and muscles that are therefore limited in movement. It may result in loose stools and/or mucus or phlegm in the lungs along with coughs when intestines and lungs are affected by too much earth. The spiritual source *hun* (wood) may become stagnant. It easily leads to obstruction of the free flow of *qi*, change and transformation along with decreased vitality, sluggishness and purposeless behaviour.

EARTH TOO WOODY

The wood aspect of *Jia* overwhelms the great movement earth and causes overactivity and stimulation of the spiritual source *yi* (earth). This results in confusion, lack of concentration, being unable to stop thinking and excessive movement and feelings of arousal. Earth-related channels that can be affected are stomach, spleen, liver, small intestine and heart constrictor.[6]

WATER TOO EARTHY

When water is dominated by earth, the flow of *qi*, fluids and *xuè* are easily disturbed. Due to stagnant flow of *qi*, there may be the tendency for laziness and people have difficulty creating and executing plans. Because of a weakened *zhi* (will/water), people like to be inspired by the willpower and drive of others.

EARTH TOO WATERY

Earth that becomes too watery turns into mud. The *yi*, associated with con-centration and memory processing, becomes inert. The coldness of the watery

---

5   See the chapters on earthly branches.
6   See the chapters on earthly branches.

earth constricts and disturbs transformation and transportation of *qi*, causing the whole body to become malnourished. These people benefit from warmth and movement. It is advisable to keep the *qi* moving when, due to illness or injury, people have to sit or lie down.

'*Ji*, Sp in earth' treat with '*Jia*, Gb in earth'

EARTH TOO EARTHY

There is a high chance of too much dampness. This may result in heaviness and stagnation on all levels possible. Physically it may lead to fatigue, a heavy feeling in the body, sticky bowel movements and so on. Mentally it may cause obsession due to stagnation in thinking; emotionally, it may cause resentment, selfishness and self-centredness and the desire for sensations: no matter what, as long as it produces emotions and feelings! On a spiritual level (*yi*), people mainly desire to be practical. Vague philosophies are often rejected; the spiritual must be physically felt and have practical meaning. This is often found in singing or dancing.

FIRE TOO EARTHY

The fire of the spleen is necessary for digestion, transportation and transformation. As with the previous imbalance, stagnation can occur, due to too much dampness and earth. This easily causes insomnia when the heart-*shen* becomes too earthy.

Chronic cases of 'fire too earthy' cause socially disturbed behaviour. It is as if people are seeking contact with the world through dirty and fogged windows. The *shenming* (spiritual brightness) becomes dull and the mind is no longer clear.

An overactive spiritual source *yi* (earth) can result in obsessive behaviour that likewise leads to a stronger focus on physicality and less on spirituality and thought processes. This kind of behaviour is further reinforced and results in decreased creativity, intuition and intelligence when the fire is unable to support earth. Increasing emphasis is being placed on intellect and mental scientific thinking. It can lead to serious illness when, due to a reverse *sheng* flow from earth back to fire, the heart-*shen* mandate is disoriented.

EARTH TOO FIERY

It affects the digestive system and the *yi* when earth is overheated. People tend to eat a lot, but still stay slim. They are easily irritable due to a lack of focus and presence and they like to be alone frequently, especially when confusion arises (it takes energy to process events, emotions and thoughts).

'YI, LIV IN METAL' – 'GENG, L.I. IN METAL'

People born with 'Yi, Liv in metal' have the ability to adapt to changing, some-times unpleasant, circumstances. All of a sudden it can be enough and they take an adamant stand. The challenge these people face is to master the qualities of 'Geng, L.i. in metal': the path of self-knowledge and clarity.

For people born with 'Geng, L.i. in metal', the challenge is to stay flexible, to adapt to the changing world and support others, without crossing their own borders. These people may, for example, find it difficult to adjust mentally and emotionally in life and may also experience physical and spiritual rigidity. In its treatment, one can only focus on the great movement, because great movements are expressed in all areas of existence.

'Yi, Liv in metal' treat with 'Geng, L.i. in metal'

WOOD TOO METALLIC

Growth and vitality of wood are subdued by the constricted dryness of metal. People may have problems with muscle strength and coordination as well as sugar balance and the immune system (wei qi). In addition, the limiting physi-cality of metal (the spiritual source po) overwhelms the free flow of qi and the hun. It may cause fits of anger and outbursts of creativity when wood likes to break through its limitations.

J.D. van Buren stated that the qi of the heavenly stem should not be addressed directly. In the case of 'Yi, Liv in metal' the liver channel should not be treated directly. Only very rarely, when the constriction in the liver becomes chronic and other options have failed,[7] might one sedate Liv-4, Zhong Feng, sealed centre.

However, I have found a gentler option; in general, the passive great move-ments regain strength through the use of the channel luo point. Needling Liv-5, Li Gou, drain of calf, with people born with 'Yi, Liv in metal', is harmless to the innate qi. However, a solo use of Liv-5 is not recommended as it may provoke a strong emotional response. In general, but especially in cases of emotional imbalance, it is advised to combine Liv-5 with Gb-37, Guang Ming, bright light. In cases of timidity, stagnation of free flow of qi with fusing pulses of liver and gallbladder, it is advised to combine Liv-5 with Gb-40, Qiu Xu, eminent region. In cases of uncertainty and weakened self-image it is indicated to needle Liv-5 with Gb-34, Yang Ling Quan, fountain of yang.

---

7   Like acupuncture points on the L.i. channel. This seems sensible, especially since the deep qi (Chapter 38) of this channel is also wood. However, this approach might lead to more tension. Then it is better to first deal with the free flow or qi in the liver itself.

METAL TOO WOODY

Wood overpowering metal may cause a perception of being possessed. It is as if people are guided by a force that entered them from the outside. Those people feel unable to control their instinctual forces and feel relieved by the use of alcohol or drugs, which is of course counterproductive in the long run.

The possible wood-*po* domination may give rise to irritability, resentment, blame and anger based on feeling worthless and expendable. The hitherto inner physical-emotional-mental organization can become chaotic. When 'metal too woody' affects the natural balance between the great movements fire and metal, ideas can practically no longer be executed. People feel desperate; it seems everyone and everything is against them.

Prior to a '*Yi*, Liv in metal' unlike *qi* treatment the creative impulse emanating from the great movement fire must be softened.

EARTH TOO METALLIC

Dampness is crucial for transformation and transportation. Too much metal dehydrates and hinders the functions of earth. Too much metal in earth affects the spiritual source *yi*, which can cause rigidity and sluggishness in engagement. People have difficulty in changing and thinking. Processing input (thoughts, feelings, circumstances, conversations and so on) and memory deteriorate. A malfunctioning earth can affect the digestive system and cause malnutrition.

METAL TOO EARTHY

Usually, the earth phase nourishes the metal phase and people feel supported at first. However, an excess of earth and dampness can become physically and behaviourally limiting. Physically this is reflected in dampness in tissues and on a spiritual level in dampness in the earth-*po*; stagnation causes worries and feelings of regret. People are easily obsessed and have poor self-esteem.

'*Geng,* L.i. in metal' treat with '*Yi,* Liv in metal'

METAL TOO METALLIC

Too much metal leads to dryness, constriction, stagnation, hardness, stiffness, sharpness and stringency with less nuanced behaviour. Physical problems such as stiffness, dry skin, tight connective tissue and reduced organ mobility are often in the foreground. Greed and possessiveness, or the opposite, indifference and generosity, occur. Too much metal can cause everything to be collected and stored, but can also lead to everything being given up and given away.

The emphasis on the seven *po* causes material and physical orientation, in which animal instincts play a leading role. Emotionally, people quickly and unconsciously go into fight, flight or freeze mode or unconsciously choose denial to defend their feelings of insecurity. Treatments are only feasible if there is a sense of safety (great movement earth) and social and introspective interactions (great movement metal) are possible.

The metal-*po* dominates; underlying feelings of shame, disappointment, guilt, sadness and fear determine the behaviour; it can range from introversion to overly defensive. In most cases, relationships are characterized by twists and turns and breakups.

METAL TOO WOODY: SEE 'YI, LIV IN METAL'

WOOD TOO METALLIC: SEE 'YI, LIV IN METAL'

The great movement metal tends to subdue the great movement wood and affects all wood, including the *qi* of the liver, whereas the unlike *qi* 'Yi, Liv in metal' is crucial for 'Geng, L.i. in metal'.

The flexible vitality of the easily adapting *qi* of 'Yi, Liv in metal' is essential for 'Geng, L.i. in metal' to be in balance. Without these features, the metal *qi* will mainly turn inward and harden.

> Truly complicated living conditions have left a 44-year-old 'Geng, L.i. in metal' patient at her wits' end. She has to file a lawsuit against her ex-husband for the health care of her children, she has a huge amount of stress at work due to reorganization and in her close circle of friends a number of people are fatally ill. Her childhood was uncomfortable. She wielded no power but had to move with the whims of her family. She has never learned to stand up for herself, which is exactly what she feels she needs to do now. She has trouble falling asleep and sleeping through the night, due to the heat of her body.
>
> Upon inquiry, there were several symptoms of 'empty heat': dry stools, dry mouth and a warm body, especially at night, a rapid pulse with yin insufficiency. In more detail the pulse diagnosis showed yin insufficiency, especially of the liver, spleen and kidney *qi*, fire was generally overactive and large intestine constricted tight.
>
> 'Empty heat' does not usually develop within a fortnight, it arises after long periods of yin deficiency, sometimes years of struggling with exhaustion. Her current circumstances were apparently the straw that broke the camel's back. While her *wei qi* (liver) and her mental-emotional backbone (spleen) are weak the heat of 'empty heat' is used to keep herself afloat. She feels trapped in

her emotions and does not know how to defend herself against the intense feelings and 'attacks' of her ex and the 'betrayal' of life.

The constricted, tight pulse of the large intestine is a sign of yin insufficiency with cold or pain. In her case, it is her innate *qi*, which means that she is ill in her 'own' *qi*. This is an important fact: It may take longer to restore health when people are ill in their 'own' *qi*. It means she lacks her innate strengths, namely a good defence system against external pathogenic factors. In addition she lacks a certain amount of introspection and self-knowledge.

Most of her complaints can be healed by treating liver *qi*, the unlike *qi*. The unlike *qi* restores the influence of the great movement on the heavenly stem. Some acupuncture points on the liver channel nourish the yin in general and can generate the much-needed relaxation. 'Empty heat' should decrease as a result of the treatment.

Before discussing the treatment further I would like to draw your attention to two other aspects of the liver. Falling asleep is a change in state of consciousness which is governed by liver *qi*: the *qi* that enables people to adapt to changing circumstances.

The effect of the treatment on resilience is better understood when the concept of the liver axis is understood. This topic, with the explanation of the related liver points, is covered in Chapter 43.

The treatment: Liv-3, *Tai Chong*, Liv-13, *Zhang Men*, on the left side, and Cv-10, *Xia Wan*.

Not much needs to be said about Liv-3. When treated on the left side, Liv-13, the *hui* point for the *zang* and the *mu* point of the spleen, affects life-oriented *qi*.[8]

Cv-10 affects the kidneys, strengthens empty *qi* and transfers *wei qi* and fluids to the kidneys. Together with Liv-3 and Liv-13 it boosts self-confidence.

During treatment, the patient fell deeply asleep. When she woke up ten minutes after the needles were removed, she shared that she had had a very clear dream about her father. We did not enter into the dream at that time. Instead I asked her to just do things that day she was really looking forward to. Two weeks later she shared that she had slept well since and felt ready to face the world again.

---

8   Liv-13 on the right affects form-oriented *qi*: when disturbed *qi* has led to changes in form.

'*BING*, S.I. IN WATER' – '*XIN*, LU IN WATER'

The innate water–fire interaction in '*Bing*, S.i. in water' seeks its way to the outside world, while '*Xin*, Lu in water' connects with the authentic source within. Despite a well-integrated awareness, the challenge for people born with '*Bing*, S.i. in water' is to connect to the authentic source. People born with '*Xin*, Lu in water' are challenged to live a socially acceptable life based on honesty and truth without feeling they are losing their own values.

'*Bing*, S.i. in water' treat with '*Xin*, Lu in water'

FIRE TOO WATERY

It greatly affects the *shen* when the great movement water overwhelms the heavenly stem *Bing*. It affects the way the *shen* coordinates and organizes and may cause disorders in the clarity of mind, senses, movements, thoughts, feelings, perceptions and will. When clouded perceptions settle in the heart-*shen*, the quality of blood changes. This affects the accuracy of memory, especially long-term memory, but also the perception and assessment of reality. Sometimes people seem to live in their own created reality and it is difficult to get through to them. And although everyone lives in their own created reality in many ways, when fire becomes too watery it seems as if freedom of thought and perception are lacking. The touchstone of the truth then lies only in one's own perception of reality, because one's own truth is leading and everything that does not meet it is ignored or rejected.

WATER TOO FIERY

The most notable effect is a fiery willpower. The *zhi* drives people forward: Goals must be achieved, projects must be completed and the agenda is full. The drive pushes away all fears and insecurities until burnout occurs and fears become all the more intense. Prevention is necessary, but is difficult, because the always active personality seems unstoppable. The combination of the two fundamental forces water and fire is life-giving and inspiring but can bring people to the brink of existence and can lead to deep depression and other serious diseases. A healthy relationship of water and fire has the potential to experience intense spiritual development and fulfilment.

EARTH TOO WATERY: SEE '*JIA*, GB IN EARTH'

WATER TOO EARTHY: SEE '*JIA*, GB IN EARTH'

'*Xin*, Lu in water' treat with '*Bing*, S.i. in water'

METAL TOO WATERY

Too much water in metal causes a disturbed internalization of experiences and a restless foundation. There is just too much moisture; long-lasting dampness and excess fluids, deterioration, decay and reduced *wei qi* occur and allow external pathogenic factors to enter the channel system. Too much fluid and coldness may cause complaints in the lung, intestines and, if this persists, may result in swollen joints and stiffness of the spine. In addition it may lead to inertia, aloofness, timidness, shyness, increased introversion and the need for more protection and defence. It can also cause feelings of resentment and anger and strengthen assertiveness in response to the dominance of the water-*po*, which causes uncertainty, fear and loneliness.

The cold water may attract heat causing unexpected rebellious movements, which, for instance, cause heartburn, more pain due to stagnation, vomiting, coughing of phlegm that is accompanied by inner tension in the thorax and abdomen, fits of anger, grief and sadness.

WATER TOO METALLIC

The coldness of water and the dryness and constriction of metal can obstruct the movements of water, *jing* and *zhi*. This causes the will (*zhi*) and *jing* to become hard and rigid. The powerless and withdrawn *jing* is unable to support the *shen* and causes a disturbed maintenance of the body and reduced happiness in life and may affect the desire to live.

The lack of movement of water is often offset by engagement in sports, dancing, sex or anything else that keeps *qi* moving, especially since 'frozen' water cannot nourish the wood. With these addictive behaviours it may take quite some time for these people to find a healthy alternative. Putting pressure and stress on these people may lead to the desire for perfection and more limitless behaviour, which causes the natural power of the *jing* to be further depleted.

Breaking through substantial rigidity through crying, anger or any other emotion that softens the rigidity leads to a temporary solution. Such a break-through is the right time to remind the person of authentic intuition that all people possess, but especially those born with '*Xin*, Lu in water'.

Point of attention: A pulse that is constricted can be easily missed due to the severity of the constriction.

WOOD TOO WATERY

Water is the mother of wood. Initially the water supports and people feel quite good and vital. When the amount of water becomes too large, it obstructs rather than supports. Vitality is smothered and the free flow of *qi* is slowed down until it blocks. Symptoms arise: pain at the flanks, moodiness, irregular periods, globus sensation and so on.

The balance between the *hun* and *shen* is possibly disturbed. An obstructed *hun* results in depression, lack of creativity, imagination, dreaming, disturbed sensitivity. It may cause restlessness, a chaotic mind, confusion and unsettled-ness when the coldness of water attracts heat and the change between behaviours becomes unpredictable.

WATER TOO WOODY

Active wood in water causes more desires, passions, overwork and so on; here the *zhi* (will) is overused. But there is more: When the *zhi* turns inward it causes people to keep talking about past experiences. They might talk about their difficult childhood, about problems at work, about problems with their partners, about the violent world and so forth. This behaviour is not aimed to solve problems, just to talk about them. Exchanging ideas can be interesting but it doesn't solve problems and people remain tense and emotional about their experiences. The power of their evoked sensations is as strong as the power of the wind and drives the movement of emotions within them. People may calm down when they learn to observe their self within its environment.

Being able to feel the cooperation of the kidney-*jing*-essence and the *zhi*-will with the heart-*shen*, the basis of the desiring consciousness, is the first step towards emancipation and individualization. Therefore, besides the treatment of the unlike *qi* 'Bing, S.i. in water', treatment should be accompanied by balancing 'Ding, Ht in wood' and *jing qi* which is best done through a balancing treatment of 'Gui, Ki in fire'.

'DING, HT IN WOOD' – 'REN, BL IN WOOD'

It is hard to put up with the burden of setbacks for the sunny nature of people born with 'Ding, Ht in wood'. They prefer to avoid misery but life can put people inexorably in front of it. The challenge for these people is to internalize the radiant sunny nature and look into the abyss of the self where the power for regeneration can be found. People born with 'Ren, Bl in wood' are challenged to bear their burdens by propagating humaneness and cordiality. When they succeed, the bliss of their passion becomes the vehicle of communication.

'Ding, Ht in wood' treat with 'Ren, Bl in wood'

Both 'possibilities' of 'Ding, Ht in wood' disturb the relationship between the shen and hun.

FIRE TOO WOODY

'Fire too woody' causes the shen to become restless. People are easily excited and may even be manic and limitless in behaviour and expectations. They can be carried away with enthusiasm so that they no longer realize that they are exhausting themselves. Unfortunately, the depletion of jing often leads to serious illness. Only supporting the jing is not enough, first the balance within the great movement wood must be restored.

The most notable symptom of 'fire too woody' is talkative behaviour in times of stress. In addition unlimited activity and lack of rest is observed, justified by feelings of compassion for others.

When the fire breaks out, it flows to metal, especially into the lungs. The fire-po becomes dominant, leading to more nervousness and excitement. Pain in the area around Lu-1 is the first indication of outbreak of fire and foreshadows grief that even may lead to depression if left unchecked and untreated.

The fiery character of the pulse is more evident than the wood. Advice should therefore focus on the fiery qualities.

WOOD TOO FIERY

The behavioural image is similar to the previous one: The fiery hun may cause aggression, irritability, restlessness and a tendency to burn out. People are very goal-oriented and keep working until something is finished. People are full of plans, but not all of them are realized. Making plans and having expectations and creative ideas is a sport in itself.

Point of attention: the increase in fire attracts water. This may cause cysts, joint swelling or disturbances in lymph flow. In some cases polyps and cysts appear near areas of bone marrow as a result of an outbreak of jing qi.

Wood too fiery can be observed by a scattered pulse (San Mai): floating, wide and without a root. Increased pressure on the artery makes the pulse irregular, more scattered and chaotic, and when the pressure is increased more the pulse is almost impossible to define.

A scattered pulse (a possible sign of fire too woody or wood too fiery) goes along with severe exhaustion of the *jing qi* and/or *yuan qi*.

'*Ren*, Bl in wood' treat with '*Ding*, Ht in wood'

WATER TOO WOODY: SEE '*XIN*, LU IN WATER'

WOOD TOO WATERY: SEE '*XIN*, LU IN WATER'

METAL TOO WOODY: SEE '*GENG*, L.I. IN METAL'

WOOD TOO METALLIC: SEE '*GENG*, L.I. IN METAL'

'*WU*, ST IN FIRE' – '*GUI*, KI IN FIRE'

Usually, the unlike *qi* offers the solution to balance the great movement; however, with the great movement fire it is more complicated. In many cases '*Gui*, Ki in fire' causes a great urge for activity and depletion of the *jing qi*, as does '*Wu*, St in fire'. The challenge for people born with '*Wu*, St in fire' and '*Gui*, Ki in fire' is to keep the *jing* collected.

Since the *zhi* (will) causes the *shen* to interact with the *jing*, it is worth exploring the development of the will. This includes the will of the baby, the adolescent, the will of thinking and feeling, the will of the adult, the will of wisdom, the wisdom of the will and so on. This subject cannot be covered in detail here. What is essential to this chapter is that if, in adulthood, the will remains focused on the achievement of goals, the *jing* can be exhausted. This is evident from poor concentration and memory and is accompanied by dizziness and absentmindedness.

'*Gui*, Ki in fire' may direct the *zhi* inwardly to connect with the true self and the manifestation of the emanation *zhen*. This may lead to acceptance of impermanence and limitations of existence but, above all, it can yield the awareness of and discrimination between the power of desire and the power of silence.

The challenge for people born with '*Gui*, Ki in fire' is to discover the internal path of creativity that comes with playfulness and timeless experiences. Timelessness is not even the right word; these are events in which time plays no role at all. I often ask patients born with '*Gui*, Ki in fire' what they enjoyed most as a child. Sometimes it takes a while, but the forgotten pleasure of it sparkles in their eyes when they start talking about it. Remembrance of it and actually doing it is often the key to the internal path of creativity and helps to encourage people to make space for happiness.

'*Wu*, St in fire' treat with '*Gui*, Ki in fire'

EARTH TOO FIERY: SEE '*JI*, SP IN EARTH'

FIRE TOO EARTHY: SEE '*JI*, SP IN EARTH'

'*Gui*, Ki in fire' treat with '*Wu*, St in fire'

WATER TOO FIERY: SEE '*BING*, S.I. IN WATER'

FIRE TOO WATERY: SEE '*BING*, S.I. IN WATER'

METAL TOO FIERY

The precarious relationship between fire and metal is briefly discussed in the section 'Fire too woody' with '*Ding*, Ht in wood'. Fire and metal need each other – metal is the objective material world in which the subtle aspect of fire, the *shen*, can express and reflect itself. In addition heat is badly needed to prevent the metal from hardening. Without the warmth of fire, the instinctual forces of the seven *po* would consolidate and become unmanageable. However, too much fire in metal is harmful and causes disorder. People lose their fixed daily structure and basic instincts tend to become disoriented. It makes people feel lost. This emotional condition is described as a feeling of no longer being in control of the body and social relationships.

First people suffer from breathing problems with stagnation in the upper burner, later from stagnation in the middle burner. When the fire grows stronger through stagnation, structures lose their strength and vitality and stagnation turns into emptiness. People become short of breath, get diarrhoea, can no longer maintain their physical strength and feel like they can never get better.

The very first requirement is to restore the balance of the great movement fire by treating '*Wu*, St in fire' rather than treating the lung and other organs related to the stagnation and emptiness. It enables people 'to say no' to the useless and unwanted and 'say yes' to the useful and desired. People might have been able to discern the useful and the useless, but they regain the power to take a stand with a balanced great movement fire.

FIRE TOO METALLIC

Fire that becomes too metallic first causes feelings of self-assurance. It is as if a difficult theory and its usefulness are suddenly understood. This is the influence of strong metal on fire and we need that! (I hope it happens at some point while reading this book.)

But fire becomes obstructed when metal overwhelms fire, which causes symptoms and diseases in several areas: the digestive system, the blood circulation, the heart-*shen* – it affects the relationship with others – the circulation of fluids and so on.

Practice has taught me that *san jiao* in particular is the most vulnerable to too much dryness. It causes, for instance, dry eyes, constipation, epicondylitis and so on. For people born with '*Gui*, Ki in fire', these types of diseases should first be treated at the level of the great movement fire – of course, only when pulse diagnosis confirms an imbalance in the stomach *qi*. It should be noted again that constriction of the *san jiao* pulse is often missed due to a possible high degree of constriction. The pulse is then incorrectly diagnosed as thin or absent.

A FINAL NOTE

People may express themselves more in their unlike *qi* than in their 'own' *qi*. For example, people born with '*Ding*, Ht in wood' may express behaviour related to '*Ren*, Bl in wood'. This can even lead to one or more of the 'four possibilities' of '*Ren*, Bl in wood', such as wood too watery and metal too woody. It might indicate a deep weakness of the innate *qi* '*Ding*, Ht in wood'. '*Ren*, Bl in wood' as a survival strategy was chosen to overcome or endure a traumatic situation. Usually deep psychological trauma, in which the individual has been deeply touched in their being and identity, is at the root of this imbalance. They probably needed a childhood survival strategy that can be treated, preferably in collaboration with a psychologist, but it may take a long time for the 'own' stronger innate *qi* to return.

PULSES AND ADVICE[9]

Too much earth in the pulse shows as yielding, soft, slightly thick with a denser centre.

Advice: Salty and more bitter foods to dry the dampness.

Too much metal in the pulse can manifest itself in different ways: It is either very light and empty upwards and disappears quickly or can be sharp, constricted, flat or hard. There is dryness and lack of yin, *xuè* or fluids.

Advice: Wood disdains constriction. Apply sweet flavours to soften and harmonize the *qi*.

Too much water in the pulse feels soft and a little elastic; on the surface it is a little hard and thin; in the depth it is more rapid and hard on pressure and disappears slowly.

Advice: Salty and bitter foods to dry and descend the *qi* and warming foods against the cold of water.

Too much wood in the pulse leads to a pulse that comes up quickly and firmly and is more flexible than constricted.

Advice: Healthy acidic, astringent flavours to gather the *qi*.

Too much fire in the pulse moves the *qi* in all directions, mostly upwards. It may feel sharp on the surface (earthly fire) or slippery on a deeper level (heavenly fire).

Advice: Pungent food to disperse, sour food to astringe, bitter food to purge and disperse and an overall cooling diet.

Further advice: Water disdains the dryness of fire. It is advisable to give food and flavours that lubricate, such as pungent foods.

---

9   For dietary advice the following are advised: Chapters 3, 4, 10, 22, 23 of the *Huang Di Nei Jing Su Wen* and Chapters 36, 56, 63, 65 of the *Ling Shu*.

PART II

The TWELVE EARTHLY BRANCHES and DEEP *QI*

I'm told that when one is good at discussing the law of heaven,
he must be able to verify the law of heaven to man.[1]

---

1   *Huang Di Nei Jing Su Wen* Chapter 39, translated in Bing, Wu and Wu 1997, p. 91.

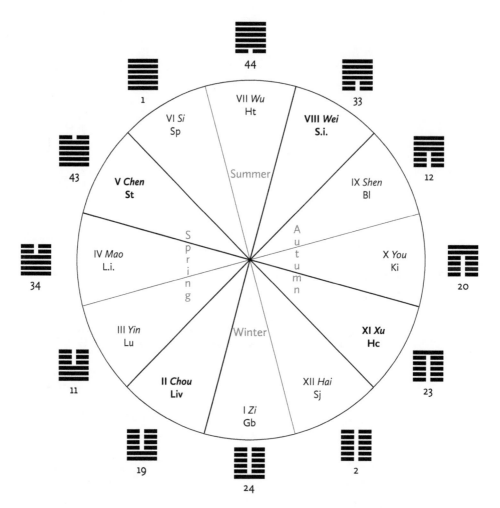

Figure II.1 Earthly branches, seasonal qi and deep qi with related hexagrams

Figure II.1 shows the order of the twelve earthly branches with their Chinese names in pinyin, the place they have in the seasonal cycle and the twelve tidal hexagrams.[2] The earthly branches *Chou, Chen, Wei* and *Xu* mark the transition from each of the four seasons to the next.

2 See Appendix II.

CHAPTER 23

INTRODUCTION

The earth and humanity are suffering from climate change, hunger and wars. I have often wondered how it is possible for the body to be so beautiful and strong. It is usually in a fairly healthy state, even though people often do not take good care of it. Diseases are warded off, our human self-healing ability leads to recovery, while humanity's heart suffers and the world seems to be getting sicker. Or do the world and humanity as a whole have the same capacity for recovery as the *qi* system?

If we take the view that human behaviour is harmful both to the world and humanity, it makes sense to study how the behaviour of the organs and channels of our *qi* system balances the suffering human being ('earth and humanity'), restores health and provides balance and tranquillity to the body functions, despite the unhealthy behaviour of so many humans. Although there are serious diseases and pandemics, the promotion of health of the body's *qi* system is usually quite successful! Sometimes though it needs the help of a practitioner of a medicine that affects *qi*. I strongly believe that human beings can contribute to the health of the earth and humanity by pursuing health in themselves. It's worth a try.

YEAR

The second part of this book discusses the meaning and development of the cycle of the twelve earthly branches and channels. Each year, month, day and hour is assigned a heavenly stem and an earthly branch. In this book we mainly focus on the heavenly stems and earthly branches of the year.

We calculate the *qi* configuration of a year from the day of the Chinese New Year. For instance, the influences of earthly branch *Yin*, lung, start from 1 February 2022 till the next Chinese New Year on 22 January 2023.

Table 23.1 Earthly branches of the year

Zi	Gb	1924/1984	1936/1996	1948/2008	1960/2020	1972/2032
Chou	Liv	1925/1985	1937/1997	1949/2009	1961/2021	1973/2033
Yin	Lu	1926/1986	1938/1998	1950/2010	1962/**2022**	1974/2034
Mao	L.i.	1927/1987	1939/1999	1951/2011	1963/**2023**	1975/2035
Chen	St	1928/1988	1940/2000	1952/2012	1964/2024	1976/2036
Si	Sp	1929/1989	1941/2001	1953/2013	1965/2025	1977/2037
Wu	Ht	1930/1990	1942/2002	1954/2014	1966/2026	1978/2038
Wei	S.i.	1931/1991	1943/2003	1955/2015	1967/2027	1979/2039
Shen	Bl	1932/1992	1944/2004	1956/2016	1968/2028	1980/2040
You	Ki	1933/1993	1945/2005	1957/2017	1969/2029	1981/2041
Xu	Hc	1934/1994	1946/2006	1958/2018	1970/2030	1982/2042
Hai	Sj	1935/1995	1947/2007	1959/2019	1971/2031	1983/2043

MONTH

Each year basically has twelve lunar months – from new moon to the next new moon.[1] Each month refers to an earthly branch. Many books start counting from spring with the earthly branch *Yin*, lung, but the cycle of earthly branches begins in winter with the earthly branch *Zi*, gallbladder. The cycle begins with the invisible growth in a seed deep in the earth in winter and finds its peak with the adult plant showing its splendour in summer. The first half of the year cycle is governed by six earthly branches, *Zi*, *Chou*, *Yin*, *Mao*, *Chen* and *Si*. They embody the yang half of the cycle that describes growth and flowering. The second, yin, half of the cycle is governed by the earthly branches *Wu*, *Wei*, *Shen*, *You*, *Xu* and *Hai*. The *qi* withdraws from physical revelation and returns into the seed in winter.

The flow of the cycle of the earthly branches rises and falls around the vertical axis of winter–summer (equivalent to the direction North–South). This is different from the cycle of heavenly stems, which starts in the East with *Jia* and *Yi* and withdraws in the West with *Geng* and *Xin*. The cycle of heavenly stems circulates around the horizontal axis spring–autumn and the direction East–West. The horizontal axis symbolizes the created physical revelation on

---

1   Because the lunar month has fewer days than the solar months of the Western calendar, an extra month is inserted every few years, making one extended 'month' which serves to match the solar and lunar calendars.

the earth. The vertical axis begins in the North and symbolizes the essence of a human's response to its origin, which is the Universal Spark of heaven.

It is noteworthy that almost all channels are related to more than one phase of the *wuxing*. For example, the gallbladder relates to sunrise, spring and wood. In the cycle of the earthly branches and Chinese hourly clock it relates to midnight, winter and water. It presents its third quality as a *shao yang* channel which belongs to midday, summer and fire.

As another example, the small intestine relates to the end of the summer and fire. It transforms *qi* from summer into autumn. As a *tai yang* channel it relates to winter and water.

The heart channel, however, is unique. It relates to fire in the five phases, seasons, six divisions (*shao yin*) and the cycle of the earthly branches. The special character of the heart is recognized by the philosopher Mencius when he says that noble people consider their nature, rooted in the heart, as benevolence, righteousness, ceremonial insight and wisdom. He continues that these four virtues are reflected in a clear and bright face and lead to a supple back and limbs. The message of the heart and its virtues are expressed in the whole body and its physical characteristics can be observed. No words are needed, he says.

In this context, the discussion in Chapter 9 of the *Huang Di Nei Jing Su Wen* is most interesting. It states that 'since ancient times the roots of life are consistent in communication with the heavens and those roots are yin and yang'. A little further on, it says that '*the heart is a root of life* which has control over the changing spirit, which glory is manifested in the face'. This is a distinctive comment. Normally, water and kidneys, and not the heart, store the *jing* and are seen as the root of life. In Chapter 9 of the *Huang Di Nei Jing Su Wen* the kidney is said to be *the root of sealed storage and pure qi*. In other words, the chapter emphasizes the important relationship between the heart and kidney in five phases theory.

The vertical axis of water and fire is just as important for the cycle of the earthly branches, although here it is not related to kidneys and heart but to the gallbladder and heart. This cycle starts in water, earthly branch *Zi*, gallbladder, expands to fire, the earthly branch *Wu*, heart, and decreases again to return to water, the earthly branch *Zi*, gallbladder.

CHAPTER 24

SEASONAL *QI*

Table 24.1 Seasonal *qi* in one year

XII	*Hai, san jiao*	Winter	Water
I	*Zi*, gallbladder	Winter	Water
II	*Chou*, liver	Winter	*Earth*
III	*Yin*, lung	Spring	Wood
IV	*Mao*, large intestine	Spring	Wood
V	*Chen*, stomach	Spring	*Earth*
VI	*Si*, spleen	Summer	Fire
VII	*Wu*, heart	Summer	Fire
VIII	*Wei*, small intestine	Summer	*Earth*
IX	*Shen*, bladder	Autumn	Metal
X	*You*, kidneys	Autumn	Metal
XI	*Xu*, heart constrictor	Autumn	*Earth*

Each season has a relationship with three different earthly branches, the last of which accompanies the transition from one season to another, and is therefore connected to the earth phase. This is different to the concept of the five phases in which the spleen governs the last eighteen days of a season. The spleen supports the complete cycle of seasons from the centre. In the cycle of the twelve earthly branches four different *qi* govern the transition: The liver governs the transitions from the last days of the winter to spring, the stomach from last days of spring to summer, the small intestine from the last days of summer to autumn and the heart constrictor from the last days of autumn to winter. These four earth-related earthly branches ensure smooth transition from one season into the next. The treatment of these earth-related earthly branches takes place during the first days of the following seasons, because it is only then that it can be determined whether the transition has taken place properly.

In winter the *qi* withdraws inward and is stored in a small protected place, causing the normal pulse to be inside, sunken, strong at the bottom, denser and sometimes even constricted.[1] It is important to realize that the inward moving *qi* in winter does not only come from the kidneys and bladder, as we know from *wuxing* theory. It is also caused by the *qi* of the gallbladder and *san jiao* related to the earthly branches *Zi* and *Hai*, respectively. When the pulse in the winter feels weak and yielding and has a rapid rate, the receding movement of autumn and winter has not gathered enough *qi*; if someone has a weaker constitution, disease is expected to occur within a few days. If the constitutional *qi* is stronger, illness can appear one to even two seasons later.[2] The weakened gathered *qi* of winter is a poor breeding ground for the strength needed in spring and the liver earth-related *qi* will not be able to provide a smooth transition. People may suffer from spring fatigue, muscle pain, hay fever and spring flu.

The three months of spring generate growth out of the stored *qi* of winter. A pulse in springtime that rises too slowly or too quickly can be the result of a disturbance in the seasonal (wood) *qi* of the gallbladder, liver, lungs and large intestine. If this is discovered at the beginning of spring and it is understood that it is caused by disturbed winter *qi*, the liver earth-related *qi* must first be treated to guide a good transition from winter to spring. Living against the rhythm of *qi* of spring can cause diseases in summer due to coldness.

The three months of the summer generate growth and blossoming and the formation of shapes. The summer pulse must rise quickly and go slowly. If this pulse is disrupted, the fire-related *qi* of the heart, small intestine, heart constrictor and *san jiao* as well as the spleen might be involved. If summer lasts longer than expected according to the calendar, in the first days of autumn the earth-related *qi* of the small intestine needs to be treated. Living against the rhythm of *qi* of the summer can cause intermittent fevers in autumn.

The autumn pulse should be light and empty upwards, sometimes even small and rough; the *qi* and *xuè* turn inward. If the pulse remains too yang and superficial the metal-related *qi* of the lung, large intestine, kidney and bladder may be involved. If autumn lasts longer than expected according to the calendar, during the early days of winter the earth-related heart constrictor needs to be addressed. Living against the rhythm of *qi* of the autumn can cause shortage of *qi* with digestive problems in winter.

---

1 Staying indoors by a warm fireplace or heater in winter creates too much dry heat that amplifies the rising *qi* of spring and summer. It may cause tonsillitis and sinusitis in spring or summer.
2 This pattern applies to all seasons.

SEASONAL *QI* IN THE CHINESE HOURLY CLOCK

The earthly branches with related channels divide the year into twelve lunar months. The day is divided into twelve periods of two hours. The flow of *qi* in these cycles of twelve different *qi* is subject to tidal conditions. Every month and every two hours, another earthly branch is in a state of high tide, while the earthly branch related to the opposite month and the opposite two-hour period is in a state of low tide. So when the earthly branch *Zi*, gallbladder, is active and dynamic in winter, the opposite earthly branch *Wu*, heart, is passive and more static. The same pattern can be seen in the daily cycle for the time between 11 p.m. and 1 a.m. and 11 a.m. and 1 p.m.

In the seasonal cycle and organ clock, the earthly branch and its channel nourish their successor in the next season and two-hour period. So *Zi* nourishes *Chou* which nourishes *Yin* and so on. This order of earthly branches explains that, for example, the fire point Sp-2, *Da Du*, nourishes the heart, in contrast to the theory of *wuxing* where fire generates earth according to the *sheng* generating cycle.[3]

Method of high and low tide

A number of techniques have been described to treat the flow of the earthly branches and channels through the 'seasons of the day'; one of the techniques is the 'high tide low tide' method. Though this method is being used clinically, in my opinion it is not practical and rather symptomatic in approach because it focuses mainly on complaints and often neglects the wholeness of the human being.

Constitutional acupuncture focuses not only on the complaints and symptoms but on the whole person by taking into consideration all the different correspondences and mutual relationships that determine the totality of the human being.

During the high tide of an earthly branch and channel, all acupuncture points on that channel are open for treatment. For instance, all points on the spleen channel are open between 9 and 11 a.m. This can be useful if the practitioner knows that the spleen needs to be treated.

However, the practice of constitutional acupuncture is different. In a case of spleen *qi* disturbance, the practitioner of constitutional acupuncture will focus on the spleen's partner in the *wuxing*: the stomach. Another method treats the

---

3   I assume from this point that the reader is already familiar with the theory and dynamism of the Chinese months and organ clock.

opposite *qi* in the annual or daily cycle, in this case *san jiao*. These methods are called 'like *qi*' and 'unlike *qi*' treatments, respectively.[4]

The method of high and low tide is beneficial when complaints always take place at the same time in the day or month. For example, people who urinate every night between 3 and 5 a.m. – due to the state of high tide lung *qi* at that time, there is naturally lung *qi shi*, while at the same time there is a bladder *qi xu* due to the state of low tide. The bladder is not strong enough to hold the urine. Due to the dynamic relationship between lung and bladder, the insufficiency of the bladder becomes more evident during that time.

However, in constitutional acupuncture we choose to treat the lung between 3 and 5 *p.m.* In this way, the bladder *qi* is strengthened, partly because lung *qi* is unlike *qi* of the bladder and partly because lung *qi* governs fluids which at that time has more influence on the bladder function.

Method of the reinforcing mother point: Treating insufficiencies

This method uses the principles of the five phases and the Chinese hour clock.

The treatment principles are as follows:

- Diagnose the insufficient *qi*.
- Find the mother of the insufficient *qi* in the *wuxing*.
- Reinforce the *qi* of the mother to treat the initial diagnosed insufficient *qi*. The mother nourishes the son.

An example: Kidney *qi* is insufficient. The mother of kidneys is lung.[5]

The best way to treat the lung *qi* is when the high tide of the lung decreases. Treatment aims to prolong the high tide period. The best time for treatment is just after high tide, when lung *qi* slowly decreases.

High tide of the lung is between 3 and 5 a.m.; the time of treatment should be between 5 and 6 a.m.[6]

The point indicated is the tonification point of the lung, Lu-9, *Tai Yuan*, great abyss.

---

4   See Chapters 39–43.
5   Yin feeds yin and yang feeds yang in the *wuxing sheng* cycle. In a case where the bladder *qi* is insufficient treat the large intestine and so on.
6   That is quite early for the patient and the practitioner, but not impossible if the complaints justify it. Although it is less effective, you can also choose to treat twelve hours later.

In short:

Find the insufficiency	Kidneys
Find the mother in five phases	Lungs
Find branch time (*first hour*) after the mother	Large intestine time between 5 and 6 a.m.
Treat tonification point of the mother	Lu-9

This example describes how the vital *qi* of the earthly branch *Yin*, lungs, can be used to effectively treat the kidneys during the high tide of the earthly branch *Mao*, large intestine, when the *qi* of the lung is already decreasing.

Method of the reducing son point: Treating excesses

This is a method that I do not fully support because caution is advised with sedation, especially when there are no external pathogenic factors; sedation might also sedate constitutional and essential *qi*. Yet, for the sake of completeness, this method is described here.

The treatment principles are as follows:

Find the excess	Bladder
Find branch time during high tide when the *qi* is still rising (*first hour*)	3–4 p.m.
Treat the sedation point on the excess diagnosed channel	Sedation of Bl-65

This method treats the excess of *qi* directly with the aim of reducing the *qi* when it is still rising at high tide time. The five phases are not taken into account in this method. It is a method that works well, but in constitutional acupuncture we focus on strengthening and hence balancing the *qi*. Excess bladder *qi* is always accompanied by insufficiency elsewhere, for example in related channels such as in the lung (unlike *qi*), kidneys (like *qi*) or spleen (*wuxing*, spleen not controlling bladder).

Method of accelerating the *flow* of *qi*: Treating excesses

This method is used in cases of excess *qi* at high tide in one of the channels.

> A female patient suffers every single morning. When she wakes up, she has an enormous amount of snot and saliva in her nose and mouth and often sneezes violently. In addition she suffers from sore, red and irritated eyes and, surprisingly to her, she is very hungry every morning. The symptoms disappear completely in a few hours.

It is striking that the patient feels much better twelve hours later. There are no other symptoms than a slightly bloated, distended stomach in the afternoon. Pulse diagnosis confirms excess stomach *qi* in the morning between 7 a.m. and 9 a.m.

The treatment principles are as follows:

The excess of stomach high tide is treated during the increase of the high tide, which is the first hour of its two-hour period. The reinforcing mother point is the tonification point of the preceding earthly branch channel. This point is treated during the first half of the excess (stomach) high tide channel time with oblique insertion with the *flow* – clockwise turning for a yang channel and anti-clockwise turning for a yin channel.[7] The aim of the treatment is to accelerate the pace of the *flow* of *qi*, which flattens the peak of high tide excess. This has a sedating effect! The high tide excess peak is no longer reached because the *qi* is forwarded to the next channel at an accelerated pace.

Summary:

Find the excess	Stomach[8]
Find reinforcing mother point (tonification point)	L.i.-11, *Qu Chi*, crooked pond
Treat during first half of the excess high tide time	First half *Chen* time, between 7 and 8 a.m.

Insertion is oblique *with* the flow,
Clockwise technique for a yang channel
Slowly in, manipulate carefully on expiration,
Quickly out and close the hole.

The intensified flow of *qi* through the earthly branch *Mao*, large intestine, accelerates the *flow* of *qi* in the channels. It reduces the excess of stomach *qi* during *Chen* time.

---

7   Looking at humans with the arms up, all yang channels flow from top to bottom and all yin channels from bottom to top. Viewed from above, the direction of flow of the yang channels is clockwise. Looking at the same flow from below, it is an anti-clockwise movement. To further clarify this phenomenon, you can hold your index fingers together in front of your chest. Make a circle with the joint index fingers by first turning them away from you and then turn back again. The right hand now makes a clockwise movement and the left hand an anti-clockwise movement. It is exactly the same movement, but the perspective from which the direction of the flow is viewed and treated is different.

8   See Table 24.2.

ANOTHER EXAMPLE

A male patient suffers from chest tension, mouth ulcers, pain around the navel, hot flushes in the face and yellow coated red tongue (fire and earth). Pulse diagnosis confirms excess heat in the small intestine. The unpleasant feelings and red face increase between 1 and 3 p.m.

Find the excess	Small intestine[9]
Find reinforcing mother point (tonification point)	Ht-9, *Shao Chong*, little rushing
Treat during first half of the excess high tide time	First half *Wei* time, between 1 and 2 p.m.

> Insertion is oblique *with* the flow,
> Anti-clockwise technique for a yin channel
> Slowly in, manipulate carefully on expiration,
> Quickly out and close the hole.

Oblique insertion – in this case anti-clockwise manipulation for a yin channel – accelerates the pace of the *flow* of *qi* and results in sedation! The excess high tide is not reached because the *qi* is transmitted at an accelerated pace to the next channel, in this case to the bladder.

The intensified flow of *qi* through the earthly branch *Wu*, heart, accelerates the *flow* of *qi* in the channels. It reduces the excess of small intestine *qi* during *Wei* time.

Table 24.2 Reinforcing mother and reducing son points

	Reinforcing Mother Point	Reducing Son Point
I *Zi* 23–01 Gb	Sj-3	Gb-38
II *Chou* 01–03 Liv	Gb-43	Liv-2
III *Yin* 03–05 Lu	Liv-8	Lu-5

---

9   See Table 24.2.

IV Mao 05–07 L.i.	Lu-9	L.i.-2
V Chen 07–09 St	L.i.-11	St-45
VI Si 09–11 Sp	St-41	Sp-5
VII Wu 11–13 Ht	Sp-2	Ht-7
VIII Wei 13–15 S.i.	Ht-9	S.i.-8
IX Shen 15–17 Bl	S.i.-3	Bl-65
X You 17–19 Ki	Bl-67	Ki-1
XI Xu 19–21 Hc	Ki-7	Hc-7
XII Hai 21–23 Sj	Hc-9	Sj-10

Method of reducing the *flow* of *qi*: Treating insufficiencies

A male patient suffers from a poor appetite with dull feelings in the upper abdomen. He feels weak and tired, especially in the morning. To enjoy the day, he has to stay in bed till at least 9 a.m. His limbs constantly feel heavy and painful.

Pulse diagnosis confirms that the stomach *qi* is insufficient, which is more evident between 7 a.m. and 9 a.m.

The treatment principles are as follows:

The deficient high tide (stomach) is treated during the second half of the reduced high tide, when the *qi* of the stomach is already decreasing, by needling the reducing son point, the sedation point. Using oblique insertion against the *flow* of *qi* – anti-clockwise turning for a yang channel and clockwise turning for a yin channel[10] – the pace of the *flow* of *qi* is reduced. It is the aim to slow down the pace of the *flow* of *qi*, which builds the peak of high tide and results in tonification!

Summary:

Find the insufficiency	Stomach[11]
Find reducing son point (sedation point)	St-45, *Li Dui*, severe mouth, hard bargain
Treat second half of the insufficient high tide time	Second half *Chen*, stomach, between 8 and 9 a.m.

Insertion is oblique *against* the flow,
Anti-clockwise for a yang channel (with yin channels the manipulation is
    clockwise)
Slowly in, manipulate carefully on expiration,
Quickly out and close the hole.

The earthly branch *Chen* is used to strengthen the reduced *qi* of the stomach at earthly branch *Chen* time.

From hours to months

To my knowledge, this treatment principle is only described in relation to the hours. I have been using this technique for many years with great success on the cycle of earthly branches and months.

Hay fever, often described as caused by insufficiency of the *qi* of the lungs, kidneys, spleen and liver, is mostly due to liver *qi* insufficiency, often caused by insufficiency of the kidneys and *du mai*. As a preventative treatment I have supported kidney *qi* in the autumn during the second half of the earthly branch month *You*, kidneys (after 13 September and before 28 September in 2020[12] in the northern hemisphere).

This technique aims to reduce the flow of *qi* in the kidneys (which results in tonification!) by treating the reducing son point Ki-1 on its tendo-muscular

---

10 See previous footnote.
11 See Table 24.2.
12 In 2020 the earthly branch *You* month started on 30 August and lasted until 28 September. There are multiple apps and sites on the internet that provide information about the correct dates of the earthly branches and months.

location opposite to Bl-67, *Zhi Yin*.[13] The needle insertion is oblique against the flow, in the direction of the tip of the toe or in the direction of Bl-67.

In addition, during the hay fever season (which begins from about Chinese New Year), the *qi* is initially ruled by the month of the earthly branch *Yin*, lung. An excessive reaction of the mucous membrane of the nose may be treated with the reinforcing mother point during the first fourteen days after the Chinese New Year (the first half of the month *Yin*).

Treatment principle: Liv-8, *Qu Quan*, spring at the bend, oblique insertion with the flow. Liv-8 is a point on a yin channel, which means that a careful anti-clockwise manipulation on expiration is indicated. This treatment can reduce the excess reaction in the lung channel.

---

13   I use this example because it is the only exception regarding the location of the acupuncture point. The vital aspects of this channel are more approachable at this location.

DYNAMICS OF THE EARTHLY BRANCH *ZI* 子²

**WINTER AND WATER *QI*, THE VIRTUE OF THE SEED
SEASONAL POINT: GB-43, *XIA XI***

To you Rat, I give my seed and the honour of sowing it.
Every seed will become a plant and multiply a million times,
But you will have no time to see it grow.
You are like a small child, determined, without a plan.
You are the starting point, renewing the Idea.
You are the governor of the Gallbladder.

Your life means action, providing people with good judgement,
assertiveness, decisiveness and determination. For your
good work, I give you the virtue of Self-Assertion.

But beware. It is not your task to feed and develop or to doubt the
Idea or to use your qualities for other reasons; then you will be the
cause of unreasonable anger. Furthermore you will show signs of poor
judgement, indecisiveness and a lack of self-assertion even becoming a
hypochondriac, or you may overcompensate, becoming a self-satisfied
person complaining about all the mistakes other people make. You
have a sensitive sense of justice; the world seems wrong to you.

---

1   The title of each of the chapters on the meaning of earthly branches starts with the name of the earthly branch, followed by the corresponding seasonal *qi* with the essential qualities of the earthly branch. It is followed by an acupuncture point that represents these qualities.

2   Born in 1924, 1936, 1948, 1960, 1972, 1984, 1996, 2008, 2020, 2032 after the Chinese New Year.

So use your qualities well.[3]

The Chinese character Zi 子 represents a small child, a starting point of life. Its energy is present at birth or in a seed, in a germ from which life can sprout. This image symbolizes the first regeneration of vegetation which is still invisible to the naked eye. Zi depicts the returning of the principle of life, hidden in the seeds, in the depth of the winter, in the coldness of the North. The seeds contain all elements to become a fully grown plant in the summer. Zi is connected to midnight when the sun reaches its deepest position; it is the turning point in the cycle to enable qi/the sun to rise again in the morning/in the East.

The flow of qi in the channels begins in the North, in the winter and midnight, in the depths of essence, where water reigns under the guidance of the earthly branch Zi and the gallbladder channel.[4] Yang rises from North to South, then descends again to re-gather in the North. The movement of qi revolves around the North–South, water–fire axis.

THE VERTICAL AXIS AND HORIZONTAL PLANE

The earthly branches vertical axis (water–fire) is perpendicular to the horizontal plane of the cycle of heavenly stems. The horizontal plane of the heavenly stems refers to the manifestation of life *on* earth. The vertical axis of the earthly branches is the inner reaction, the human response to the creative qi of the heavenly stems.

Every person is unique and yet we are all essentially equal. Everyone has their own self and yet we were all conceived from an egg and a sperm cell. Everyone has their own consciousness and *shen* and yet we are all part of the consciousness and spirit of the earth.

As soon as the ego and the psyche develop, differences arise that evoke power and powerlessness and, as soon as we are born to a family, in our own culture and nationality the same thing happens. Our experiences and perspectives can be very different and yet we are all connected to the same source of life force. We are brothers and sisters of the collective consciousness of the earth and, in that

---

3   To highlight certain essences of the qualities of the earthly branch and its related Chinese astrological animal, the description of the earthly branches starts with a short poem by the author of this book. The poem was written when I remembered in a flash a story my teacher told me long ago, in which the twelve astrological animals were once called to the Buddha to receive their character and place in the Chinese calendar of the enlightened Master. The original myth is about *Yu Huang Shangdi*, the Jade emperor, inviting twelve zodiac animals to visit the deity in heaven. In my poetic inspiration I made that the Buddha.

4   And the twelfth earthly branch *Hai* and the *san jiao* channel.

sense, we could know how to meet as equals on the horizontal plane, each with their own personal zenith and nadir, heaven and earth, South and North point. Partly we are equals, partly we are fundamentally different from each other.

The twelve earthly branches are the background principles for the twelve main channels that flow from the hands to the feet and back,[5] so that each human being is a reflection of their individual zenith-nadir. The more we live in harmony with the universal and personal heaven and earth, the more likely our actions are to become authentic and true to the self. The twelve earthly branches and the *qi* in the channels support human beings to focus on that.

Heaven is not something outside of us that rules over us; heaven is anchored deeply in everyone's being as that in which we are all equal and recognize each other. In the depths of our being, the earthly branch *Zi* connects with that in which we are equals, which is, at the same time, the source of our differences.

The concept of the earthly branches demonstrates the importance of the alignment of personal psychological patterns (that is, from which people live, think, feel, talk and act) with the universal source. The earthly branch *Zi* is the invisible seed from which that alignment arises.

THE DYNAMICS OF THE BEGINNING

Suppose that this is the very first time you read about constitutional acupuncture. You are already an experienced practitioner but you feel the need to learn something new. You want to add knowledge to be able to treat your patient a little differently, hopefully better.

Or imagine that you follow a strict set of habits every day, first brushing your teeth and then taking a shower, or first eating your breakfast and then getting dressed. One day you feel so annoyed with yourself and your habits that you plan to take a different approach. You no longer want to be guided by old habits.

Or imagine that you have just treated a patient who is feeling physically and emotionally overloaded and blocked in his emotions due to the fear of what might happen with his relationship. You have given him a great treatment, massage and acupuncture. He is now able to look to the future with a completely new perspective.

These are all circumstances related to earthly branch *Zi* and the gallbladder channel: feeling the need for change and looking forward to it. The

---

5   The flow of *qi* starts in the *san jiao* channel of the left hand and goes to the head. The *qi* continues on its way to the legs via the gallbladder channel, rises again via the liver channel to the thorax and reaches the hands via the lung channel after which the other channels follow the same circuitous path, eventually ending with the heart constrictor channel at Hc-9.

transformation is based on the essence of what has been learned or experienced. The earthly branch *Zi* shields and reveals change and first ideas for renewal.

For those born with the earthly branch *Zi*, there is the innate capacity to change, to be able to regenerate and renew, even after severe illnesses. *Zi* means the ability to live multiple lives in one life, to change from one job to another, or to have several functions at the same time. But there is a pitfall. The more people try to control the process of change, the more blockages might occur in the gallbladder channel. An open mind with confidence, courage and contentment are essential for good health and free flow of this channel.

Treating the earthly branch *Zi*, the gallbladder, opens the inner door to relaxation and supports the insights and efforts of the patient to change.

ZI, HUMAN NATURE AND VIRTUE

In order to mature, humans have an inner compass of truth that must be nurtured and nourished. This seed of virtue, like other seeds, must be given sufficient 'water' in the form of guidance, reinforcement, education and inner attunement and openness to what feels right and correct.

For centuries, the Chinese people had a rather negative view of human inclinations and human nature. Morality came from and was influenced by the outside world and therefore human tendencies and the nature of people had to be taken into account in ethical rules. The Mohism school of thought[6] used punishment and reward to change and perfect the nature of humans, while the Legalists attempted to steer human conduct in the right direction through laws and regulations with punishments only. They assumed that people were bad by nature and therefore had a disruptive effect on society. The paradigms of these schools of morality, which compete with Confucian moral thought, have not gone unnoticed. For example, perverse or pathogenic *qi* is still seen as 'not correct' and treated by 'punishment', that is, an attack to remove the pathogenic *qi* rather than to enhance the innate strength of the patient.

Over time, Chinese society underwent a major change and people began to look at themselves differently; this happened due to the ideas of the philosopher Mencius. Mencius assumed that the seeds of virtue exist in every person from birth onwards and that the growth of these seeds and their maturation would be enabled by accepting and allowing intuition and inner impulses. This was a revolutionary way of thinking. Mencius didn't oppose moral rules. Rules and

---

6　There were four main schools of philosophy and society during the Spring and Autumn and Warring States Periods: Daoism, Confucianism, Mohism and Legalism.

regulations were needed to distinguish good from evil. Following the rules only because of the rules, however, was discouraged because this type of behaviour could lead to abuse of the rules and having an excuse for immoral behaviour and harm of others.

It was a major change in Chinese thinking that nourishment of the seeds of virtue could come from inner qualities and not only from external social morality. The way people communicated with their family and friends, and thereby with everyone else, was able to flow from their inner nature rather than from the rules and regulations of society.

In general, people need to find their place in society with all its rules and regulations, but the origin of our compassionate nature lies deep down in each human's being. An important role in the process of growth and development of virtues (that feeds inclinations) is undertaken by the *qi* of the innate seed (North) and the compassionate heart (South), which in turn improve the *qi* for correct living, thinking, feeling, acting and talking.

My teachers – also the five phases and French acupuncture-oriented ones – taught me to start a treatment with nurturing and nourishing innate strength. Constitutional acupuncture according to the heavenly stems and earthly branches fits very well with this premise. It is only advisable to counteract and disperse a pathogenic factor when the innate power turns out to be too weak. Preferably, a practitioner of constitutional acupuncture begins to strengthen the root and core of weaknesses.

Nourishment and development of the seed into maturity is founded upon the *qi* of earthly branch *Zi* in the North at the deepest point where life returns, begins and returns again. *Zi* pictures the seed of compassion. It can be nourished by 'water', bringing forth intuition and inner impulses that ultimately lead to a mature and compassionate heart. The initial state of the seed has to be accompanied by guidance and support of the following earthly branches, so that it can enable us to grow and develop into the compassionate beings that we really are.

SEASONAL POINT: GB-43, *XIA XI*

Gb-43 is the water point on the gallbladder channel and is called *Xia Xi*, which is translated as narrow ravine. It is also known as harmonious stream. A harmonious stream in a narrow ravine represents the seed quality and compassionate nature of the earthly branch *Zi*. The *qi* is still hidden but harmonious, small and determined, confident, decisive and compassionate. Another translation of *Xia Xi* comes into its own here: noble mountain river.

Gb-43 tonifies yin in general, especially in winter, and directs the flow of *qi* back to the root. Especially in the summer, it roots the *qi* and it is indicated in all cases when the heart-*shen* is overheated with symptoms of rising heat and stagnation in the upper burner.

CHAPTER 26

DYNAMICS OF THE EARTHLY BRANCH *CHOU* 丑[1]

**WINTER AND EARTH *QI*, THE VIRTUE OF
FLEXIBILITY, ADAPTABILITY AND SUPPORT
SEASONAL POINT: LIV-3, *TAI CHONG*, GREAT SURGE**

To you Ox, I give the power to create matter from the seed.
To support growth of young plants.
You have a difficult task which needs patience.
You are like a young plant, with a plan to reach for the light,
determined to advance and to be flexible when needed.
You are the governor of the Liver.

Your life means growth, knowing how to plan effectively and being
flexible to adjust to different circumstances. You are characterized by
your personal drive and good understanding of the moral standard.

For your good work I give you the virtue of Flexible Power.

But beware. This power is flammable. When you use your flexibility
for other reasons than reaching for the light, it will harm you. It will
cause irritability, expressing anger. Your flexibility will cease, becoming
stubborn, with a poor ability to cope with your world. You may
experience signs of depression with the tendency to hyperventilate.

So use your qualities well.

---

1   Born in 1925, 1937, 1949, 1961, 1973, 1985, 1997, 2009, 2021, 2033 after the Chinese New Year.

The renewal of life in the seed during the time of *Zi* is sprouting and receiving support from the *qi* of the earthly branch *Chou* 丑. This Chinese character portrays two half-opened hands that bind together. It shows the bonding and cooperation of two principles, left and right, yin and yang. There is combined power that supports plants to grow in two opposite directions, up and down. The seed roots to become stronger, to seek water and nutrients, and from the seed sprouts a trunk that seeks a way up, to the light of the sun.

The awakened and renewed consciousness is rooted in earth and ascends to heaven. The hands are half open to symbolize the relaxation necessary to guide life to future expression in a new world. The guidance of the *qi* of earthly branch *Chou* is only successful when it senses and perceives the environment well. Adaptability and flexibility characterize the guidance for growth and transformation, which is only possible when everything is properly sensed and noticed. It demonstrates the importance of the senses in general. Growth of the senses of perception is governed by the earthly branch *Chou*. The sense of touch that guides development, action and reaction starts in the embryonic stage during the second week of pregnancy; the other senses begin to develop from the fourth week on.

CHOU, EARTH: THE MEETING OF YIN AND YANG

Earth is a third means: the meeting and interaction of yin and yang belong to the action of the earth phase. Its dynamics are involved in change, transformation, transition, as are also the capacity to distinguish, coordinate and balance.[2] It holds the space where two different forces meet and merge, in this case the universal life-*qi* in the seed that meets the forces of physical growth. The interaction of yin and yang creates a balanced consciousness in the centre of the earth phase. This becomes a fixed pivot point from which the upward and downward movements in the seed can take place.

Similarly, on one hand consciousness contacts the universal *qi*, the unity and wholeness behind everything; on the other hand consciousness reaches out to the manifested physical world in which everything is in opposition and division. Within the central pivot space of the earth, the still hidden life-*qi* develops further in the spring into concrete visible actions and manifestations.[3]

The way the seed, a symbol of unity and wholeness, breaks up and expresses its motivation to grow and transform with flexibility is a process guided by the

---

2   This also applies to the earthly branches *Chen*, *Wei* and *Xu*.
3   The third earthly branch *Yin*.

qi of the earthly branch *Chou*: Life reaches out and up to the light and roots down into the earth to seek nutritional power. Life in form is possible because of its vitality and perception.

> *Dao* gave birth to one.
> One gave birth to two.
> Two gave birth to three.
> Three gave birth to the ten thousand things.
> The ten thousand things carry yin and embrace yang.
> They achieve harmony by combining these (two) forces.[4]

CHOU AND GROWTH

The condition of the pivot space held by the four earth-related earthly branches determines the character of every development of consciousness, growth and change. This applies to physical, emotional, mental and spiritual changes. The earthly branch *Chou* and the liver are mainly involved in initial changes, where this energy is aware of the possibilities of growth and changes. Unfortunately, when dysfunctional, it may also lead to illnesses.

Stagnation of the earth *qi* of the earthly branch *Chou* causes reduced growth and development, which may be accompanied by symptoms of heat.

> I have treated young people who struggled to keep up at school. They suffered from learning difficulties and reduced development. Their problems were easily resolved with simple treatments and advice influencing the field of this earthly branch *Chou*. The recovery of the flow of *qi*, mostly by calming and moving treatments of liver *qi*, together with support of self-confidence, brought very quick results. In addition I advised avoiding sour food such as yoghurt and butter milk. These foods constrict *qi*. Avoiding sour restored the guidance of the earthly branch *Chou* and the liver *qi*. It supported patients to keep up at school and feel emotionally safe with their peers.

Stress, frustration, social media, coffee, alcohol and the like are causes of disruption of the balanced *qi* in the inner space that may result in stagnation of earth with symptoms of unrooted *qi* and reduced growth. There might be symptoms of restlessness, (subdued) anger, muscle cramps and pains, sighs, anxiety and

---

4   *Dao De Jing* Chapter 42, Wu 1989.

hyperactivity. These symptoms are compensation mechanisms for the lack of movement due to the stagnation of the earth space in the earthly branch *Chou*.

CHOU AND CHOICES

Weakness of the earth *qi* of the earthly branch *Chou* forces people to make choices in the external world or they can focus on rooting and connecting to the inner essential and authentic source in themselves. The latter can make social communication more difficult. Conversely, when people just focus on outward choices, self-knowledge and reflection may become obstructed.

It is noteworthy that both solutions to support earth are similar, regardless of choice. The weakness and stagnation of the earth requires attention and nourishment which result in desires and longings. Instead of seeking healing through silence and attentive awareness, the desire to be someone else prevails. People with weakness of this earthly branch may have unattainable ideals or imitate role models and follow gurus on whom they depend for their growth and development. The weakness of earth can lead to addictions and can be offset by overeating, especially sweets and carbohydrates.

The correct *qi* of the earthly branch *Chou* shows in steadfastness, correct timing, patience and perseverance, pliability, focus, purposefulness and relaxation. It brings change, growth and movement with flexibility, adaptability and guidance without being forced to do so.

The earthly branch *Chou*, liver, supports the manifestation of the separated forces of yin and yang, which are eternally entangled and reveal the motivation and expression of life. *Chou* is largely responsible for the movement of *qi* throughout the body and the free flow of *qi* and *xuè*. It provides fluids, *wei qi* and nutrition when and where needed. The liver *qi* moves up or down, in or out, fast or slow, carefully or abundantly. The flexibility of these movements requires a stable, harmonious fixed pivot point that is balanced and in which peace prevails: the earth quality of the earthly branch *Chou*.

In the event of a disruption of liver *qi*, regaining a balanced earth space is the very first step towards healing. Meditation, yoga, *qigong*, mindfulness and a calming diet that harmonizes the earth of the liver *qi* with treatment of Liv-3 are advisable, of course always checked and balanced with the constitutional *qi* and pulse diagnosis.

SEASONAL POINT: LIV-3, *TAI CHONG*

Liv-3, *Tai Chong*, great surge: This *yuan source* point vitalizes the free flow of *qi* and movement. Its function is to balance yin and yang in the liver, to regulate liver *qi* and to build fluids in the liver. Liv-3 leads to clarity of the mind, which becomes full of cordiality and courage. In addition, the greatness (*tai*) of the source (*chong*) nourishes and moves and mobilizes *qi*.[5]

Liv-3 is the earth point and represents the balanced pivot space of consciousness of the earthly branch *Chou*. It builds a bridge of encounter between the nourishing *qi* of earth below and the vitalizing *qi* of heaven above.

People with the earthly branch *Chou* in their birth chart should have flexible, adaptable, moving *qi* at their disposal. However, these people often seem to struggle with their innately strong liver *qi*. How is that possible?

Unfortunately, society and the Western diet do not assist with maintaining a healthy balance for those with this constitution. Society seems to value fixed agreements, habits and compulsion more than the lively and spontaneous character of the earthly branch *Chou*, so that even these people feel compelled to adapt to rigid social values. They adapt at their own expense and are much stricter on themselves than they would actually like. This puts pressure on flexibility and adaptability. The tensions created may be further exacerbated by processed food that eventually damages and hardens the liver *qi*. Emotionally, these qualities lead to uncertainty and pent-up anger that makes people ill at a deep level: the level of their strong innate liver *qi*.

---

5   Liv-3 is contraindicated in asthma – when exhaling is difficult, with signs of heat and fire. It may cause more heat and reduce the mother (stomach and spleen) to nourish the lung.

CHAPTER 27

DYNAMICS OF THE EARTHLY BRANCH *YIN* 寅[1]

SPRING AND WOOD *QI*, THE VIRTUE OF COMMUNICATION
SEASONAL POINT: LU-11, *SHAO SHANG*, LESSER *SHANG*/METAL

To you Tiger, I give the opportunity to awaken life,
You are the shelter where heaven and earth meet respectfully.
You provide the first contact between the seed and its surrounding.
Your action is to receive and to give peacefully,
Without asking why or how.
You are the governor of the Lungs.

Your life means freedom based on a firm structure. You
provide people with a good opportunity to have an easy
social interaction, with a social self-confidence.

For your good work, I give you the virtue of Peace.

But beware. If you influence the process between heaven and earth
to benefit yourself, it will harm you. Life will become constricted
and condensed, to bring you guilt, grief, sadness and despair.
You suffer from an inadequate social life, which can develop into
emotional and physical claustrophobia or into overconfidence.

So use your qualities well.

---

1   Born in 1926, 1938, 1950, 1962, 1974, 1986, 1998, 2010, 2022, 2034 after the Chinese New Year.

The days get longer. The scents of the first sunny daffodils, crocuses and snow-drops announce spring. Plants sprout from the ground, buds are about to burst. They stand proud in the light they were looking for. People enjoy the vital power of spring, the warm sun and fresh air. Life is very visible and tangible.

The hidden forces in the seeds of *Zi* are transformed, further developed and supported by *Chou* to become young plants that perceive the light of the sun. The plants open their leaves. Flowers turn towards the sun, just like the lungs do after birth when cosmic breath-*qi* is inhaled for the very first time.

The Chinese character *Yin* 寅 shows a roof, the symbol for heaven. It covers a person who politely lowers their hands; the two hands meet under a shelter and pay respect. This symbolizes that people visit and greet each other in the spring, welcoming, celebrating and paying respect to the renewed awakened life that comes in tune with the rhythm of heaven.

Unlike the half-opened hands and bundled strength of the earthly branch *Chou*, the two hands of *Yin* meet to welcome and shape the new. The character *Yin* reflects the image of the encounter of the *da qi* (cosmic *qi*) and *gu qi* (earthly *qi*) meeting under a canopy[2] to create *ying* and *wei qi* that flow in and around the channels.

Any kind of encounter and communication is an expression of manifestation of the earthly branch *Yin*; it ranges from shaking hands to non-verbal communication. The quality of communication expresses the quality of the underlying lung *qi*. The power of shaking hands, the eyes looking down or looking straight in the eye, which can be based on courage, pride or confidence and so on, express the power of the underlying quality of the lung *qi*.

YIN AND *CHOU*, LUNG AND LIVER

The lung channel emerges from Cv-12, *Zhong Wan*, central venter in the middle burner.[3] It touches and penetrates respectively the large intestine, the stomach and the lungs after which it joins the throat at Cv-22, *Tian Tu*, heaven's prominence or celestial chimney. Then it emerges and becomes palpable at Lu-1, *Zhong Fu*, central treasury. The trajectory of the lung channel[4] starts in earth (Cv-12) and reaches out to heaven, expressing the basic principle of the meeting of yin and yang.

---

2   The lungs occupy the uppermost position among the internal organs and are known as the canopy of the organs.
3   *Hui* point of the *fu* and a front *mu* point of the stomach and the middle burner.
4   Many Chinese medicine books start with the lung channel. It is the channel of spring and Chinese New Year. However, the flow of *qi* of the earthly branches and channels starts hidden in the North, with *Zi*, the gallbladder, the returning of *qi* in the winter.

Cv-12 primarily harmonizes the central part of the body. The start of the lung channel in the earth area goes along with the balanced pivot earth space that was discussed with the earthly branch *Chou*. From the space of Cv-12, the *qi* of the lung channel moves down and up, similar to the growth of the plant during the earthly branch *Chou*. It roots in the large intestine and flows up to the stomach and passes the diaphragm to meet the lungs and throat at Cv-22. This acupuncture point controls the exit of *qi* to the chest similar to the first green buds and flowers that touch the light of the sun in spring. The *qi* of the lung at Cv-22 determines the power of the voice, the clarity of creative thoughts and all other forms of the creative expression of innovation.

Cv-22 is a window of the sky point that supports free communication with the universal spirit. It opens the connection with creativity that, when received by the heart-*shen*, is expressed in speech. Eloquence means that Cv-22 is open. Reluctance to speak or not be able to tolerate changes and innovations means Cv-22 is closed.

The lung channel emerges from both the harmonizing *qi* of the earth qualities of Cv-12 and the earthly branch *Chou*, liver. The connection to the liver channel is especially important because it partially contributes to the movements of the diaphragm. Sadness, grief, anxiety, guilt and shame, in particular, can stagnate the movement of the diaphragm. In Chinese medicine, these emotions are assigned to the lung *qi*. However, the support of liver *qi* is indispensable and conditional for the recovery process. Grief and similar emotions that stagnate the diaphragm require the Cv-12 area and liver to be addressed prior to treatment of the lung. A supportive arm around the shoulder, words of comfort, finding a quiet and peaceful place in the self are expressions of support for the balanced pivot, earth space of the earthly branch *Chou*. It is the ground on which the lung channel rests. It can, of course, be assisted by treating the liver channel with, for example, Liv-3, *Tai Chong*.

PROPER BREATHING AND RELATIONSHIPS ARE HEALING REMEDIES

Being present and alert, vitalizing each other and being able to communicate are essential aspects of a lively reciprocal relationship. This goes hand in hand with the vital *qi* of the lung which generates feelings of freedom and implies that the only authority is the love of the *shen*. Freedom in this context does not mean that one can do whatever one likes; on the contrary, it is not based on will and desires at all. Instead, freedom is based on an inner order of the heart-*shen* and a reciprocal relationship is therefore characterized by independence, benevolence and love.

The lungs provide the roof of the house of organs and ensure purity of exchange between heaven and earth. When the heart-*shen* is harmoniously aligned with the lung,[5] there is peace and no conflicts or power issues arise. There is no place for conditions, preferences, self-enrichment, comments, explanations or other skills of mental origin; the lungs, just like heaven, give and receive. Breath is the heavenly emanation that contains the power of life and is present in every living being. Limitation of this principle leads to conflicts and diseases.

The earth space of the earthly branch *Chou* supports mature emancipated relationships characterized by independent exchange of compassion and love. The more peaceful and balanced the earth space of the earthly branch *Chou*, liver, the more the authenticity and individuation of both partners is supported. This emerges from self-knowledge, flexibility, adaptability and the capacity to grow. It lays the foundation for trust in what IS instead of feelings of uncertainty about the future and the desires those evoke. It shows respect for everything, whether liked or disliked, everything is allowed to be present and is welcomed. It is said that when the earth is open, people dare to take risks. I believe that this is true when people take risks based on freedom of movement in the present and not based on willpower and purposefulness. If earth is stagnant, it can lead to excessive worry and panic attacks.

The more restless the earth space of the earthly branch *Chou*, the greater the dependence on a partner or others to feel safe. This is an important factor in diagnosis, as the underlying nature of lung disease may come from a malfunction of liver *qi*. Troubled diaphragm breathing and other lung complaints may be based on disrupted relationships (earth pivot of *Chou*), which often causes insecurity.

> This reminds me of a patient of about fifty years of age. Her symptoms almost all indicated a disturbance of the lung *qi*. She suffered from eczema, shortness of breath when tired, occasional attacks of hyperventilation, loose stools alternating with constipation, and recurrent throat infections. While recording her medical history, she exhibited an extraordinary compulsiveness regarding her diet, the use of supplements and sport activities. She looked young for her age, though her face had a dull non-emotional expression. She thought she looked old and ugly, explaining her rigid behaviour towards her eating habits. This actually annoyed me a little bit and I wrote in her file that she was a control freak. Only when I read the file later did I see how I had

---

5   This is expressed in the balance between *xuè* and *qi*.

judged her and I felt ashamed. It did not feel right to project my aversion to my own controlling behaviour onto clients through bias. To find out the reason for her compulsiveness I intended to examine her more objectively at the next appointment.

When we continued the conversation during the next appointment, she was very open and shared that the relationship with her partner was unsatisfactory. She felt dependent on her friends and work and focused mainly on her health through diet and sports to experience some happiness.

I started to understand that her compulsiveness was a compensation for the stagnated earth *qi* of the liver. This idea was confirmed with her pulse diagnosis: a tight liver pulse with an underactive lung pulse. I had missed these signs the first time due to my own biased attitude.

Tightness can be caused by coldness, pain or yin insufficiency. However, it is also a sign of too much metal and dryness that obstruct the earth.

Using Liv-3, followed by two acupuncture points on the small intestine and kidney channel,[6] the earth of the liver *qi* was liberated and her breathing became calmer. At the next appointment three weeks later, she shared, with a big smile, that it was much easier for her to deal with her compulsiveness. Her symptoms disappeared after a few more treatments.

SEASONAL POINT: LU-11, *SHAO SHANG*, LESSER *SHANG*/METAL

Lu-11, *Shao Shang*, is the *jing well* point and wood point. *Shao Shang* means lesser metal. It suggests that there is a better or more significant metal. The word *Shang* does not appear in the name of any other point on metal-related channels but in the *jing well* points Lu-11, *Shao Shang*, and L.i.-1, *Shang Yang*, which is translated as metal yang. It is therefore interesting to discuss this word *Shang* a bit more.

Sometimes, *Shang* is translated as 'merchant', an intermediary that carries out transactions between multiple parties. As described in Chapters 70 and 71 of the *Huang Di Nei Jing Su Wen*, *Shang* means the musical tone that relates to metal. It has the sound of gongs and bells, a heavy, solid sound.[7] In general,

---

6   Unlike *qi*; see Chapter 46.
7   There are five types of sounds that each correspond to one of the five phases: *Jue*, the sound for wood that belongs to spring and resonates with awakened life. *Zhi*, the sound for fire and the summer that touches the heart. *Gong*, the sound for earth and late summer and the centre, that makes you broad-minded. *Shang*, the sound for metal and autumn that resonates with integrity and righteousness. *Yu*, the sound for water and the winter that makes a balanced flow of *qi*. Every sound has a greater and lesser aspect. Lesser *Shang* can also mean the yin-type metal sound.

sounds are ways to communicate, such as speech, playing music and singing. Sounds are intermediate forces and, like merchants, not impartial.

Sounds have meaning: soft or hard, pleasant or sharp, high or low; sounds are ways in which the inner emotion behind communication is expressed. In addition it helps people determine localization; when walking in the street, we listen to the noise and therefore the location of buses and cars. We have learned to determine whether they are driving towards us or away from us. Sounds support us to determine our position in a space and to make decisions. They are important objective tools that influence our subjective sensations. Sounds play a role in determining likes and dislikes, defensive and offensive actions and so on. Decision-making is better implemented by the use of L.i.-1 than Lu-11.

L.i.-1 is a metal-related *jing well* point opposite to Lu-11, which is a wood-related *jing well* point and therefore has lesser metal. As a result, Lu-11 breathes *qi*, new life, into consciousness and dynamizes *qi* that can take root in the body. The full metal aspect of L.i.-1, that inexorably chooses between beneficial and non-beneficial, is involved in making decisions.

Pain from stagnation of *qi* that manifests in the pulse as tightness can be treated with sedation of L.i.-1. I have noticed over the years that this stagnation is often caused by the inability to make difficult decisions. Needling L.i.-1 can restore clarity that creates emotional space to make a decision.

Lu-11 and L.i.-1 are both known for their influence on the throat, the organ that produces sounds and speech. They are often sedated in cases of (wind) heat in the lung. Nevertheless, it is advisable to be careful with Lu-11 sedation, since it also sedates the wood quality of the lung and thus the vitalizing influence of the earthly branch *Yin*.

CHAPTER 28

DYNAMICS OF THE EARTHLY BRANCH *MAO* 卯[1]

SPRING AND WOOD *QI*, THE VIRTUE OF ACCELERATED GROWTH AND LUSHNESS
SEASONAL POINT: L.I.-3, *SAN JIAN*, THIRD SPACE

To you Rabbit, I give the courage to strive forward,
To let go of the experiences of the past.
Your door is always open to new movements and excitements.
You mirror life's foundations as feelings and emotions,
which assemble in the 'brains' of the belly.
You are the governor of the Colon.

Your life means growing fast into the future. You give people the
great strength necessary to let go of the experiences of the past, and
the fulfilment within by that which you experience from without.

For your good work, I give you the virtue of Courage.

But beware, if you become greedy, addicted to the fulfilment,
your life will become full of anguish, desperation, grief and
guilt. You will lose the insight that everything relates to
everything else, and will think only of your future gain.

So use your qualities well.

---

1   Born in 1927, 1939, 1951, 1963, 1975, 1987, 1999, 2011, 2023, 2035 after the Chinese New Year.

The Chinese character *Mao* 卯 depicts open doors. It symbolizes that resistance and caution have disappeared. Spring is at its peak. The freedom and vitality of the earthly branch *Yin* continues in *Mao* as strong and quick development and growth.

With the drive to manifest a strong, lush shape, *Mao* pushes the *qi* forward and upward. The plant grows upward with enormous force. When in nature the sunlight touches the plants and the trees, the palette of all the different colours of green seems to emit bright light itself. In people, the *qi* of spring comes to the fore in the form of enormous willpower and the desire to be proud when goals are achieved.

Emotions of guilt and regret can disrupt the earthly branches *Chou* and *Yin*, giving *Mao* a restless base that can render the will powerless. Being blamed or dominated by someone can negatively impact people's vitality and growth, decreasing willpower as well.

YIN AND *MAO*, LUNG AND LARGE INTESTINE

Along with the heart, the lungs embody heavenly *qi*. The upper burner[2] (with the lungs) focuses on subtle and refined forms of *qi* used for the channel system. The elimination of waste in the upper burner takes place through exhalation and vaporization of body fluids by perspiration. The classics compare this process in the upper burner with mist. Humans build physical, social and cognitive self-awareness through subtle forms of vitalization and communication through the earthly branch *Yin*, lung.

In contrast, the large intestine, along with other organs in the lower burner, embodies the earthly *qi*. The lower burner transforms, separates and excretes and is more concerned with maintaining the body through metabolism and elimination of waste through faeces and urine. These functions include processing emotions and feelings. The earthly branch *Mao* and the large intestine realize, metabolize, eliminate and reinforce (individual) feelings and emotions of the self.

SHAME AND GUILT

Shame and guilt start to develop around the age of eighteen months when the child experiences separation from a group or family. The intense feelings

---

2   Although the lungs are located in the upper burner and the large intestine in the lower burner, they are coupled in the metal phase and seasonal *qi* wood.

of shame and guilt can be evoked by an unexpected laugh about something seemingly insignificant such as the cute behaviour of children. Of course, disagreements between parents and illness of one of the parents can also cause feelings of shame and guilt.

Shame has a social frame of reference. It is an emotion that is related to the norms and values of a group or culture. The consequences of shame are therefore more localized in the upper burner (social ego), while other emotions, especially guilt, are more localized in the lower burner (individual ego).

Every emotion is felt in the heart, yet the heart prefers to be empty and to be open to heavenly alignment. It therefore transfers the *qi* of emotions to other organs. In cultures where social honour and shame are important, it is especially the *qi* of shame that is transferred from the heart to the lungs and the heart constrictor. It may stagnate at these locations and therefore deplete the *qi* present. Should the *qi* of shame instead remain in the heart, it would affect the heart-*shen*. For people who are victims of sexual abuse and rape, shame often remains in the heart and damages the heart-*shen*.[3]

Shame is an emotion that isolates and stagnates and exhausts the *qi* in the upper burner and the diaphragm. Treatments should therefore focus on the relationship between heart, heart constrictor and lung in order to balance the *qi* of protection and communication. It should be noted, however, that in response to shame people sometimes adopt an artificial personality that appears to be unproblematic, so that the wounded self can remain hidden.

The range of situations in which guilt plays a role is enormous. In the context of this book, it is important to discuss the *qi* of guilt and guilt feelings in relation to the earthly branch *Mao*.

Shame damages the essential being, the heart-*shen*, whereas guilt harms the ego. Feelings of guilt emphasize and are indicative of a damaged ego, for example a failed action or failure to achieve a personal goal.

Guilt can be social or individual but, in contrast with shame, guilt feelings are easier (not easy) to treat than shame. Courage is needed to look at and work on the ego tricks that block growth and freedom of the mind. Guilt is a deep-seated emotion that, upon perception through the heart-*shen* and when no inner forgiveness and reconciliation has taken place, sinks to the lower burner where it mainly affects the large intestine and kidneys.

---

3   The heavenly stem *Ding*, heart, is involved. Pulse diagnosis shows an insufficient heart pulse that responds positively to treatment, but only for a short time. It becomes insufficient again within a few days. The unlike *qi*, the heavenly stem *Ren*, bladder, displays the same image. These patients may benefit from acupuncture treatments, but also need to be treated by a psychotherapist in order to help process the trauma.

Due to the general moving quality of emotions, such guilt might first lead to frequent defecation and urination, but eventually it causes foul smelling stools, possibly constipation and stagnation of fluids due to the particular stagnant nature of guilt. When feelings of guilt persist, the *qi* of the large intestine and the kidneys weaken and stagnate; the heart-*shen* can no longer release the sensations to the lower burner. Consequently, the heart-*shen* stagnates, causing it to overflow. Symptoms are characterized by heat such as palpitations, insomnia, mental restlessness, vivid dreams, dry cough and so on. It creates the need to dissipate heat through perspiration. When this situation persists the body starts to purge heat via the large intestine and kidneys with symptoms such as loose foul-smelling stools, possibly diarrhoea and frequent urination with a strong smell.

Feelings of guilt are often unconscious or denied. Compensation mechanisms and denial strategies can cause people to become addicted to work, passions and excitements, tension and stress but also to do well and to be compassionate. In addition they may become more materialistic as a compensation for the weak large intestine *qi*, but particularly to cover the feelings of guilt and pain. Because physical and emotional boundaries are constantly being exceeded, this behaviour can ultimately lead to burnout and chronic fatigue.

Feelings of guilt and shame are acquired emotions that determine the character of a person, partly because of their influence during the development of the personality in childhood.[4] Guilt and shame are so rooted in upbringing, education and culture that often as adults we no longer know that they are the driving forces behind behaviour. This is mainly due to emotions such as underlying feelings of inferiority, self-hatred, anger, grief, regret and remorse and so on. It should be borne in mind that suppressed guilt and shame are powerful incentives for protest and anger.

In Chinese medicine, anger is mainly related to liver *qi*, but anger, rage and heartless behaviour due to guilt and shame often stem from the release of the stagnant *qi* of the large intestine and the lung.

In order to regain the authentic power of the earthly branch *Mao*, large intestine, the inner psycho-emotional space must be investigated and freed from the stagnation of guilt and penance in order to regain freedom of space for the heart-*shen*. This requires courage,[5] which can be enhanced with treatment of the *shao yin* division.

---

4   Temperament and character are part of the personality. Temperament is the natural part of the personality conveyed by the pre-natal *jing*. Character is the reflection of life experiences. Temperament is rooted in the kidney yang essence, character in the kidney yin essence.

5   The word 'courage' derives from the Latin 'cor', which means 'heart'.

Courage doesn't necessarily mean fighting someone. On the contrary, it is about understanding and working on your own frustrations, obsessions and patterns, in order to communicate better from the power of one's own essence (*shao yin*). A dictionary definition of courage is the 'ability to do something that frightens one; bravery or strength in the face of pain or grief'. This definition describes the power of the earthly branch *Mao*, large intestine: the doors are open completely and the motto is continuous growth. This is the only purpose, no matter what, even if it scares or hurts. Opening the doors of guilt and shame requires courage, but the results are enormous strength and authenticity.

SEASONAL POINT: L.I.-3, *SAN JIAN,* THIRD SPACE

L.i.-3, *San Jian*, third interval, is a *shu-stream* and wood point. L.i.-3 is most commonly used to disperse or sedate *qi*; it dispels wind heat from the head, throat, teeth, eyes and mouth. It frees the surface and is used for various skin diseases.

In general, *shu-stream* points on yang channels have a strong influence on the respective channels. As wood points they activate the moving, flexible and outgoing *qi*, especially in cases when people suffer from feelings of heaviness with joint pains.[6]

L.i.-3 is particularly beneficial for treating symptoms due to stagnation and dampness. It is, for instance, indicated for cramps and for late menarche in young girls due to both dampness and stagnation.

L.i.-3 is beneficial when there are feelings of guilt, when stagnation has occurred in the lower burner. L.i.-3 supports the flow of *qi* in the lower burner and thereby provides support to the heart-*shen*. It releases the blockage in the lower burner that has affected the heart. A specific symptom of this type of stagnation is the constant need to lie down and the desire to fall asleep.

The positive effect of L.i.-3 on the heart-*shen* can be further supported by L.i.-15, *Jian Yu*, shoulder joint (when needled in the direction of Ht-1, *Ji Quan*, highest spring). This combination moves the stagnation and provides mental clarity. This treatment is especially recommended when people also feel confused due to exhaustion.

---

6   *Nan Jing* Question 68.

CHAPTER 29

DYNAMICS OF THE EARTHLY BRANCH *CHEN* 宸[1]

**SPRING AND EARTH *QI*, THE VIRTUE OF CENTRAL
STABILITY AND TRANSFORMATION
SEASONAL POINT: ST-36, *ZU SAN LI*, LEG THREE MILES**

To you Dragon, I give my compassion and the
honour of showing it to the world.
You are like the moon, reflecting the light of the sun.
You are the axle of a spinning wheel.
All and everything turns, but you.
You are the centre desiring energy from heaven and earth.
You are the governor of the Stomach.

Your life means concentration and meditation through centralization.
You show compassion and sympathy, knowing how to nurture
yourself and others well. You receive what is yours and take
a resolute stand, resisting what does not belong to you.

For your good work, I give you the virtue of Stability.

But beware, your good work easily makes you boastful. Then life
will become controlled by obsessions or greed and addiction.
Furthermore, it brings you excessive pensiveness and insecurity.

So use your qualities well.

---

1   Born in 1928, 1940, 1952, 1964, 1976, 1988, 2000, 2012, 2024, 2036 after the Chinese New Year.

The earthly branch *Chen* is very much in the moment. It is fully aware of past experiences and future purposes, but does not lose its presence in the moment. In nature, the earthly branch *Chen* connects the vital life of spring with the abundance of lushness in the summer season. It provides nutrition and support to ever-changing life.

The Chinese character *Chen* 辰 is usually translated as the sprouting at the end of spring, but it means more. *Chen* is also associated with a woman bending forward, while she conceals her 'shame' or menstruation. Others describe *Chen* as pregnancy, expansion and thunderstorm. The common denominator of these translations is the state of near fullness; a state where something is about to break out. Transformation and the new are on their way.

Chen belongs to the earth phase. Like other earth-related earthly branches *Chen* facilitates the meeting and separation of yin and yang movements: The plants move up to the light of the sun and at the same time they seem to bend their flowers towards their roots that nourish them – plants let their heavy flowers hang down a bit. At the level of humanity, *Chen* is the ability of consciousness to be aware of the ever-present cause of strength and vitality in the present.

STABILITY AND TRANSFORMATION

In previous chapters we discussed the central space of earth with the earthly branch *Chou*. It connects the original oneness of life in the seed with the dual world of existence. In comparison with the earthly branch *Chen*, the earthly branch *Chou* is yang motivating, supporting *qi* to improve growth. *Chen* is yin in character, it balances, receives and responds. It organizes the present and supports the continuation of the cycle of life by implementing the past in the now.

Feelings such as pleasure, disgust, empathy, sympathy, rejection, acceptance are often based on feelings and thoughts from the past, habits, expectations, desires and even addictions. The magnitude and strength of the yin central earth space of *Chen* is present in every living being and depends on the evolutionary state of the living form. *Chen* is an instinctive force in plants and animals. The strength of *Chen* in humans manifests as the awareness of past feelings and thoughts as a means of guiding action in the present. Yet it is also the awareness of conscious freedom in every moment. *Chen* is the field of transformation in which interaction of past and present takes place.

These qualities make *Chen* important for food intake. Food, in the broadest sense of the word, can only be absorbed if it is changed and adapted in such a way that once eaten it can be digested and absorbed optimally so that the living form feels safe, satisfied and stable.

A weak earthly branch *Chen*, stomach, makes people feel less at home in a changing society. They often struggle to meet the demands of society. It can lead to overload and the inability to say no to social demands. People feel insecure and conservative because any unexpected change is stressful since they cannot express their personal preferences (or even know what they desire). Such people stick to old habits and create a social network that provides them with stability. Opinions and advice from others, including practitioners, will not be accepted until the healthy *qi* of the stomach and inner stability have returned. A healthy lifestyle and diet are necessary adjustments, but implementation of these adjustments is only fruitful when the stomach *qi* is improved.

Usually, malfunction of *Chen*, stomach, causes digestive and behavioural problems due to mental instability and uncertainty. This is often accompanied by a risk of dependence on others, which is especially important to know to ensure the practitioner's independence. Strengthening the stomach *qi* makes people free and open with an independent inner stability.

It is especially through openness and vulnerability that *Chen* invites engagement with the environment. The root of stability comes from the wholeness of heaven and is revealed in the human energetic field in a central earth space where yin and yang meet and merge. The central space can be the human identity between the self and the outside world, the ego between self-image and reality, the present moment between the past and the future and, physically, it refers to the spine, the central axis of the human body.

Instability in the present moment causes insecurity and fear. Instability in identity causes disrupted engagement; people have no idea what to do with life. Instability of the vertebral column can give rise to scoliosis, back pain, unstable joints and neurological symptoms. Instability of the ego shows in a restless mind, emotional distress, worry and pensiveness. Not infrequently these physical and emotional problems come together.

A disturbed ego easily reflects inward and is associated with malfunction of *Chen*, stomach. Unfortunately, the weakness is often compensated for by excessive willpower, overdrive and desires. This can lead to migraines, exhaustion, high blood pressure, back pain and so on. A balanced *Chen* causes people to experience life as it is and not as it is hoped, expected or otherwise desired; there is no place for expectations, regret, judgement or rejection and instead stability and acceptance give rise to inner confidence.

Instabilities in *Chen*, stomach, might be diagnosed and treated with St-42,[2] *Chong Yang*. The pulse felt on St-42 shows the state of yin and, specifically, the

---

2   Scoliosis and a suffering ego may be treated with St-42, Sp-6, Liv-3, Gb-39.

state of stomach *qi*. The central earth space in *Chen* pursues no purpose other than being in accordance with heaven to ensure transformation, harmonization and nourishment of the flow of *qi* in the entire cycle.[3] This requires the stillness and stability of the central earth space in *Chen*.

CHEN AND HARMONY

The way of heaven is to benefit, not to harm.[4]

The way of heaven diminishes when there is too much and supplies when there is too little.

The way of humans is different; they take from those who do not have enough, to fill to those who already have too much.[5]

As people age, this quest for life and harmony – the way of heaven or the way of humanity – becomes more relevant to people born with the earthly branch *Chen*.

SEASONAL POINT: ST-36, *ZU SAN LI*, LEG THREE MILES

St-36 is the earth and *he-sea* point on the stomach channel. The *qi* enters a deeper level to gather with the stomach organ.

What else can be added to everything that has been written about this point? It is probably the most described and used point in the history of acupuncture. St-36 fits into the image of *Chen* being attuned to the heavenly order of the three burners: heaven–earth–human. The effect on the three burners is mentioned in Chapter 20 of the *Huang Di Nei Jing Su Wen*, and – without explicit mention – the text gives voice to the functions of St-36:

Heaven is one, earth is two and man is three, and three times three is nine, which corresponds with the nine distant areas of China. There are three regions in man and each region is symptomatic of three parts of the body, in determination of life and death, in order to deal with one hundred diseases and to strike a balance between deficiency and excess, and finally, to get rid of disease.[6]

---

3   The four earth earthly branches are *interconnected* and work together, but individually bridge two adjacent earthly branches, so that all of the twelve earthly branches are involved in generating transformation.

4   *Dao De Jing* Chapter 81, Wu 1989.

5   *Dao De Jing* Chapters 77 and 81, author's notes.

6   *Huang Di Nei Jing Su Wen* Chapter 20, Lu 1990, p. 136.

St-36 gathers the cosmic order and stabilizes the relationship heaven–earth–humanity throughout the body to stimulate the production of *qi* of the *san jiao* which in turn stimulates the production of *wei qi* and *ying qi*. The beauty and power of St-36 is outstanding. Many say that it never hurts to use this point, but in my opinion that is incorrect.

The effectiveness of the earthly branch *Chen* comes from yin and emptiness instead of from yang and fullness. Movements, and thus thoughts and emotions, should take place around a point of emptiness, openness and vulnerability. It is characterized by perseverance and strength rather than giving in and weakness. As it says in the *Dao De Jing* Chapter 11: 'Thirty spokes are connected in the hub of a wheel, but the wheel works thanks to the hub hole.'

Emptiness is not nothingness; it brings order, balance and stability. The meaning of bringing order refers to the 'natural way', which is a silent mind without intrusion of the personal will and desires and without conflicting circumstances. Life is received as it is presented.

But silence of the mind can be frightening. Being in silence can lead to uncertainty and loneliness but most of all to fear of nothingness. I have treated people who had panic attacks from facing emptiness because they felt that they had no longer any ground under their feet. One of my patients said: 'It feels that the ego becomes diffuse and disappears.'

These disturbing emotions can be so strong that they motivate people to compensate for the anxiety, for example by demanding attention, looking for debate and discussion, gathering a huge amount of knowledge, constant thinking, social media or similar stimulations: anything, as long as people do not have to experience silence and emptiness! Unfortunately, trying to avoid anxiety leads to more and more anxiety and neurotic behaviour.

> Worth mentioning is a patient who had complaints from heavy work overload: He suffered from migraines, back pain, nervousness, exhaustion and insomnia. He cried when he shared his complaints with me.
>
> During the treatment I advised him to do nothing for half an hour a day. He looked at me with fearful eyes and said: 'What should I do?' Doing nothing was no option for him. He told me that he was too scared. He was afraid to have time because emotions would then reveal themselves and become too intense for him. With some insistence on my part, he started doing nothing for one minute a day. It was terribly difficult for him but, after a while, things slowly got better and he could 'do nothing' for 30 minutes; just stare out of the window without it having any function. He began to like to 'do nothing'

and he had more time to perceive himself and discover what feelings were coming. This reduced his overload.

In these cases treating St-36 is not recommended. It can cause unsafe feelings of emptiness, resulting in overwhelming experiences of deep-seated emotions. Only when people are ready to face their emotions is St-36 indicated and can then profoundly change their perception of thinking and feeling!

The preconditions for treatment and healing of such a disturbed emotional life are a peaceful *shen* and the capacity to be in the present moment: the core quality of the earthly branch *Chen*.

St-30, *Qi Chong*, rushing *qi*, or *Qi Jie*, street of *qi*, is not a seasonal point but in these cases it often works better than St-36, especially when there are *shen* problems, panic attacks, and depression due to stagnation of *qi* due to long-term heartbreak and identity crises.

A FINAL NOTE

It is remarkable, and so beautiful at the same time, that children live unconsciously in the present with playful ease. Adults seem to have to consciously learn to live in the present. Perhaps presence and serious attention aren't the only keys here, but rather playfulness.

CHAPTER 30

DYNAMICS OF THE EARTHLY BRANCH *SI* 巳 [1]

SUMMER AND FIRE *QI*, THE VIRTUES OF SOLITARINESS AND ORGANIZING
SEASONAL POINT: SP-2, *DA DU*, GREAT CAPITAL/ORGANIZATION

To you Snake, I give the power to spread my Idea.
You are the ambassador of heaven on earth,
To organize the inner world as the outer world.
You are devoted and in service to your world.
You are the flower of consciousness.
You are the governor of the Spleen.

Your life means creation through transformation of the
heavenly energy based on ordination. You show discipline
and order; by these you will know how to organize your
internal reality. Your strength comes from concentration
and meditation through self-contemplation.

For your good work, I give you the virtue of Positivity.

But beware, if you forget the love through which you work,
your discipline and order will change into fixation and blockage,
showing as excessive pensiveness and obsessions, intractable
habits and dogmatism. Then you are especially focused on
negative experiences, which can develop into melancholy.

---

1   Born in 1929, 1941, 1953, 1965, 1977, 1989, 2001, 2013, 2025, 2037 after the Chinese New Year.

So use your qualities well.

It is summer. The plant is in full splendour and blooms with beautiful colours. The life forces, hidden in the seeds in winter, now show themselves in full glory. The woods have a high density of foliage and abundance of vegetation. The form forces enjoy the summer!

The *Si* 巳 pictograph depicts a fully formed embryo and a snake.

A fully formed human embryo – *Si* – contains all the qualities needed to follow the human path on earth. Humans determine the direction of the path of life themselves. But there is always a choice between a life in accordance with the order and virtues of heaven or not. *Si*, spleen, represents the order of heaven in humans which shows in the government of all cyclical 'climatic' movements (in humans and otherwise).

The earthly branches *Si* and *Chen* are the earthly representatives of heavenly *qi* on earth and in humans. The related *qi* of the stomach and spleen organize and coordinate the channel system in line with the *qi* of heaven and earth, nature, climate, diet, feeling and emotions.

Si and *Chen* prepare the conditions for the yin (second) half of the cycle of earthly branches. This decline of form manifests with the release of the life forces when plants begin to lose lushness. Solidity of the form will slowly change into fluidity of life.

During the second half of the cycle, yin qualities such as susceptibility, vulnerability and receptivity replace motivation, movement, growth and development. These yin qualities often feel unnatural and seem difficult to master. Yet they arise in order to give strength rather than weakness and indulgence.

SI, THE SPLEEN, AND THE ONENESS OF HEAVEN

Si belongs to fire and the emanation *heng*. It represents the ever-penetrating consciousness of the oneness of heaven that lives in all that exists and thus co-influences the nature of the *shen*. During the time of *Si* and *Chen* human consciousness is influenced by the order of heaven. This reveals as human order and stability organized from and built on receptivity, emptiness, openness and sensitivity. The yin qualities of the spirit and the mind are extremely important for the consciousness to receive the *qi* of heaven via the great movements and heavenly stems.[2] The more stagnation in *Si*, spleen, the more inaccessible the

---

2   All movements on earth are arranged by the *qi* of heaven via the great movements and heavenly stems.

shen and the more inflexible humans are in assumptions, expectations, feelings, thoughts and ideas. Over the years it has become clear to me that treating with heavenly stems and earthly branches begins and depends on the quality of the patient's earthly branch *Si*, spleen.

SI, THE SPLEEN, AND OPENNESS

Openness, receptivity and vulnerability can provide insight into certain emotions and habits that actually hide the uniqueness and freedom of the self. Recognizing these emotions and associated 'programmed' patterns can clear the veil. This brings people closer to recognizing reality and actuality: the authenticity and the truth of the circumstances. Above all, openness of character brings a person closer to the uniqueness of themselves and others as solitary authentic beings. Being alone and authentic are not synonyms for loneliness and fear; on the contrary, they can bring love, connection and compassion that turn loneliness (associated with fear) into togetherness.

SI, THE SPLEEN AND KIDNEYS

Life is radiant in summer; people sit in the sunlight in the garden, meet friends and go out, go on vacation and live 'the good life'. Being out and celebrating life fills people with warmth. Summer is seductive, both literally and figuratively. What people desire is mostly on offer and is satisfied. But, beware, too much outgoing behaviour can deplete the kidneys, especially kidney yang.

In the cycle of earthly branches and the Chinese hourly clock, the spleen implies fire, warmth and cordiality. Symptoms and diseases associated with spleen *qi xu* may arise when people exhaust themselves too much and too often. This is due to exhaustion of the fire of the spleen that is empowered by the fire of kidney yang. When depletion persists, eventually symptoms and illnesses develop due to kidney yang *qi xu*: soul pain, loneliness, fear and feelings of being gagged.

Just as flowers in summer come from the seeds of winter, conversely, consciousness based on openness will bear fruit in the depths of one's being; the ego is connected to its origin in which the memory of the true self and the mandate of heaven is received in the pre-natal *jing*-essence and is stored in the kidney yang.[3] A sense of freedom of the soul is not external; it is an inner realization

---

3   Kidney yin nourishes the body, controls growth and deals with reproduction and development through life. The memory of our life experiences is stored in kidney yin.

that comes from the *jing*-essence as the foundation of consciousness. This is where treatment and self-cultivation can start. Although self-cultivation is less addressed in the summer, it is precisely this sense of inner freedom that is the quintessence of soul healing.

Leon Hammer, one of my teachers, once told me that 'the *shen* is the ongoing inspiration of man, but love resides in the water as a potential realized and expressed by the heart'. Self-knowledge, openness and emptiness are the keys to open the gates of love that reside in water.

It is hopeful and positive that nowadays many people live gently, sensitively and open-heartedly, but many are still being raised to be strong and tough, to go for the highest and defend a position, to appear untouchable. It would be encouraging if there was more appreciation for everyone's uniqueness and yin character, even in cases of disagreement.

THE SNAKE AND THE IDEA

The first sentence of the poem of *Si* says: To you Snake, I give the power to spread my Idea.

The question might arise: 'What Idea and with what purpose?'

To understand this, we must discuss the snake as a symbol of summer and winter.

In China, the snake is regarded as a mystical animal that can transform into a human being. A famous drawing from the Tang Dynasty depicts the legendary figures Fu Xi and his sister and wife Nü Wa. Each has a human torso and the lower body of a snake; their tails are intertwined. Fu Xi carries a square[4] in his left hand and Nü Wa carries a compass[5] in her right hand. The picture symbolizes the meeting and merging of heaven and earth. The half-human half-snake sages show the conscious union of still differentiated elements in the revealed physical world (summer).

The snake is also the animal of the North and winter, the place where all forces merge into unity, the place of the eternal source of *qi*.

On the one hand, the snake symbolizes the undifferentiated forces of winter that are subjective, silent, unconscious, latent, spiritual, creative, and, on the other hand, the reunification of differentiated forces in the summer that are objective, manifest, conscious and physically creative.

The conscious experience that the outer expression of summer is based on

---

4   A symbol for earth.
5   A symbol for heaven.

the unconsciousness of the inner being of winter (in other words that the mind and spirit, *shen*, are based on the authentic *jing*-essence) leads to the natural way, the Idea that leads to authentic freedom of the *shen* with an active and awake consciousness. This is founded on self-knowledge and deep-rooted understanding of heaven and earth, yin and yang, inside and out, winter and summer, but above all on the experience of and reconciliation with the inner light and love in the *jing*-essence. Sp-1, Sp-2, Sp-3 with Sp-4 opens awareness in that direction and are therefore useful in supporting patients with depression.

SEASONAL POINT: SP-2, *DA DU,* GREAT CAPITAL/ORGANIZATION

Because of the coherence between Sp-1, *Yin Bai*, Sp-2, Sp-3, *Tai Bai*, and Sp-4, *Gong Sun*, Sp-2, *Da Du*, great capital, must be discussed together with the three other points. The coherence is mainly reflected in the use of the word white – *Bai*: Sp-1, *Yin Bai*, hidden white, Sp-3, *Tai Bai*, supreme white. *Bai* also appears as part of the Chinese character *Du* in Sp-2.

Bai represents the light of the sun, the ultimate symbol for heaven and yang that spreads its bright white light in the morning. In Sp-1 light is received and reflected, present yet hidden (yin). Sp-2, great capital, shows the bright illumination of light that brightens togetherness and organization of a capital (form/yin). The further radiation of light manifests and expresses itself in the world (the body) in Sp-3, supreme white. Sp-4 represents the ambassador of heaven on earth/in the body. It spreads the light of heaven and organizes the earth and the body in alignment with heaven.[6]

Si is the pinnacle of yang, the outcome of growth and thus the result of the light of the rising sun. At the same time, it is the pinnacle of yin as the full and complete expression in the form: the starting point of intense internalization of the self. The encounter of the two opposing qualities corresponds with *Si* as the representative of heaven on earth. The meeting of yin and yang gives *Si* the possibility to organize the inner world in alignment with heaven and the outer world.

Bright white light in this context[7] refers also to the bright white light of the rising planet Venus in the East in the morning, and its setting in the West in the

---

6   Sp-4, *Gong Sun*, was the other name of the Yellow Emperor, the ambassador of heaven on earth. Sp-4 is the opening point of the *chong mai* which guides the transition of pre-natal (the Idea) to post-natal (the phenomena). Sp-4 transfers pre-natal *qi* to post-natal *qi*.

7   The mystical nature of symbols can be explained in different ways, and they are true in all senses.

evening.[8] Just as the planet Venus reflects the bright light of the sun, humans reflect and internalize[9] the light of the sun through receptivity and openness.

The reflection (yin) of the bright white light of the sun (yang) in the planet Venus provides the clarity of mind that allows the recognition of the uniqueness of the self and of others in the self. It shows that the self is not a separate wholeness. It consists of the ego's inner experiences and the experiences of impressions of everything around the ego through the human mind. This applies to every human and all egos: The self is an omnipresent, limitless fact!

Sp-2 is indicated when people are unable to adequately deal with our restless world. This shows itself as mental or physical lethargy, mental retardation and lack of concentration. Sp-2 helps people to get closer to themselves and to maintain their centre and balance. It brings more proportionality, stability and a sense of togetherness.

---

8   The planet Venus can be observed just before sunrise in the East as the morning planet or just after sunset in the West as the evening planet.
9   The planet Venus belongs to the phase metal and symbolizes letting go and internalization.

CHAPTER 31

DYNAMICS OF THE EARTHLY BRANCH *WU* 午[1]

SUMMER AND FIRE *QI*, THE VIRTUE OF LOVE
SEASONAL POINT: HT-8, *SHAO FU*, LESSER MANSION

To you Horse, I give the opportunity and power to serve.
You meet Man; to love and to work in harmony.
You are the origin of love and joy, struggle and opposition.
You show both sides of every action.
You are essential to the understanding of the Self.
You are the governor of the Heart.

Your life means attunement with your world, characterized by joy
and happiness based on high self-esteem, awareness and confidence.

For your good work, I give you the virtue of Love.

But beware, if you become selfish, you will experience a joyless
life. You will try to overcome your low sense of self-esteem with
a hysteric or euphoric attitude based on a hidden loneliness.

So use your qualities well.

The heat seems to be taking its toll. The first signs of coming autumn are visible.
The leaves and flowers begin to fall on the ground. The very first decline of the

---

1 Born in 1930, 1942, 1954, 1966, 1978, 1990, 2002, 2014, 2026, 2038 after the Chinese New Year.

proudly flowering plants and the beginning of the struggle for survival begins as early as mid-summer.

The Chinese character 午 depicts a pestle that symbolizes hitting, crushing and grinding. It is time for major transformations now that yang has reached its peak. The first signs of yin, hidden deep in the earthly branch *Wu*, arise from the excess of yang. The plants protect themselves from too much heat. The process is similar to the return of yang that announced itself in the earthly branch *Zi* in winter; then it was caused by an excess of yin.

The yin in the summer begins to absorb the heat of summer, through which the plant can protect the seeds in the future, in winter. The collected warmth increases the chances of survival in the winter but comes at the expense of the vitality of the plant: Its leaves and flowers start to fall.

The form perishes and life regains its potential. If the yin is too weak in the summer, the plant will have to struggle to survive in winter. In clinical practice this phenomenon can be observed in patients who exhaust their fire-related channels in the summer, especially when it is too hot, while paying little attention to the preservation of yin. They may then fall ill in autumn or winter.

THE VERTICAL AXIS *ZI–WU*

The entire cycle of the earthly branches is built around the vertical axis of *Zi–Wu*. This means that the cycle of earthly branches is resting on the opposing initiating forces of yin and yang, water and fire. Yin and yang are the revealed fundamental principles that regulate the cosmos through opposition and cooperation, but both stem from oneness; they are therefore two presences of one and the same principle and essentially equal to each other.

As growth comes from the hidden seed of the earthly branch *Zi* in winter, decline appears at the highest peak at the time of the earthly branches *Wu* in summer. But, mystically, the growth and decline of life are equal.

Yin and yang, growth and decline, activity and receptivity and so on are the opposing forces that attract and complement each other. Because of their mutual cohesion and tension, everything moves and nothing is stable. This notion is made practical in the open hourly point system *Zi Wu Liu Zhu*:[2] a system in which an optimal time for an acupuncture treatment can be found and points on the twelve channels are selected based on the 'openness' of a point at a specific day and time. *Zi* and *Wu* are the first and seventh earthly branches

---

2   The most well-known 'open hourly point acupuncture' system based on heavenly stems and earthly branches.

representing the North–South axis, the winter and summer solstices. *Liu-Zhu* means flowing and pooling, or to flow and to pour into. Thus *Zi Wu Liu Zhu* means the time-bound rising and falling flow of *qi* and *xuè*, which flows out of *Zi* and reaches its maximum in *Wu* after which it returns to *Zi* again.

THE EGO AND DUALITIES

'You have to set high goals for your career. To get there you have to make the optimal study choice. You have to get high grades. Besides your studies, you have to do a lot to get as far as possible later. You have to maintain a good social network otherwise you will be excluded,' said a student in a study on the mental health of young people. King Willem Alexander of the Netherlands probably had such students in mind during his Christmas speech (2019): 'As free people, we want to get the best out of life and blame ourselves if that doesn't work. We mirror ourselves to others, set the bar high and like to present a perfect version of ourselves.'[3]

The ego is raised to feel the need to compare and therefore chooses to validate itself by building a clear picture of itself. 'You are better than me.' 'I should have done better, next time I will beat you.' 'The mind is worse than the heart.' 'You should have known better.' 'I wish I was more spiritual.' And so on.

Dualities such as 'me and you', 'my family and the rest of the world' and also 'past and future', 'happiness and suffering' and so on are important issues of the ego. The ego builds its identity as an individual being by using the experiences of interactions it has had with the ever-changing world. It also confirms itself in experiences it has with thoughts, feelings and consciousness and takes its place in the world by aligning the awareness of the present moment with past experiences and future expectations. The actual place of a healthy and balanced ego lies exactly between past experiences and expectations for the future. Past and future are, as it were, the living pillars on both sides of the ego.

You can even say that duality and ego are almost interchangeable elements: What applies to duality applies to the ego. When the ego fights for good, it fights against evil. When the ego focuses on togetherness, it combats divorce or separation. With each choice, the opposite is disputed but the rejected part demands attention, which maintains and strengthens it! The experience of duality separates the perceived world into understandable parts by which the ego strengthens its identity. Although it is changing, in Western culture it is not self-evident that the ego acquires a place in the world through togetherness and unanimity.

---

3   Translation by Joan Duveen of Giesen 2019.

The ego's freedom can be limited due to traumas, bad experiences and expectations built on these experiences of the past. This orientation leads to actual conflicts and frustrations in the present. The coordination between the ego and its pillars (past and future) is often not very successful. The ego may linger in strong emotions from the past or focus heavily on expectations in the future. Conflicts of the ego take place due to misunderstandings in the experience of time and create imbalance in the present. The uncomfortable side effect of this is that the ego can no longer clearly look at the nature of the conflict in the present because fear of the future, shame and guilt, and past traumas mask the clear view of the present.

The question arises as to whether the ego can escape the prison of time and duality. Are we able to find an experience of unity by resisting opposing forces through meditation or detachment exercises? Just as the principle of duality cannot be challenged, the principle of ego cannot be challenged. Any struggle to let go of the ego intensifies the tension in the reality of duality in which it lives.

Contemplation and meditation can give relaxation and tranquillity. That is useful and pleasant, but the experience is often still rooted in a dual reality. Meditation techniques focused on breathing are also in a dual reality as long as the part of the ego observes breathing. Many meditation techniques have been described, but actually there are no words that describe timeless, thoughtless, non-conceptual meditation; any spoken or written description confirms the world of duality. The key phrase might be 'attentive awareness', in which there are no thoughts and no movements. This state can enable the ego to transcend duality temporarily; temporarily because human beings simply cannot function in the world without an ego. Attentive awareness may still be part of the reality of everyday life, but it may not be compatible with conditioned or compulsive behaviour.

It seems likely that the state of duality leads to conflicts in the ego because the ego does not simply surrender. It proves its identity by means of dualities. Learning to distinguish and accept the opposite forces rather than separating and judging them is the first step to changing the perception of opposing dualities and perhaps this can facilitate conflict resolution. This process begins with the benefits of the power of yin instead of yang: sensitivity and receptiveness, rather than action and reaction. This can lead to acceptance and collaboration of polarities.

YIN–YANG AND THE NATURAL STATE

It is a misunderstanding that the Daoists value yin[4] more than yang.[5] Yin and yang have the same value, but because Western culture is mostly yang, appreciation for the yin is more noticeable. But it is the acceptance of both that can lead to something Daoists call the natural state. It can be a lifelong calling to practice acceptance of both growth and decline, strength and vulnerability, and so on. It is on this path which inner freedom can be found through what Daoists call the 'natural state' in which the ego connects with the permanent rather than the temporary. Perhaps that permanent aspect of the revelation of life is the secret of love.

Being in the natural state is a path full of obstacles, because people may, for instance, call the student on this path selfish or self-centred. This is understandable because inner soul work can keep you pretty busy. Learning to deal with the judgements of others and yourself is a quest in itself. In addition this path touches on experienced trauma and early psychological survival mechanisms. These traumas and survival mechanisms are often no longer necessary, but still have power over the ego. Terminating the power of these requires understanding and courage along with a lot of time and energy. Being open to and owning experienced traumas and being able to gradually place these traumas in the past without confusing the ego in the present make one's attention focus more on the current environment and current state of the self. Through time, care, vulnerability, sensitivity, openness and love instead of conflict, the ego learns to recognize the actual world and the people in it (and vice versa), so that the focus of the ego in the world changes – possibly into a more peaceful self.

A PERSONAL PERSPECTIVE

This path, which once begun never ends, has made me more tolerant and gentler. As the mind became clearer, I saw more of what really IS instead of what I hoped or expected to see, which also meant that I gained more insight into the differences between sentiments and love.

What I used to call love was accompanied by all kinds of emotions and sentiments in which ambitions and desires were hidden.

Over the course of my life, love became something that can hardly be properly recorded in words: For me, there is love when it evokes a feeling of peace and uplift of the soul, including moments/events of decline, stagnation,

---

4   Yin is the source of receptivity, sensitivity, vulnerability, gratitude, service and the like.
5   In Confucianism yang is valued more than yin.

unpleasant sensations and even death. Love is not the opposite of death, hatred or indifference, love encompasses all that exists. Love has no opposite dualities and transcends time and thought.

Love became clearer to me when I was allowed to be present with dying people. Love is essentially life that emerges at conception and is especially visible in the eyes of the newborn and releases at death. I still remember all the encounters in which people said goodbye to earthly life and loved ones. It happened without sentiment but with grace and in great peace. Everyone in the room lost the sense of time and felt elevated by the presence of impersonal love. Similar experiences happened when I was present at the birth of my own children and some of my patients' children. The more times I witnessed birth and death, the more insight I gained about what love might really encompass.

DYNAMIC DUALITIES OF THE EARTHLY BRANCHES AFFECT THE PHASE EARTH

The dynamic dualities in the cycle of the earthly branches, better known as the opposites in the Chinese hourly clock, shape the evolution of the ego by balancing opposing forces. In particular, the cooperation of the duality *Zi* and *Wu*, gallbladder and heart, balance and strengthen the central earth space, the ego, the central driving force of humans. But when the ego is primarily focused on conflict or is obsessively seeking harmony and de-escalation, the earth and earth-related channels are affected and should be addressed first. Unlike *qi* treatments[6] can even (unintentionally) reinforce behaviour that is based on conflict. This may be the result of a hardening of a soul desperate for safety, which is usually due to an imbalance in the earth-related earthly branches *Chen*, stomach and *Xu*, heart constrictor.[7]

LIFE AND FORM[8]

The growth and blossoming of plants and trees in the first half of the cycle of the earthly branches are often seen as expressions of life (yang), whereas they are actually form (yin) expressions of a life principle: The plant is increasingly taking shape (yin) and manifests its right to exist.

Due to their expression in the form, life forces limit their own possibilities. After all, life forces intrinsically have infinite possibilities, but once they are

---

6   See Chapter 43.
7   See Chapter 38.
8   Life forces (yang) dominate in winter (yin) and the form forces (yin) dominate in summer (yang).

caught and solidified in the form they become limited in their expression: A flower is limited to its own special shape and colour, just as all people who are limited within their own specific shapes and possibilities. Within that, everyone has their own unique potential. This concept means that disturbed expression of individual possibilities, such as not being able to find a hobby, work or life goal, must be approached by addressing the initial principles of the beginning of life in the earthly branch *Zi*, gallbladder: the foundation of returning yang, the initial life-*qi* expression into form/manifestation.

During the yin (second) half of the cycle of the earthly branches, the structure of the plants diminishes and decay leads to death. Decline starts during the earthly branch *Wu*, heart, when the form forces weaken. The life forces and fluids return to the roots, to the essence of water. This process regenerates and enhances the potency of the plant.

The constantly reduced strength of the form forces in autumn and winter plays a causal role in increased strength and freedom of the life forces. Deterioration of forms goes hand in hand with an increase in the capacity of the life forces, which shows as an increase in yin behaviour such as increased sensitivity and vulnerability. Decline and decay are gifts rather than weaknesses. They depict the centripetal movement of the increasing life forces that may unlock the gates of yin. This concept means that difficulties with ageing and vulnerability are treated initially through the earthly branch *Wu*, heart, the founder of yin, the source of free life forces and authenticity.

Furthermore, acupuncture treatments applied to yang-oriented people should focus on the yin half of the earthly branches cycle that starts with *Wu*, heart.

YOU ARE THE BEST!

Many people struggle with decline as they get older. Accepting decline as a normal consequence of life is a first step in the process of accepting transience and giving up the fight for everlasting youth.

Ignoring aging is especially true for our Western society where concepts of growth, success and 'blossoming' are dominant. People wish to avoid aging and often choose to be medically treated to feel young and vital forever. This type of conduct is often activated and rewarded from childhood: 'You are the best, you are gifted' and 'Well done! You are highly intelligent.' Parents, schools and society seem(ed) to emphasize rapid development and have more respect for autonomy, individuation and exploration than for being lazy, dreamy and playful and remaining dependent.

This kind of upbringing can easily come at the expense of the development of sensitivity and reciprocal interactive relationships between parents and children. Fortunately, in recent years there has been more focus on providing emotional support and parents are more involved in the development of their children instead of just cheering for the results. There seems to be a little more attention and appreciation for natural growth through making mistakes, dreaminess, laziness, doing nothing, boredom and just playing.

Yang (motivating) upbringing and the demands of society that emphasize form and appearances can cause many types of physical-psycho-emotional diseases, both individually and in the social context. The desire for everlasting youth and strength is accompanied by excessive attention to excellent performance and matter-oriented behaviour, which easily exhaust the pre- and post-natal *qi* and *xuè*.

We see people, even teenagers, with excessive stress and burnout along with severe pains or even aggression and unscrupulous conduct. The receding life-giving principle, a consequence of the continuous form-oriented behaviour, results in diseases caused by disruptions of *qi* and *xuè*. The recovery begins only with the recovery of *Wu*, heart.

Stagnation that evokes heat can cause conduct that separates rather than connects; egocentrism, anger, intolerance and especially diminishing spiritual inspiration and reduced togetherness result. It is common these days to see patients between the ages of 30 and 45 who look well groomed and sporty, who have a great position in a large company, work hard, make a successful career and are enthusiastic, but on the other hand have health symptoms with insomnia and unfortunate relationships due to an incapacity for vulnerability, sensitivity and mutuality in relationships. They are exhausted and have complaints due to *jing qi xu*, because they have no time to contemplate, have insufficient sleep and are unable to do nothing.[9] This decline is apparent in all layers of the being: physically, emotionally, mentally and spiritually.

AGING IS AN OPPORTUNITY

Inner spiritual wisdom may happen when life forces return inward and are well maintained. By accepting normal deterioration of form forces and embracing aging – having less focus on formality and appearance without losing decorum and respect – life forces are released and turn inward and are less attached to

---

9   The *jing* regenerates the life forces during 'not-doing'.

form. Self-reflection, self-knowledge, surrender and acceptance cause the ego to become more authentic, which may lead to emancipation and individuation.

Removing the veil from the vital original spirit (the innate heavenly and earthly nature, *shen* and *jing*) is a turning point from which consciousness then expresses itself in a loving peaceful authentic way with a greater eye for reality and actuality, because desires and fears have disappeared. The ego may become peaceful and may embrace aging and death instead of grief and sorrow.

This process starts with an acceptance of the power of susceptibility, openness, receptiveness, sensitivity and vulnerability (yin) through which life (yang) finds its expression through the inner being rather than through a focus on form and matter. This is the source of gratitude and the heart of joy.

What applies to aging also applies to serious illnesses or intense emotions. Diseases and traumas are doors through which people can come into contact with the life forces within, the forces that develop the heart of the self. The forces of yin can find and open these doors and can turn out to be profound turning points. In almost all cases this insight only becomes clear afterwards. Sharing this knowledge prematurely (for example as a practitioner) before true insight and understanding have arrived or during a painful and sad period of discomfort can lead to rejection, frustration, disappointment and anger.

HOPE

Fortunately, people increasingly feel the need to become aware of the forces of life, as in *qi*-awareness exercises, mindfulness training, meditation, breathing exercises, practising stillness, being in the present moment, yoga and through seeking acupuncture treatment. This interest can create conditions for regeneration. It can restore the unhealthy balance between yin and yang in human behaviour.

SEASONAL POINT: HT-8, *SHAO FU*, LESSER MANSION

Ht-8 is a well-known point for reducing heart fire, along with symptoms arising in the heart channel, throat, tongue and mouth as well as in the bladder (due to heat descending to the lower burner).

Sedation of Ht-8 reduces the performance-oriented competitive conduct we have discussed before. It should be noted that sedation of a heart point should go hand in hand with tonification, for example Ht-6, *Yin Xi*, yin cleft, to avoid heart and *shen* insufficiency. Ht-6 is indicated when somebody is less creative, less focused and less clear-minded because the heart *qi* is stagnant or underactive. The heart cannot distribute blood, which leads to malnutrition, and the heart-*shen* cannot guarantee the wholeness of the being.

Ht-8 tonification regulates heart *qi*. It opens the heart, focuses the mind and opens creativity. Ht-8 makes the heart receptive to internal and external impressions for which the heart must be ready. Receptiveness cannot be enforced.

When people are unable to experience emotions and lack motivation Ht-8 should be preceded by Cv-14, *Ju Que*, great gate, the front *mu* point of the heart. It strengthens self-esteem and the desire to live. Bl-44, *Shen Tang*, spirit hall, is indicated when people isolate themselves or are heartbroken due to *xuè xu*.

When the heart recovers, people discover creative forces that know no boundaries. The ego should then learn to relate to new shapes and directions that reveal the wonder of life.

CHAPTER 32

DYNAMICS OF THE EARTHLY BRANCH *WEI* 未[1]

**SUMMER AND EARTH *QI*, THE VIRTUE OF CAREFUL
TRANSFORMATION AND RENEWAL
SEASONAL POINT: S.I.-8, *XIAO HAI*, SMALL SEA**

To you Goat, I give the power of understanding.
You penetrate the deepest depths,
To transform and reorganize what is yours.
Outside you show beauty and joy like a tree in full bloom.
Inside you support your essence for renewing life.
You are the governor of the Small Intestine.

Your life means understanding of the process of renewal providing
people with a sense of freedom and creativity. They can express
joy thanks to your care and endless support. Your sharp sense of
discrimination is expressed by a disciplined use of your mental
faculties together with a fluent, powerful use of language. For
your good work, I give you the virtue of Perseverance.

But beware, if you become too dominant or arrogant, your joy will
change into worries, you will live a life lacking in spontaneity. You will
try to overcome this by showing the tendency to intellectualize your
emotions and experiences and by compulsive talking. You will lose
your sharp sense of discrimination: Your care will become suffocating.

---

1   Born in 1931, 1943, 1955, 1967, 1979, 1991, 2003, 2015, 2027, 2039 after the Chinese New Year.

So use your qualities well.

The Chinese character *Wei* 未 depicts a large tree in full bloom. The extra branches at the top of the character symbolize maturity and maturation. The first scents of fruit announce the end of summer.

Most fruits have seed formation: a reproductive process and a survival mechanism in seed-bearing plants. Seeds are embryonic plants that are still enclosed in a protective skin. They contain the information necessary for the next life cycle of the plant. Seeds are the core from which life returns in the time of the earthly branch *Zi*, gallbladder.

For people, seeds are the essential lessons, the harvest of experiences that affect the present and the future. The earthly branch *Wei*, small intestine, represents the present moment, the ever-changing bridge that connects the experiences of the past with the future. The constant factor in change is the earth of the earthly branch *Wei*, which accepts the past and does not try to influence the future. *Wei* represents the reality of the moment.

THE EARTH OF THE EARTHLY BRANCH *WEI*

Earlier, with the second earthly branch *Chou*, we discussed a central space of earth from which two opposing movements germinated, yin and yang. Yin took root, yang expanded and awakened the third earthly branch *Yin*. With the fifth earthly branch *Chen* we discussed a similar process. It resulted in a space of stability that served as a reference point for movement and change. With the increase of yin, a similar earth space becomes present in the eighth earthly branch *Wei*.

From the seeds in winter grew plants and flowers. Life is collected in new seeds within the fruit and is linked to the future, to continue and secure a new life cycle. The fruits protect their valuable content until the space is given, at the right time, to release the seeds to ensure fertilization. The earthly branch *Wei* offers this space and generates the correct conditions for fertilization and transformation. The earth space of *Wei* is best described as a damp space, an atmosphere that creates a prerequisite for transformation. Damp is water that comes into contact with the heat of fire. The heated water with damp accelerates the movement of *qi* and creates an environment in which solid forms can be transformed into subtler forms.[2] This transformation applies to forms, but also to the more subtle realms; thoughts, for example, transform into ideas, some

---

2   Needed for digestion of food and distinguishing and separating pure and impure *qi*.

feelings change the state of consciousness. Any dominance of dryness and heat in the small intestine hinders these possibilities of transformation.

Four planes or directions converge in the earthly branch *Wei*: past, future and inner, outer. The interactions of the four planes may lead to extroverted activities and plans for the future or to introverted attachments to the past, to extroverted behaviour that keeps the past alive or to introverted artistry that creates images of the future, and so on.

We rarely stay focused on the present. In fact we mainly live in the illusion of thought, because we keep thinking and talking about what has happened or what is going to happen. The earthly branch *Wei* draws attention to the present and for that very reason contributes strongly to physical-emotional-mental-spiritual health.

Problems related to the earthly branch *Wei*, small intestine, often deal with (re)finding a living relationship between traumatic events from the past and the present, so that the view of the future can become bearable. Traumas are solidified emotions that can keep people trapped in the past. However, traumas are also the seeds that bear essential lessons that may help people grow. Healing traumas and growth of the self becomes challenging without the damp-earth condition of the small intestine.

In addition to the stagnation of the self in time awareness in Western culture, there is also current tension in the attunement between the inner personal world and the external social world. People with *Wei* issues feel they have to make choices or that circumstances force them to act. However, the key to health does not lie in making the 'right' choices, but in finding the balance in the centre, in the *qi* of the earth of the small intestine that gives a sense of freedom of spirit, mind and being.

THE COLLABORATION OF THE BRANCHES *WU, WEI* AND *SHEN,* HEART, SMALL INTESTINE AND BLADDER

Wu provides openness, sensitivity, susceptibility and vulnerability. *Wei* creates the space that allows gentle perseverance, to take the time to receive and absorb the world and act clearly. Gentle considerations characterize the continued increase in yin power, which continues to accumulate in the ninth earthly branch *Shen*. This yin power forms the basis for intuition and the art of putting things into perspective.

Wei is the bridge from outer behaviour to inner presence, from the learned to the practised, from making mistakes to success, from impressions to understanding. The damp, yin, earth space of *Wei* is a necessary transformative step to create a field in which the order of heaven has a landing place that inspires and transforms experiences, knowledge, skill and events. It is the breeding ground of intuition for the following earthly branch *Shen*, the bladder.

CAREFUL BUT THOROUGH

The importance of increasing yin shows in gentleness, caution and in taking small and careful steps. Yin behaviour is thorough, persistent and should be supported by adequate rest and healthy nutrition. Problems in the field of *Wei*, small intestine, are best served by an approach that incorporates these yin characteristics.

A healthy earthly branch *Wei*, small intestine, is necessary to be able to process emotional experiences from the past, to integrate such experiences and possibly implement new strategies. *Wei* also supports the ability to distinguish between acquired or hereditary behaviour. This distinction is important in order to learn to differentiate between (innate) temperament and acquired structures of character of the person involved. Because temperament comes from the hereditary *jing*, this distinction gives insight into (im)possibilities for change in character and behaviour.

Human behaviour associated with *Wei* is constructive, adaptable and obedient to present circumstances. Due to its presence in the present, time is recognized as a friend and not as an enemy. People born with *Wei* should take their time to adapt because, even in difficult times with intense emotions, they can build on inner peace and a clear mind. They know that rushing doesn't work. The processing of emotions takes time but, in the end, precisely by taking time, they are slowly softened and lessons learned are thoroughly integrated.

The small intestine pulse should be nicely formed and moderately superficial. Past traumas that affect the present are felt on the small intestine pulse as tight or tense and slightly deep. Treatment of the small intestine supports the trauma healing process.

In addition to processing the past, people benefit from doing something completely unknown in the present, because the present is in fact unpredictable and unknown. Through the refreshing quality of the new, people learn to focus on the mystical side of the present.

SEASONAL POINT: S.I.-8, *XIAO HAI*, SMALL SEA

S.i.-8 sends *qi* inward into the small intestine organ. However, treatment of S.i-8 is not the best-known point to treat the small intestine organ. S.i.-8 is known for its benefits for the channels of the stomach and small intestine. It also creates the damp condition needed for transformation and renewal. The 'small sea' aspect of S.i.-8 supports yin earth qualities, such as receptiveness and calmness, that support transformation. Renewal only comes when people process the past and can connect with the present.

S.i.-8 is preferably used in combination with S.i.-7, *Zhi Zheng*, upright branch. S.i.-7, the *luo* point of the small intestine channel, derives *zheng*, upright *qi* from its connection with the *yuan source* point on the heart channel. S.i.-8 along with S.i.-7 calm the mind, moisten the body, strengthen the essence and bring grounding. Together they therefore provide the conditions needed for a balanced transformation. This treatment requires an accurate diagnosis before use in order to prevent damp stagnation.

DEATH CYCLE

S.i.-8, the earth point of the small intestine channel, is contraindicated if the fire is too weak. In this case it may reinforce the reverse *sheng* relationship between the phases earth and fire. It may be the beginning of a sequence of movements called the death cycle. Diseases and symptoms can progress in this cycle through the five phases as follows: reverse *sheng*, *ke*, *ke* and reverse *sheng*.

For example, diseases related to the organs and channels of the phase earth evolve into diseases and complaints of the fire phase (reverse *sheng*). Thereafter, problems arise in the metal (*ke*) and wood (*ke*) phase, followed by death due to diseases related to the water phase (reverse *sheng*). When diseases start in organs and channels of the phase metal, the phases earth (reverse *sheng*), water (*ke*), fire (*ke*) are successively affected, after which the patient dies due to problems of the wood phase (reverse *sheng*). This cycle can develop within a few days, but it usually takes more time, even years.

The description of some other small intestine-related points might offer more understanding on the topics of bridging past and future, inner and outer transformation and of the central space as a landing place for the order of heaven.

For example, Cv-4, *Guan Yuan*, gate of *yuan qi*, is the front *mu*-point of the small intestine where the *qi* gathers internally. Cv-4 aimed to the past and internal state[3] tonifies kidney yin and yang and the *jing*. It roots the quality of the *yuan qi*, in other words it roots human beings in their basic principle (the seed), being connected to the original source (see its name). In addition Cv-4 is

---

3   This depends on the other points chosen in the same treatment.

the meeting point of bladder and kidney with *chong* and *ren mai*. It relates to the essence and connects internally to the womb and *bao mai*.[4]

Cv-4 aimed to the future and external state[5] meets the post-natal *qi* of the stomach and spleen. In addition, it tonifies *qi*, *xuè*, all five *zang* and regulates menstruation and conception, the lower burner and small intestine.

In conclusion, Cv-4 roots a person in depth and essence and assists functions in expression of the post-natal creation. Incorrect alignment with yin, the essence and the heart *qi* results in post-natal conditions that uproot yang *qi*. It may help to treat S.i.-8, which is especially important in cases of overactivity and fullness of *du mai* with agitation of the heart *qi*.

S.i.-1, *Shao Ze*, lesser marsh, is the *jing-well* point of the small intestine channel where the flow of *qi* arises from the heart channel. The moisture of the marsh (*Ze*) is an important precondition for the transformative qualities of the small intestine *qi*. S.i.-1 is used in cases where the small intestine is unable to receive and discern, leading to reduced transformation. This results in fullness and stagnation below the heart with heat and stagnation in the orifices and mental fog.

S.i.-6, *Yang Lao*, nourishing the old, ensures purity of mind and calms people so that stable decisions can be taken on the basis of individual independence. In addition S.i.-6 opens the path to spiritual maturity. It is characterized by spiritual freedom and mobility.

S.i.-16, *Tian Chuang*, heavenly window, represents the influence of heaven in people. It brings the yang of heaven down to humans. S.i.-16 influences speech and the ability to think. This point focuses the mind and supports the mental discernment necessary for thinking and clear speech. S.i.-16 teaches people to think first before speaking. They become more cautious as they gain insight into the effect of spoken words. S.i.-16 roots the yang of heaven and opens to the qualities of yin and earth. It grounds new perspectives, new visions and new mindsets based on well-considered decisions.

---

4   *Bao mai* is the channel that connects the heart with the womb. The *bao luo* connects the womb with the kidneys.
5   This depends on the other points chosen in the same treatment.

CHAPTER 33

DYNAMICS OF THE EARTHLY BRANCH *SHEN* 申 [1]

AUTUMN AND METAL *QI*, THE VIRTUE OF A TURNING POINT
SEASONAL POINT: BL-67, *ZHI YIN*,
ARRIVAL OR EXTREMITY OF YIN

To you Monkey, I give vision and the power of discrimination.
You save what is good and needful.
You let go of the unsuitable.
You give hope in times of standstill.
You are the hidden power behind new ideals.
You are the governor of the Bladder.

Your life means survival, especially in times of misfortune.
You are successful because of your intuition and your good
sense of humour. You show freedom of emotional and
creative expression and you have the power of letting go
of inappropriate feelings. Furthermore you show no sexual
repression. This is the way to overcome times of misfortune.

For your good work, I give the virtue of Humour.

But beware, if you become dogmatic and unreceptive, forgetting
your sense of humour, your actions will end in failure. You become
conservative, hanging on to outmoded feelings and being unreceptive

---

1   Born in 1932, 1944, 1956, 1968, 1980, 1992, 2004, 2016, 2028, 2040 after the Chinese New Year.

to new ones. You become repressed in your emotions, creativity and sexual expressions and unaware of your blocked situation.

So use your qualities well.

The lifeblood of the trees and plants retreats to the core in autumn; the outward expression ends. The plants wilt, the form slowly disappears, parched leaves whirl through the air, the trees feel the power of autumn winds. Disappearance and death seem to be the only possible outcome. Life has withdrawn from the revealed form but still has not lost its radiance and, despite the decline, plants and trees show beauty with silence and hidden strength. The consciousness is already preparing for the manifestation of new forms in spring. Hidden and hardly visible to the naked eye, a new life cycle quietly starts in the stillness of the earthly branch *Shen*.

The beautiful colours and scents of autumn in the woods and fields seem to be calling us. We enjoy walks in the magnificent light of autumn.

As people get older and arrive into the autumn of their own life, most people experience resistance and feel sad or angry that it is no longer as it used to be. What can we learn from nature? Where are the human equivalents of beautiful colours, scents and the beauty of light as we age, when the lifeblood and physical forces retreat?

HEAVEN AND EARTH, OUTSIDE AND INSIDE

The Chinese character *Shen* 申 depicts two hands that firmly enclose a rope or a body. This idea of two hands was discussed earlier with the characters of the earthly branches *Chou* and *Yin*. In *Chou*, two hands bind together to support growth of young plants, and in *Yin* two hands meet each other under a shelter, showing respect and welcoming the awakening of life. With the earthly branch *Shen*, the closing hands encircle a vertical body suggesting the cooperation of two alternative principles that engender new life.

The vertical body is a symbol that represents the inspiration and initiation of life that comes from heaven and reaches the earth and humanity. This might be the reason why the character *Shen* can be translated as 'lightning'. It is the light of the yang of heaven that is received in the yin, earthly world of humanity and is hidden in the depths of everyone's being.

Shen means to stretch, to express, to apply, to trust, to restrain or to report. As part of the character heart-*shen* 神 it could be translated as 'from heaven extending to all living entities'. *Shen* describes a combination of two different movements: It focuses outward to the world and reports inward to the heart-*shen*. In fact, I believe that with mutual relationships, when people see, feel and experience each other, the *shen* of two or more people together create an interconnected *shen* that exists in itself as a reality. It is the relationship, the projection of everyone's reality and the inner experiences that merge together and bring about the collective *shen*, making it an important fact to consider in any treatment approach.

INTUITION

Intuition is a force through which people perceive and come to know the essence without reasoning. It comes from the heavenly spark of light that is present in everyone.

The sensitivity and responsiveness of the previous earthly branches have developed further into the earthly branch *Shen* as intuition, which imparts the art of putting things into perspective. This intuition, an inner awareness, is similar to the awareness of the joy and beauty of autumn – the colours, scents and autumn light. The experience of intuition is a realization of an inner light. It is congruent to the time when the life forces turn in and illuminate the core.

In the spring, the earthly branch *Yin* awakens life that vitalizes and makes the external world flourish. During the period of the earthly branch *Shen*, the time is right for an internal awakening that happens in the silence and depth of everyone's being.[2]

Intuition is the natural channel that opens one up to the virtues of heaven such as compassion, justice and universal moral principles. These qualities may manifest when people can let go of ego issues and find the freedom to be authentic, accessing the courage to face their fears, so that they regain an open connection to the internal 'heaven'.

Proper treatments of the earthly branch *Shen*, bladder, and the process of conscious inner intuitive awakening can at first evoke emotions. The burden of past experiences covering the source of intuition might initially feel too overwhelming and difficult to process. This initially may cause additional solidification of emotions. Sadness, fear, despair and so on need to be treated and liberated first. It is better not to talk during *Shen*, bladder, treatments, because silence and stillness and the 'simple' act of observing breathing might lead to

---

2   The opposing dynamics of autumn and spring illustrate human destiny and raise typical human practical issues that need to be addressed. The opposing dynamics of summer and winter evoke issues of essence and love that people can also learn to deal with.

new insights. It may be that people suddenly know exactly what's needed, as if a lightning bolt suddenly brings clarity and healing.

The earthly branch *Shen*, bladder, guides the search for the essence and develops the 'inner senses' through which people can draw emotional and rational conclusions. Unfortunately, when the ego is in trouble or looking for recognition, it uses these features as well; the ego uses intuition to gain a position. Yet, the true power of intuition is empathy. People who suffer from complaints related to the bladder channel, such as a slipped disc with pain on the dorsal side of the leg, or have neck and headaches, and so on, are often victims of unempathetic behaviour from others or from themselves.

The challenges for people born with the earthly branch *Shen* often include making difficult choices. Life seems to turn against them and manoeuvre them into difficult circumstances over and over again. For those who turn inside and listen, fighting windmills,[3] doubt, sadness and despair can turn into hope and joy. When this life lesson of 'ego-difficulties-reaction versus intuition' comes back again and again, a good sense of humour is indispensable to help gain access to intuition.

The path to intuition starts off with being still and turning inward, which allows the 'evaporation' and release of the conditions, habits and thoughts and other form (ego) principles. This condition of release can also be achieved by workouts or long walks. Through the effort, the ego relaxes and detaches itself from all its thoughts and habits.

SEASONAL POINT: BL-67, *ZHI YIN*, ARRIVAL OR EXTREMITY OF YIN

Zhi Yin, Bl-67, should be discussed with *Zhi Yang*, Gv-9.

In Gv-9 the extremity of yang *qi* arrives for distribution. It can be used in cases of fullness of yin and emptiness of yang, such as fullness in the chest, diaphragm, stomach with pain in the chest and back, together with aching shins and tired legs, depression, asthenia, with feelings of discouragement.

Bl-67 marks the end of yang in the bladder *qi* and the beginning of yin in the kidney *qi*. This acupuncture point is indicated when water or kidney *qi* is sluggish and without momentum or purpose. This condition is often accompanied by pain in the neck and head or other types of stagnation in the upper burner area. Treatment of Bl-67 opens a yin source that generates dynamic intuitive changes.

---

3   Like Don Quixote.

People with *Shen*, bladder, problems benefit more from inner attunement to perceive intuition. It is noteworthy that people born with the earthly branch *Shen*, bladder, are aware of their intuition but often, due to social or relational pressure, do not listen to it. Intuition makes people less dependent on standards and protocols, including those of the practitioner.

Independence is crucial for a human's individual relationships and also for our relationship with heaven. This independence is reflected in the free expression of feelings and the taking of individual responsibility, in order to individualize and distinguish personal consciousness from others. Conscious differentiation can lead to conscious integration and lead to a healthy collective consciousness. Bl-67 activates this path of consciousness.

CHAPTER 34

DYNAMICS OF THE EARTHLY BRANCH *YOU* 酉[1]

**AUTUMN AND METAL *QI*, THE VIRTUE OF
REVERENCE AND COMPLETION
SEASONAL POINT: KI-7, *FU LIU*, RETURNING CURRENT**

To you Rooster, l give the power of self-preservation.
You seek lonely places, surveying the situation.
You work in a state of ferment creating new potential,
Based on a well-organized structure.
You have a mission to fulfil.
You are the governor of the Kidneys.

Your life means contemplation. You hold natural reverence for
life's forces and show a natural self-preserving fear. You provide
people with a positive sexual identity and the capacity for
affection with the ability to engage in emotional exchange.

For your good work, l give you the virtue of Responsibility.

But beware, if you think that people hold reverence for you instead of
the life forces, your pride will cause excessive and inappropriate fear.
You could even become paranoid, being fearful of losing your position.

So use your qualities well.

---

1   Born in 1933, 1945, 1957, 1969, 1981, 1993, 2005, 2017, 2029, 2041 after the Chinese New Year.

The green colours of leaves disappear and turn red, brown or yellow. There is less light of the sun, causing the plants to enter into a resting mode. The life juices retreat into the core. Nature sacrifices the form; fruits, seeds and grains are released for the continuation of the cycle of life.

The Chinese character *You* 酉 depicts a cider or wine press in which the precious juices of fruit and grains are extracted and fermented. Food and drink are transformed; the longer the fermentation lasts, the more salt is added, the more the pressure is increased and the more yang the result.

This process can teach us that rest, concentration and internalization in autumn and in the evening when the kidney *qi* is active contributes to the recovery of yang *qi*.

CONCENTRATION[2] AND PRESSURE

The process and strategy of fermentation is similar to practising *qigong*, meditation and contemplation. These types of exercises start with the feeling of an inner need for change. The improvement of inner yang/life-*qi* and reduced focus on the material/outer world causes behaviour to change and practising *qi*-exercises becomes a pleasant habit. I sometimes compare *qigong* and meditation to brushing the teeth or having breakfast. It doesn't feel right to skip it.

Qigong and meditation purify and strengthen the whole human being. With attentive presence and constant listening without personal will, the preservation of yang *qi* may become a reality.

The increase in pressure is gained by repetition. The pressure evoked differs from pressure due to stress, which has a negative effect. The desire to practise is due to the habit of practising and the positive feeling it brings.

OBSERVATION

Observation is usually defined as a perception performed for a specific purpose. When we focus on a specific target which causes or arises from a desire to achieve a goal, inherently something counterproductive develops, the fear of failure.

Observation that stems from the qualities of the earthly branch *You*, kidneys, however, can be described as listening without a purpose, using all the senses with attention. It is characterized by gratitude and giving space to all that exists, without judgement, purpose setting or any form of discrimination. Inner

---

2 Salt is a metaphor for concentration and focus.

listening and attention are different from what we usually mean by observation. Inner listening is yin in nature, which means that the mind observes itself and responds from inner understanding. This means that book knowledge and the like only have value when they have become internalized experiences and actually become timeless. Reverence for the self, rather than knowledge and outer appearances, is the foundation of any healthy relationship.

SLEEP

When people get tired and want to go to bed the earthly branch *Shen* is involved; the farewell of the day is led by *Shen*. Our subsequent bedtime ritual, preparing for the transformation to sleep consciousness, is a major turning point guided by the earthly branch *You*. Just as the earthly branch *Mao* causes strong outward growth, the earthly branch *You* causes powerful inner growth: regeneration of *qi* and *xuè* in the inner essence.

Therefore, it is useful to wind down from the day at sunset or just before falling asleep, to internalize the essences of experiences, to absorb the light of the day and let go of emotions and thoughts.

Inner observation and awareness of breathing as well as scanning the body can take you to the core of your being. The darkness of the night is beneficial to contact the deepest aspects of the being. The waking consciousness is passive during sleep, but the spiritual person takes the opportunity to get in touch with the yang *qi* within the yin, the life-*qi* within the time of the light of the moon – *tai yin*.

As Mark Twain says: 'Everyone is a moon, and has a dark side which he never shows to anybody',[3] to which I would like to add a statement by Carl Gustav Jung: 'One does not become enlightened by imagining figures of light, but by making the darkness conscious.'[4]

The earthly branch *You* is the gateway that leads into the darkness of the soul.

At sunrise, the inner lights may gather again into a light that shines and shares life-*qi* with all.

RESPONSIBILITY

It is easier to perceive and integrate the light of the subtle world during sunset and the darkness of the night, in the light of the moon, than it is during the day

---

3   'The Refuge of the Derelicts' (Twain 1972).
4   Jung 1968, para 335.

with the radiance of sunlight present. It is easier to train observation during yin times, especially around sunset. Observation, listening and paying attention are essential for understanding and implementing responsibility for preserving vital life-*qi*.[6]

The kidney yang is 'the storehouse of the vital *qi*', also known as *pre*-natal *qi*, or *qi* that is based on the *qi* of ancestors. The kidney yin is also the 'gateway to the stomach', known as *post*-natal *qi*. The kidneys are the underlying foundation for the stomach and spleen *qi* and contribute support to the entire digestive system.

Exhaustion caused by overstimulation of the kidney *qi* – through excessive yang behaviour – results in insufficiency of pre- and post-natal (kidney) *qi*. This is characterized by a lack of foundation and less lubrication, causing, for example, cough, asthma, dryness in the throat and tongue, lumbar pain, stiffness, pain and lack of will as well as anxiety. Treatment of kidney *qi* alone is insufficient. Personal responsibility for one's health should be the incentive not to constantly cross boundaries and to respect the importance of the inner yin force.

SEASONAL POINT: KI-7, *FU LIU*, RETURNING CURRENT

These considerations may contribute to an understanding of the functions of Ki-7, the metal/autumn point on the kidney channel. The name of Ki-7, *Fu Liu*, returning current, is often described as resuming a straight path after the strange loop that the kidney channel takes over the heel bone at Ki-4, *Da Zhong*, Ki-5, *Shui Quan*, and Ki-6, *Zhao Hai*.

Returning current means that the *qi* returns to its source, where the seed of new life resides. Ki-7 assists people to recover from difficult situations and troubles, to 'strengthen the backbone' and overcome fear.

Other names for Ki-7 are *Fu Bai*, deep lying white[5] or *Chang Yang*, glorious yang. Deep lying white is the beneficial outcome of regeneration of glorious yang through observation, introversion and introspection. In the depth of one's being, Ki-7 increases the essence of the kidney yang. It is the core quality of the emanation *li*.[6]

---

5   The colour of metal and introversion.
6   See Chapter 3.

CHAPTER 35

INTRODUCTION TO THE EARTHLY BRANCHES *XU* AND *HAI*

We may find light in the darkness
in times of despair and agony.

The organs/functions of two earthly branches, *Xu*, heart constrictor, and *Hai*, *san jiao*, do not occur in the cycle of the heavenly stems and related organs. The special functions of these two earthly branches contain deep secrets that I will try to discuss here as far as I can, but I am convinced that my understanding will deepen over time, as it has done many times over the past forty years.

Xu and *Hai* start their functions just after birth and therefore belong to post-natal *qi*. They are both organized in three sections: upper, middle and lower. Each of the three regions is subdivided into three more, allowing nine regions to operate the body. These regions of transformation are involved in the creation process in which heaven creates the earth for the benefit of humanity and all other forms of life and consciousness. Through these three areas, living beings can live in accordance with the order of heaven and earth.

Heaven has no reason for existence, humanity seeks it. The human quest to give meaning to life expresses itself in the nine regions: through the drives and rights to exist. In the beginning, these motivations are predominately self-centred and personal. As people age, depending on the health of the earthly branches *Xu* and *Hai*, the possibilities for togetherness and a 'we-society' come into focus.

CHANGE IS THE SYMPTOM OF LIFE[1]

On my Facebook page in March 2020, during the Covid-19 crisis, I published the following text on the effect of the deep transformations that were present at the time and which were partly related to *Xu* and *Hai* and include kidney *qi*, *jing qi*, the *shao yang* division.

Regularly I was asked what the Chinese calendar has to say about this Corona crisis. I don't really want to explain the technical, rational details of this now. In connection with each other I first want to say something about what people can do to increase resistance and second give some insight in what we go through according to the Chinese calendar.

Obviously, the general rules apply here, such as sufficient exercise, eating healthy – not processed – food and drink, fresh air, less stress and so on, whereby the rules of authorities such as hygiene, keeping distance, staying indoors must be followed. In addition, we can strengthen our protective/defence *qi* (*wei qi*). This is mainly produced in the lower burner (kidneys), in addition to the middle burner (stomach and spleen) and the upper burner (lungs). The lower burner *wei qi* is best enhanced by *qigong*. If you have never had any instruction in this, I suggest a 'simple' and effective exercise here.

Stand with feet parallel, shoulder-width apart. Make conscious contact with the feet and toes with the earth and root yourself deeply in the earth. Your knees are slightly bent and open without tension and the chest is open with the shoulders down and relaxed and the neck is straight. Visualize a vertical line from the centre of the earth through yourself up into the sky. The body is between earth and heaven and is relaxed. Just breathe normally, not too shallow, not too deep. For the lower burner, focus on your abdomen, when it feels stronger there, filled with *qi* and warmth, focus on the middle burner, the area of the liver, stomach and spleen, and the diaphragm, then on the upper burner, the areas of the lungs and heart. You build, as it were, the protective *qi*, based on the strength of the *qi* of the kidneys. Build the exercise in such a way that you can eventually stand for thirty minutes a day.

With humility, I would like to add the following, which is the outcome of my understanding of the calendar and could also have a beneficial effect on the protective *qi*.

It became clear to me that a few months before the Corona crisis began that many people worldwide, more so than before, were already undergoing major

---

[1] My father wrote this message on the first page of the *Yijing* my parents gave me for my eighteenth birthday.

dramatic, transformational events and developments in which fear played a particularly important role. The Corona crisis appears to be the peak of this development for the time being.

When we go through major changes, such as during this crisis in which the world comes to a halt and major dramas take place, the gateways to insight are calmness and taking care. The new comes about through change and when we see how the changing life manifests it reveals how mankind and each individual can move on. Through fear, restlessness and panic, the ego tends to rise above others and disrupts this process not only for itself but the whole of society.

From fear arises resistance to upcoming changes. However, changes, even if they are uncomfortable or insidious, characterize our existence. There is nothing in this world that is permanent, although people often live as if their life was infinite and unchanging. Despite all of our efforts, we are not able to stop what is coming. All of us together (!) can guide the transformation and try to understand it by turning inside and observe and face our own fears, which then give space to life again. By calmness, caring and facing our fears, without fighting or fleeing, our fears can disappear and when fears disappear the kidney *qi* opens and protective *qi* individually and socially become stronger.

Fear arises from uncertainty. However, certainty cannot be found in others, although it often seems so. Certainty can only really be found in self-knowledge and authenticity of the self, together with tolerance (*shao yin*, kidney-heart). Where wholeness is within, there is togetherness in the world.

Love and Light to all.

I had not predicted the severity of the Covid-19 crisis, although I had already discussed with colleagues, students and patients that if the climate during autumn and winter did not get colder, we would get a lot of flu with unexpectedly high fevers in late 2019 and the first half of 2020. The lack of withdrawal of life-*qi* in 2019 due to the long warm, sometimes damp, climate had a twofold effect. First, the lack of withdrawal of warmth did not sufficiently nourish the kidneys and the *jing*. In addition, the heat ascended, resulting in more heat and stagnation of damp in the upper burner.

This situation is dangerous for those whose kidney and *jing qi* are already weaker due to their constitution, behaviour or trauma.[2]

---

2   It turned out that people with kidney failure seemed much more susceptible to Covid-19 with relatively more deaths. This was shown by the first results of research by UMCG, Radboud UMC and Amsterdam UMC, led by Ron Gansevoort, professor of nephrology (UMCG) in August 2020 (Ortiz *et al.* 2021).

The year 2020 (*Geng-Zi*) was governed by dryness.[3] This exacerbated the stagnation and heat already present. In addition the water aspect of the earthly branch *Zi* was deficient as a result of the decreased withdrawal of fluids in 2019. People's physical status was not ready to deal with the virus's hot poison.

The upcoming problems became clearer to me in the months before the Covid-19 pandemic, when many more people than usual experienced dramatic confrontational events that depleted the *qi* of the kidneys, *jing* and heart. It was striking to me that this *qi* was also disturbed in people who did not experience intense events.

One of the most unexpected comments from my pulse diagnosis teachers was that the pulse not only reflects the current situation but also gives a prediction about the future. The general nature of the deviations in the pulses in many people heralded a major change that would affect the quality of life of all humanity.

FEAR

Usually, Chinese medicine practitioners follow the idea that fear depletes the kidney *qi* which causes the *qi* to sink. In Chapter 39 of the *Huang Di Nei Jing Su Wen* it is stated that due to fear the pure *qi* declines, causing a blockage in the upper burner. This results in a downward movement of the *qi* of the upper burner, disturbing the lower burner and overall circulation of *qi*.

In practice, however, I have observed that *qi* also ascends due to the broken relationship between the upper and lower burner. This causes the *qi* of the upper burner to stagnate and possibly even rise. This disorder in communication due to fear can be diagnosed in the heart constrictor and *san jiao*: sunken, taut, scattered, loss of root in the depth and stagnated or jumping superficially.

During the last two months of 2019 I felt these pulse qualities[4] on many patients from different countries in Europe. This kind of pulse on the heart constrictor position, when accompanied by *jing qi xu*, indicates fear of not being seen or fear of the unexpected. It includes fear of fear, fear of change and fear of impermanence and death. Felt on the *san jiao* position, along with *jing qi xu*, it indicates fear of missing out or fear of not being able to complete something.

The tragic time of Covid-19, when many fell ill and many died and were mourned, was one where the disease was clearly felt in the pulse beforehand. Despite and also because of the enormous grief, many people were confronted

---

3   '*Geng*, L.i. in metal'.
4   The heart constrictor and/or the *san jiao* along with deficiency of the *jing* and heart.

with previously deeply hidden domains of the soul; this often touched on the deep sense of the right to exist.

Deep-rooted existential traumas were exposed and demanded attention. For many, these uncomfortable feelings caused anger alongside feelings of injustice and depression. In others the deep psychological transformation led to inner peace and freedom. For many, it was a difficult, challenging time that set the soul in motion. I have also known people whose changes in consciousness were experienced as part of a collective change of consciousness of humanity, and brought with them the hope that these changes would support human evolution towards a fairer and more caring society.

CHAPTER 36

DYNAMICS OF THE EARTHLY BRANCH *XU* 戌 [1]

AUTUMN AND EARTH *QI*, THE VIRTUE OF LOYALTY AND SERVING
SEASONAL POINT: HC-7, *DA LING*, GREAT MOUND/HILL

To you Dog, I give the power to unite with Love.
You prepare the earth for the next sowing season.
You are the hinge between potency and reality.
This Love first causes decline yet is based on loyalty.
You are fully committed to the future race.
You are the governor of the Heart Constrictor.

Your life means serving, with minor, personal involvement.
You show the capacity for commitment.

You listen to the rhythm of life, giving love where needed. Sometimes
you destroy, giving the freedom to follow a new direction.

For your good work, I give you the virtue of Freedom.

But beware, if you involve yourself too personally, trying to personify
yourself with the Love, you will fail to hear anymore the rhythm
of life. Then you will show self-preoccupation with excessive self-
containment. You will lose your freedom, fearing over-exposure.

So use your qualities well.

---

1   Born in 1934, 1946, 1958, 1970, 1982, 1994, 2006, 2018, 2030, 2042 after the Chinese New Year.

It is the end of autumn and nature prepares for winter. The plants dry out, the earth is covered with falling leaves. For a while, the leaves protect the roots and the earth from the approaching frost.

Over time, the nutrients of the natural humus are absorbed by the roots, which is needed for the fertility of the earth for the next sowing season and the renewal of life in spring. Yang, life-*qi*, is almost completely withdrawn under the earth, leaving the surface of the earth listless and exhausted.

The character of the earthly branch *Xu* 戌 depicts a lance, the weapon of a guard. It represents injury and death or destruction for the purpose of protecting the new. Farmers use the plough and prepare the earth to support the fertilization process. The decay of the form of plants and the loosening and turning of the soil are destructions of the past with the aim of creating the right conditions to give new life a chance...

Like other earth-related earthly branches, *Xu* has a time-related dual character. The past needs to be released and the focus is on the future. On a human level, letting go is a radical process and it is difficult to see and appreciate the future as positive. This problem specifically affects patients with chronic diseases, such as amyotrophic lateral sclerosis, multiple sclerosis, Crohn's disease and the like. These people need to learn to cope with reduced capacity and are forced to let go of exactly what they identify with: sports, exercise, appearance, making music, eating and drinking, work and friendships, feeling healthy, the prospect of getting better, dignity and so on. The same can happen during the natural aging process, when people suffer from a decrease in strength.

LOYALTY

Fear of change or fear of the future, loss of strength and also the image of dying are just a few aspects of life that people can experience as threatening and terrible. So much so, that it is difficult for them to maintain a spiritual life. Then different things can happen, but I have often seen people develop a strong need for loyalty that mainly evokes a sense of commonality. Loyalty becomes the proof of togetherness. The following doesn't sound very empathetic, but I want to delve a little deeper into this trait of engagement. Loyalty to and from others can be selfish in nature but also at the same time create a sense of security. The resulting dependence on loyalty can last a long time, because people seem to benefit from it.

There is a pitfall: If the soul and spiritual life are not fed in any other way, loneliness and fear gain the upper hand despite the fact that people have ensured communality and a loyal environment. The first symptoms that occur in this situation are nervousness and neurotic behaviour.

In the elderly and/or in cases where nervousness prevails, the tension between loyalty and loneliness might cause illnesses due to the malfunction of the earthly branch *Xu*, heart constrictor, such as osteoporosis, dementia, heart failure and osteoarthritis. But even if people are still in the prime of their lives, family feuds where misunderstandings about loyalty prevail can be the underlying cause of the above and other diseases.

So returning to the life and death of a plant: How can we translate the end of the plant's life cycle to the human level? Loyalty of the plant is not aimed at maintaining its shape but at offering its form to give future life a chance, without any 'personal' benefit or expectation. What about loyalty and human existence?

Loyalty of the earthly branch *Xu* refers to unconditional readiness in which 'anything is possible' as long as the essence of life can prevail. I do not mean that loyalty based on selfishness or personal desires is wrong. Society, companies, relationships and friendships cannot function or exist without a personal form of loyalty. Loyalty to yourself or others can be much needed: quitting a job and leaving or staying in a relationship are examples of this. Having to let go of things is often very painful, but sometimes necessary to give the new a chance.

A girl (16, born in a year with the earthly branch *Zi*) was forced to live with her mother after her parents divorced. The agreement made between the parents, without consulting the daughter, gave her no choice. After some time it became clear that this girl was suffering and exhibited behaviour that was diagnosed as anorexia and self-mutilation. Her life was under serious threat. She decided to live with the father and visited me to treat her health problems.

Pulse diagnosis clearly indicated a conflict in the heart constrictor *qi*, which was tight and hard but insufficient. During the treatments, she brought up her loyalty conflict regarding her parents.

I explained to her the Chinese view of the relationship between the heart constrictor (the ministerial fire) and the heart (the emperor fire): For a peaceful country, the minister must listen to the emperor and not to the people in the country. The emperor is the son of heaven[2] and has been given the power to rule over everyone, to promote goodness without personal interest. In line with this concept, it means that in the body the heart constrictor must be loyal to the heart and not react to the impulses and opinions from the

---

2   Rarely a daughter of heaven such as Wu Zetian, the famous, rather cruel, Tang Dynasty empress (seventh century BCE).

environment. I asked her what she wanted for herself and how she felt about the situation.

She looked at me in amazement with wide open eyes; it had never occurred to her that her own feelings were of any importance and that she could share her feelings and ideas about her own life and that people would listen to it.

The constitutional treatment of the heart constrictor changed her awareness of loyalty and personal responsibility for her renewed life. All parties involved were initially only focused on legal frameworks, legal agreements and the physical problems of the daughter. After some time she started to speak with both her parents about the future instead of the past and everyone woke up. Gradually her parents' focus shifted from the technical and physical to what was really essential emotionally for their daughter; the mutual love between her parents and herself and the love for herself together with general happiness in relationships. This outcome is certainly not always achieved, but I have never forgotten this girl. This transformation would not have been successful without her dedication, insight and perseverance. It was especially possible due to her love of life. Not infrequently, patients are the best teachers!

Loyalty may become unhealthy when it comes at the expense of freedom. This type of loyalty often sublimates the fear of loneliness and losing someone or something. Strangely enough, this behaviour is often accepted by the 'victims' while the 'perpetrators' do not get the opportunity to face their fears.

One treatment approach, only possible when people want to learn to deal with their fears, is to treat the earthly branch *Chen*, stomach. This creates stability and an awareness of healthy intake in the broadest sense of the word. *Chen* determines the acceptance and refusal of food; it determines which food is beneficial and nutritious or unfavourable and unhealthy.

It takes courage to face fears, but it takes even more courage to tackle unhealthy choices and it requires perseverance and a clear awareness of what is being 'swallowed'.

THE HEART AND HEART CONSTRICTOR AT BIRTH

One of my teachers taught me about the physical and energetic transformations that take place during birth. After the first breath is taken by the newborn baby, a process develops where the *yuan-shen* (which resides in the heart) divides into two parts. One part of the original *shen* ascends to the space between the eyebrows, the area of *Yin Tang*, where it remains quiet, patient, watching and waiting. This part is called the essence of the *shen*. The other part stays in the heart. It is called the being, the personal *shen* or the ruler.

My teachers taught me techniques of meditation that first focus on purification of the lower burner and kidney *qi*. This was followed by breathing exercises to ascend the pure *qi* to the area of the heart. The theory states that the *qi* of the kidneys and the heart merge and conceive a new being that rises up to the essence between the eyebrows to receive enlightenment. I have no experience in this direction and I am not in a position to say anything about enlightenment.

I was taught (and confirmed through clinical practice) that the closing of the septum of the heart, as well as the changes that occur in the liver during birth, are determined by the *qi* of the earthly branch *Xu*. It 'injures' and divides the *yuan-shen*; the newborn baby releases the past and enters a new life. The newborn gets its freedom and turns away from the safe hiding place in the mother and from the resonance of the mother's heartbeat. This transformation into solitary existence is at the expense of oneness with the *yuan-shen* and ensures that humans become social beings looking for connection and perception.

In fact, the *qi* of the heart constrictor does not become active until the very first inspiration, when the newborn has left the safe place in the womb, the pre-natal shape of the heart is transformed and the lungs start breathing on their own. From that moment on, the heart constrictor functions as the loyal servant of the heart. It listens to the radiance of the being that resides in the heart and protects it. Neither the heart constrictor nor the *shen* in the heart are aware of the essence between the eyebrows. Spirituality can be defined as the heart consciousness that remembers the way to the space between the eyebrows.

THE DYNAMICS BETWEEN HEART AND HEART CONSTRICTOR

The heart constrictor (the protector of the heart) and *wei qi* belong to the natural defence mechanisms.[3] When the defence of the self against the violence and hustle and bustle of the world is overly challenged, all defence mechanisms may be overloaded. Pulses are tight or wiry, inflexible and inelastic. The yin of the heart may be closed to susceptibility and sensitivity, and the heart pulse feels tight or stagnant and slippery but weak.

Treatment of the heart with moxa on Gv-11, *Shen Dao*, divine path, opens susceptibility and the gate to love, replacing any other form of defence mechanism.

---

3   The first layer of defence is the *tai yang* division, the bladder and small intestine. The heart constrictor belongs to a deeper level of defence but can be quickly affected when emotional issues prevail.

This supports and activates the energy of love, joy, peace and happiness. Some say that a channel flows from Gv-11 to and around the heart and continues to Gv-20, *Bai Hui*, hundred meetings, to perceive the radiance of heaven and to open the heart.

When the heart *qi* is weak, the *qi* of the heart constrictor needs to protect the heart. The pulse of the heart constrictor becomes stronger and tighter, sometimes with signs of heat. This kind of protection is common for instance in people with eczema. Treatment should focus on nourishing heart *qi* and not on calming, relaxing and cooling the heart constrictor *qi*. This would leave the heart *qi* unprotected.

When the heart *qi* is strong and full and the heart constrictor *qi* is weak and empty, people are intuitively vulnerable and hypersensitive. This can be hereditary and constitutional. It is also observed in children or adults who are emotionally damaged by (sexual) abuse or by parenting lacking in boundaries. In order to create a filter against the impressions of the world it may help to optimize the heart constrictor *qi*. In addition to psychotherapy, trauma therapy, time and attention, constitutional acupuncture is a wonderful tool and support to strengthen and relax the heart constrictor *qi*.

SEASONAL POINT: HC-7, *DA LING*, GREAT MOUND

Da Ling is a large burial mound or tomb, a monument to someone who has died. This is probably why this point is often used to support people in times of mourning.

Hc-7 is the earth and *yuan source* point of the heart constrictor channel. In Chapter 1 of the *Ling Shu* the importance of Hc-7 is emphasized as the *yuan source* point of the heart channel itself and not of the heart constrictor channel.

In addition Hc-7 is a *gui* (ghost) point, *Gui Xin*, ghost in the heart. It is used in cases when damp and phlegm torment the heart. This leads to weakness and apathy along with manic depression, agitation with crying alternating with laughter, sadness, grief and even nymphomania. It is a clinical picture in which underactivity alternates with uncontrollable excess and outbreaks of heart *qi*.

Hc-7 is considered a main point to treat symptoms such as heat in the *ying qi* and *xuè* that threaten the *shen* or lead to eczema. It is recommended with emotional disorders due to rising heat that disrupts the *shen* and heart constrictor, possibly resulting in fever.

Hc-7 supports the release of problems that are actually no longer current or cannot be changed, but which nevertheless keep the psyche busy. It attunes people with their essence to help explore the inner space in which the light of heaven shines.

Hc-7 can be used when work problems do not stop and can no longer be tolerated, when there is fear of surgery or when there are constant concerns about a home situation and so on. In short, Hc-7 supports letting go to enter a new future.

Shadowy and dim!
And yet It contains within Itself a Core of Vitality
The Core of Vitality is very real,
It contains within Itself an unfailing Sincerity.[4]

---

4   *Dao De Jing* Chapter 2 (Wu 1989, p. 43).

CHAPTER 37

DYNAMICS OF THE EARTHLY BRANCH *HAI* 亥[1]

WINTER AND WATER *QI*, THE VIRTUE OF INVOLVEMENT AND HUMILITY
SEASONAL POINT: SJ-2, *YE MEN*, FLUID DOOR

To you Pig, I give you understanding of my Idea.
You are conscious of the Plan, though not capable of sharing it.
You generate change as concealed energy,
Building and caring, receptive and involved.
It is through humility that you serve.
You are the governor of the Three Heater.

Your life means involvement. You give people an emotional and physical harmony with their environment. By good regulation you show the capacity to generate and accept change.

For your good work, I give you the virtue of Humility.

But beware, if your humility is misplaced, it will show as excessive caution and an over regulated lifestyle. Your efforts to evangelize my Idea will fail every time, without understanding why. This will frustrate you and make you lonely.

So use your qualities well.

---

1   Born in 1935, 1947, 1959, 1971, 1983, 1995, 2007, 2019, 2031, 2043 after the Chinese New Year.

After the completion in the tenth earthly branch *You*, kidneys, earthly branches *Xu* and *Hai*, heart constrictor and *san jiao*, ensure the continuation of the cycle of life. The glory of the abundance of shapes in the summer has almost completely disappeared and life-*qi* is approaching its peak level, hidden in the core of the root.

The character *Hai* 亥 depicts two people, a woman and a man, hiding under a shelter. A shelter or canopy[2] symbolizes heaven that overshadows and illuminates the earth and all people on it. The heavenly influence of *Hai* is visible, reflected and embedded in all forms, in rivers and mountains, springs and valleys, human beings and animals. The act of love between a woman and a man reflects the heavenly interactive gathering and unification of yin and yang. This unification, depicted in the earthly branch *Hai*, is unique; in all other earthly branches there is cooperation or opposition of yin and yang, never unification.

Receiving the influx from heaven with the togetherness of yin and yang under a canopy during the time of the earthly branch *Hai*[3] is an auspicious symbol. It is the propitious time for planting seeds and for fertilization.

The earthly branch *Hai*, *san jiao*, the three burners, functions in line with heavenly and earthly *qi* only when both the earthly branch *You*, kidneys, and the earthly branch *Xu*, heart constrictor, function in line with the cyclical movement of the earthly branches. The latter are prerequisites for a good *san jiao* function and should therefore always be addressed with *san jiao* problems.

San jiao mediates between heart-*shen* and kidney *jing*-essence.[4] Merging fire and water is necessary to create the right conditions for a new conception, both in physical and spiritual awakening.

Dear reader,

It is conceivable that this type of text cannot be understood with a single read. This certainly applies to this subject. The way the *san jiao* appears is difficult to put into words because *san jiao* represents something outside the world of thought and time. I have spent quite a few years trying to familiarize myself with the character of the *san jiao* and this research and further understanding is still ongoing. The following text on the *san jiao* should be seen as a testimony to my study and experience up to this point and hopefully it will be accepted as a guideline.

I would like to ask you to explore these concepts with an open mind and

---

2   A canopy is a symbol for the lungs that cover all other organs, just as the sky covers the earth.
3   During the tenth lunar month or from 9 till 11 p.m.
4   The heart *qi* descends via the *bao mai* and kidney *jing qi* ascends via *bao luo* to connect in the uterus, the porch that is governed by *san jiao*.

feeling, to carry the ideas with you for a while. When you experience the resonance of these words and the meaning behind the text, it can reach the heart-
shen and *jing*-essence so that the words not only remain words and thoughts,
but can also take on meaning in your personal life and appear to be useful to
yourself and to your patients.

With warm regards
Joan

ANDROGYNOUS

The earthly branch *Hai, san jiao,* is androgynous, something that has both female
and male traits; it is a fusion of yin and yang. In this sense, it is a reflection of
the original oneness, the state where yin and yang are not yet separated. The
multitude of things that are created by the separation of yin and yang all together
constitute and represent the original oneness. The initiating and nurturing powers of the earthly branch *Hai, san jiao,* are connected to and involved in everything
that exists to ensure togetherness. They guard the unity of the body in the light
of and attunement to the original heavenly order and the Universal Spark.

The spiritual androgynous experience happens in the experience of the present moment, when past and future feelings and thoughts merge in the present.
It can be a lasting state but is mostly experienced for a short period of time
during sexual intercourse and orgasms.

The present is a continuous movement, an endless now with every possible
potential for creation to flow according to its original nature. The *qi* of heaven
and earth merge when every impulse from the past and the future comes to
rest and the natural state of the 'now' reveals itself. This is not a concept, but
appears as the realization that everything and everyone is already in their natural
state. The characteristic nature of unification and involvement in the present
moment is timeless and omnipresent, continuous and unchanging.

When needed, and without any delay, *Hai, san jiao,* merges yin and yang,
form and life. The result is fertilized by water and linked to the warmth of fire:

> From ancient times, the roots of life are in correspondence with the heavens;
> such roots are called yin and yang ... The nine divisions of China, the nine
> openings in the human body, the five viscera and the twelve articulations in the
> human body, are, all of them, in correspondence with the energy of the heavens.[5]

---

5   *Huang Di Nei Jing Su Wen* Chapter 3.

The *shen* and *jing* essences are divided and fragmented in humans, but are mystically one.

In practice, this means that *san jiao* is responsible for wholeness of the body and mind through its joining with the original oneness in the essence. Any health issue breaks up the wholeness,[6] which means that the treatment is incomplete if the *san jiao* has not been treated at least once.

The mystical root of the *san jiao* lies deeply hidden in the relationship with the *yuan qi*. It is the generator, catalyst and governor of all *qi* and *xuè* and has the freedom to interact with all forms of *qi* and *xuè* such as *ying qi*, *wei qi*, blood, fluids and the five tastes.

The relationship with all and everything cannot be explained by the course of the *san jiao* channel alone. The realization of the *deep* function of the *san jiao*[7] can be addressed through the use of acupuncture points on the *ren mai*. These points facilitate the heavenly distribution of *qi*.[8]

THE DYNAMICS OF *REN MAI* AND THE DEEP *SAN JIAO* FUNCTION

Some points in the lower burner on the *ren mai* channel activate the *deep san jiao* function.

The *ren mai* starts in the uterus just below Cv-3,[9] *Zhong Ji*, middle summit, and comes to the surface in Cv-1, *Hui Yin*, meeting of yin. This point is the nadir of the vertical axis; on the opposite side is the zenith, Gv-20, *Bai Hui*, one hundred meetings, the meeting of all yang.

In Cv-1, *chong mai*, *ren mai* and *du mai* meet. It is the solid base from which life divides, fragments and develops and is the human reflection of the oneness of heaven.

Cv-2, *Qu Gu*, bend bone, is closely referenced with Ki-11, *Heng Gu*, horizontal bone. These points give physical meaning to the living yin just obtained from Cv-1. The main function of Ki-11 is to transform yin into nutrient components and bring yin to the legs. Some sources mention Ki-11 as a special *mu* point of the kidneys and heart constrictor, with which it forms the foundation for the *qi* of the earthly branch *Hai* and the deep *san jiao* function. Cv-2 meets the liver channel, the liver and gallbladder tendinomuscular and divergent channels, the

---

6   The *san jiao* network is connected to all individual cells and their internal metabolism.

7   The deep *san jiao* function is described in the *Nan Jing*, the *san jiao* channel is described in the *Ling Shu*.

8   Some sources call it the *dong*/moving *qi*, residing between the kidneys.

9   Some sources take Cv-3, *Zhong Ji*, middle summit as the origin of *ren mai* and consider it the beginning and foundation of a good relationship with the outside world.

three leg yin tendinomuscular channels and receives a branch of *du mai*. In this way it forms a foundation on which the moving life is carried in the depth of the bend in the bone. Cv-2 supports life physically, psychologically and energetically, together with Bl-11, *Da Zhu*, great shuttle, the *hui* (meeting) point of the bones and entry point of sea of blood, which provides structure to the whole.

The foundation for life has been laid in Cv-3, *Zhong Ji*, middle summit, which bears the same name as the North Pole star, the place of the heavenly emperor and the centre of heaven. This point represents the original heavenly power in humans. The nadir of the vertical axis merges with the zenith in the sky, the influences of which enter the body at Gv-20. The opposite of Cv-3 being in contact with the outside world is Bl-67, *Zhi Yin*, arrival of yin, which strengthens yin and intuition as we discussed with the earthly branch *Shen*.

Cv-4, *Guan Yuan*, gate or *yuan qi*,[10] is one of the points where yin and yang merge, as happens in Cv-12, *Zhong Wan*, middle venter, front *mu* point of the stomach and the *san jiao* middle burner, and in Cv-22, *Tian Tu*, celestial chimney, window of the sky point, meeting point of *chong* and *yin wei mai*. These points keep the balance of yin and yang along with Gv-4, *Ming Men*, door of life. They correspond to and execute the merging of yin and yang, the reflection of the original oneness to guard the unity of the body.

The meeting and merging of yin and yang in Cv-4 and Gv-4 is the basis from which the deep *san jiao* function in *ren mai* operates. Similar actions to strengthen the deep *san jiao* function take place in Cv-12 in the middle burner and Cv-22/Gv-9, *Zhi Yang*, in the upper burner.

The *qi* of the lower burner is rooted in the *jing*-essence which can be enriched by acupuncture points like Cv-3, Cv-4 and Gv-4 through their connection with the *bao mai*.

Cv-5, *Shi Men*, stone door, is the front *mu* point of the *san jiao*. The name suggests accumulation of *qi*, as do names of other points that are at the same level: Ki-14, *Si Man*, four fullness, and St-27, *Da Ju*, big great. This place in the body shows the effect on *qi* that results from the merging of yin and yang that accumulates just before being further distributed by *san jiao*. This area shows people's identification with life and the desire to procreate.

---

10 The physical external expression of Cv-4 is in Bl-60, *Kun Lun*, mountain. *Kun Lun* is the (alternative) name for Cv-4 and Bl-60. Each in their own way, from the centre of humans and humanity, connect between heaven above and the earth below. The worldly representation of this is the Kun Lun mountains. Kun Lun is a sacred mountain range. It is an axis mundi, a world axis, the central vertical link between heaven, earth and humanity. The peak of the mountain reaches to heaven and the base is firmly grounded on the earth. The centre of the mountain is the place of humans and a focus for life forces that elevate humans above the forms. Therefore the Kun Lun mountains are considered a sacred place where gods and other mythical figures dwell.

Cv-6, *Qi Hai*, sea of *qi* or ocean of *qi*, governs the metabolism of *qi* and *xuè* in general and brings the *qi* to the chest. This point is the root of life-maintenance for the whole body.

Cv-7, *Yin Jiao*, yin crossing or meeting, is where *ren mai* meets with the *chong* and *yin wei mai*, kidney, heart constrictor and *san jiao*. As front *mu* point of the *san jiao* of the lower burner, it controls stagnations and blockages and relieves heart pains due to conflicts between yin and yang.

The deep *san jiao* function is diagnosed in the pulse in the depth of the proximal pulse (*chi* position) of the right hand, under the pulse of the heart constrictor. The qualities found there should be related to the pulse qualities of *ren mai*.

The deep *san jiao* function controls and coordinates the *qi* of the *jing*-essence and water. Just after birth it roots the fire – *heng*, the ever-penetrating consciousness – to lower areas where it is stored in kidney yang. Throughout life, *san jiao* offers the fire of kidney yang to the heart but ensures that those *qi* do not disturb the heart, allowing it to cope with the large amounts of thoughts and desires of the ego. Disturbance in kidney yang and the *san jiao* impact the peace of the fire and the *shen* of the heart.

THE INTERNAL DUCT OF THE *SAN JIAO*

San jiao is a network that represents heaven in humans and enables individualization. It establishes heavenly *qi* in the self as pure consciousness, illustrating heaven.

In 1973 Dr Guido Fisch, a physician in Zurich, Switzerland, wrote an article about the Internal Duct of the *san jiao*, a previously unknown term to many, which was accepted by Dr van Buren. Fisch acquired this knowledge from Nguyen Van Nghi (1909–1999), a Vietnamese-French physician, author and teacher. Van Nghi is considered one of the founders of Chinese medicine in the West and was a great advocate of one medicine in which Eastern and Western medicine are not seen as separate and different.

The Internal Duct of the *san jiao* describes a network of *qi* in the abdomen which guarantees purity in the lower burner. This fits in with the idea that the *san jiao* is a network, larger than just the channel. It assists the entire being from the lower burner in maintaining purity through mediation between heaven and earth, yin and yang. Points that influence the Internal Duct of the *san jiao* are L.i.-8, *Xian Lian*, lower ridge, L.i.-9, *Shan Lian*, upper ridge, L.i.-10, *Shou San Li*, arm three *li*/miles, Sj-4, *Yang Chi*, pool of yang, Cv-10, *Xia Wan*, lower venter, St-37, *Shang Ju Xu*, upper great void, St-39, *Xia Ju Xu*, lower great void, and St-42, *Chong Yang*, rushing yang.

THE *SAN JIAO* CHANNEL

The *san jiao* is activated immediately after birth when the baby sucks on the mother's breast for the first time. Suckling at the nipple of the mother's breast causes contraction of the mother's uterus and causes her *jing qi* to withdraw and to recover. In the child, suckling activates the digestive *qi* system so that the food can reach the baby's *qi*. This lays the foundation for the baby to grow and develop and it is the first step towards independence.[11]

The functions of the arm *san jiao* channel are distinct from the deep *san jiao* function that distributes *yuan qi* or *dong qi* in the body. The arm *san jiao* channel and the deep *san jiao* function seem to have nothing to do with each other, but appearances are deceptive because, in cases of insufficiency of the deep *san jiao* function, the *qi* in the *san jiao* channel becomes stronger, compensating for the shortcoming. When overactive, this leads to symptoms such as indigestion, urinary difficulties, pain and swelling in the throat, deafness, tinnitus and pains along the trajectory of the channel. This pattern can be observed fairly often.

A daytime *san jiao* pulse that is diagnosed as a 'normal' pulse is often a sign of compensation and overactivity, because the pulse of the *san jiao* channel on the superficial proximal pulse (*chi* position) of the right hand should be weaker and certainly not powerful during the day compared to the late evening and night. During the day it should not be superficial or easily observable. In the case of compensation for the deep *san jiao* function it is important not to sedate the *san jiao* channel, but to nourish the deep *san jiao* function via the *ren mai*. This treatment should immediately calm the *san jiao* pulse.

SEASONAL POINT: SJ-2, *YE MEN*, FLUID DOOR

The efficiency of Sj-2 depends on the efficiency of the left-hand Sj-1, *Guang Chong*, rushing pass, where the *qi* of heaven enters the human body.

The word *Chong* refers to the surge of *qi* that enters or flushes through.[12] In the case of Sj-1 it is the birth of *qi* in the channels. This is received through the influence of the emanation *li*, the beneficial force that is revealed in this metal point on the left hand, the yin/receiving side of the body.

Similar to the idea that heavenly *qi* is received by humans, Sj-1 is a

---

11 Sucking a teat from a bottle also activates the *san jiao* channel, but the effect on the mother does not occur. When the baby is unable to suck, massage of the area around the mouth and on Sj-1 is indicated to activate the *san jiao* channel and the *ren mai* and the related functions.

12 As in Gb-9, Liv-3, St-30, St-42, Sp-12, Ht-9, Bl-3, Hc-9, respectively *Tian Chong, Tai Chong, Qi Chong, Chong Yang, Chong Men, Shao Chong, Mei Chong, Zhong Chong.*

transformation point between the head (heaven) and the torso with the arms and legs (human).

Sj-1 is treated when there is fullness in the upper burner with symptoms such as conjunctivitis, acute diseases of the ears, eyes and throat, along with emptiness in the trunk and limbs such as shortness of breath, perspiration with weak extremities and severe cough when the patient changes position.

After the heavenly *qi* has passed through the pass of Sj-1, it reaches the water point Sj-2, *Ye Men*, fluid door. Sj-2 is a barrier in the form of a gate (*Men*). In a universal sense, this gate opens to the waters of life that shed light from the timeless into the temporal. In a limited but more practical sense, this point influences the function of the *san jiao* channel to keep the movements and *qi* in the arms healthy. In addition it supports the function of distributing fluids in the body. Sj-2 can be used in any case of fluid stagnation. It acts on all fluids in the body as does St-44, *Nei Ting*, inner courtyard.

The core function of *san jiao* and Sj-2 is to mediate between the heart and kidneys, which calms the heart-*shen* and strengthens the kidneys. The balanced collaboration between heart and kidneys contributes to humility that comes from the understanding heart and wisdom of kidney-essence.

The *qi* in the *san jiao* channel continues to flow, gaining a foothold at Sj-3, *Zhong Zhu*, middle island, to reach the pool of yang and *yuan qi* for distribution in Sj-4, *Yang Chi*.

> Then the Buddha said: Every one of you carries part of my Idea.
> Every one of you is perfect, but that you will only know, when
> all of you become One. Only then the Plan will be revealed.

CHAPTER 38

DEEP *QI*

DIAGNOSIS OF DEEP *QI*

For practitioners in constitutional acupuncture the pulse is the most important diagnostic tool. Pulse diagnosis is an art, an important but rather difficult part of Chinese medicine, first of all because it is a lifelong apprenticeship and good teachers are not always available. In addition the focus of teaching is different in the many different kinds of schools, all of which, however, have their origins in the teachings of Wang Shu He (180–270) and Li Shi Zhen (1518–1593). John Shen, and later Leon Hammer, have systematically further developed pulse diagnosis, as have J.D. van Buren, J. Worsley and others.

J.D. van Buren shared his acquired knowledge in this area with his students, based on the lessons he had received from his teachers like Lavier and Wu Wei Ping, along with the translation of a book about stems and branches he had received from Chang Bin Lee and of course his years of study and experience with patients. This particular form of pulse diagnosis, which also has its roots in the original sources, has been further developed by leading teachers in our field. However, there are only a few teachers who use the current form of diagnosis with the focus on the five phases, heavenly stems and earthly branches, in which the deep *qi* also plays an important role. Taking lessons in this form of pulse diagnosis is indispensable for the serious practitioner of this system of treatment.

J.D. van Buren was not only known for his exceptional talent for pulse diagnosis, but also for body diagnosis, another indispensable element in diagnosing patients. He had told me several times that his book on this subject was as good as finished, but unfortunately it was never published. His diagnoses were based on in-depth knowledge of the subject, an incredible memory along with profound insight combined with intuition, and not on intuition alone as some people have assumed.

Besides pulse diagnosis,[1] the deep *qi* diagnosis is focused on the complexion of the face. When the complexion of the face has an unmissable colour, it is caused by deep *qi*. Unclear, vague, patchy colours originate from the *wuxing* phases whereas an overall clear interpretable colour is caused by the deep *qi*.

Table 38.1 Distinctions between facial complexions related to *wuxing* and deep *qi*

	Wuxing	Deep *Qi*
Bladder and kidney	Dark, unclear bluish, darkish	Clear bright white
Gallbladder and liver	Greenish, unclear blue-green (*qing*)	Gallbladder: clear dark blue Liver: clear yellow
Small intestine, heart, *san jiao*, heart constrictor	Patchy red, vague and unclear	Small intestine and heart constrictor: clear yellow *San jiao*: clear dark blue Heart: clear strong red
Stomach and spleen	Unclear yellow	Stomach: clear yellow Spleen: clear strong red
Large intestine and lungs	Unclear patchy white	Clear green, blue green (*qing*)

As soon as there is an '-ish' complexion as in, for example, a whitish colour instead of a clear-cut white, it originates from the five phases. But sometimes there can be confusing combinations. A chalk white face with a darkish colour under the eyes means the deep *qi* of the kidneys as well as the five phases quality of the kidneys is involved. Another example is when a whitish complexion is combined with bright red areas on the cheeks. This may indicate that the deep *qi* of spleen or heart subdues the five phases quality of the lung. However, when that redness is more patchy it indicates that the fire from the five phases-related fire organs and channels is involved.

THE UNKNOWN KNOWN

I thought I understood the concept of deep *qi*, but the first time the depth, scope and importance of deep *qi* became more explicit to me was during an observation day in the clinic of J.D. van Buren. Usually, J.D. van Buren sat at one side of the patient and I sat at the other, both feeling pulses. Then we changed positions. Sometimes he asked me about my findings before the treatment and

---

1   In terms of understanding the relationship between deep *qi* and pulse diagnosis, I recommend that you read the Pulse Classic by Wang Shu-he (Shou-Zhong 1997) and the *Huang Di Nei Jing Su Wen* Chapters 17, 18 and 19.

we discussed the treatment afterwards, other times he just treated and I had to discover the reasoning behind the choice of points myself.

It was a female patient; her birth chart showed the great movement water and the heavenly stem *Bing*, small intestine. I don't remember what she suffered from, but I remember struggling to understand why J.D. van Buren opted for only one point for treatment: Sp-2, *Da Du*, great capital.

My face must have been a big question mark because he immediately said: 'Because of small intestine in water, the earth has too much water *qi*. This makes the spleen too watery. Feel ...'

In the spleen pulse I did indeed feel the specific quality of water, and on his directions, I could also feel this in the small intestine. 'I don't use unlike *qi* now, because this watery quality is cold and extinguishes the fire of spleen.'

He continued: 'Small intestine is fire with deep *qi* earth that became too watery. This influences the spleen that is opposite to small intestine, namely earth with deep *qi* fire.'

This lesson is etched in my memory along with the beautiful smooth pulse that appeared during the treatment. This lesson describes rules about the deep *qi* that are very different from the knowledge and rules of the seasonal *qi*.

ALL CHANNELS AND ORGANS HAVE DEEP *QI*

The classification of earthly branches with seasonal *qi* and deep *qi* is completely identical, but the meaning of the deep *qi* is different and broader. The seasonal *qi* is linked to periods of time in a day, in a month and to a specific season and has meaning over the course of the related hours, months and seasons. The deep *qi* is particularly linked to a separate property of a certain organ and channel and, unlike the seasonal *qi*, the effect of deep *qi* is relevant all year long regardless of the season, exceeding the energetics of the seasonal points.

Deep *qi* seems like a whole new idea in Chinese medicine, but looking at the pulse descriptions from well-known classical works and the teachings I received from several of the world's leading teachers, it is clear that the deep *qi* can be found in the described pulses. Deep *qi* is not a new concept, but an already known aspect within pulse diagnosis, without previously having been given a name. Sometimes it takes a while to find the relationships between the deep *qi* and the correct description of the pulse qualities. The more pulse diagnosis is practised, however, the clearer it will become. The theory is actually more difficult than putting it into practice because words cannot fully convey what the fingers feel.

However, good guidance in this area is indispensable. Therefore, I recommend looking for a teacher who has experience in pulse diagnosis. I don't believe people ever finish learning in this area, but someone with years of experience can share their understanding with less experienced colleagues. In this way we can all contribute to human well-being.

DEEP *QI* WATER

General picture: Deep *qi* water feels soft as the pulse curves around the fingers like putting your hand in a bowl of water; however, when the pulse is approached quickly it feels hard.

Sj-2, *Ye Men*, fluid door; the *san jiao* is a reflection of the original oneness within the individual essence and expresses itself through the *qi* of water. The *san jiao qi* is a pure *qi* that resides in the depth of one's being. The deep *qi* water of *san jiao* is needed for lubrication to create optimal conditions. The pulse reflects these properties as well as its hidden availability to all other *qi*.

The healthy pulse of the *san jiao*: Nicely formed, moderately superficial, thinner than small intestine, slightly watery, deeper than stomach.

Pathology: Too weak means a lack of *qi*; weak when all other superficial pulses are hard and all deep pulses but the heart constrictor are weak means insufficient sympathetic nervous system tone and an overactive vagus nerve; hard when all other superficial pulses are weak and all deep pulses but the heart constrictor are hard indicates an overactive sympathetic nervous system with insufficient vagus nerve tone; too tense or tight means nervousness with pain during the night and irritability – the load in the person's life exceeds their capacity to carry it.

Too superficial is usually associated with insufficiency of the *jing*. Too medial[2] and too close to the tendon means too dependent on the *jing*. Too lateral indicates a person who is overly dependent on the input of social impulses.

Gb-43, *Xia Xi*, narrow ravine or harmonious stream; the deep *qi* water of gallbladder expresses the renewal of the source of life through the *qi* of water. The pulse shows the availability of the *qi* of water to direct the conduct of all *qi* in line with the original essence. The gallbladder channel mainly runs on the sides of the body to allow rotation around the vertical axis, the North–South axis, which is the inner channel that aligns with and connects the *qi* and virtues of heaven and earth. Due to life's challenges, this pulse is often much more superficial

---

2   Evaluating this, it should be taken into account that the *san jiao*, heart constrictor, bladder and kidney pulses are more medially located positions, compared with the other pulses.

and stronger than it should be. This is a sign that much is being asked of the original essence.

The healthy pulse of the gallbladder: Slightly superficial, a bit short, slightly elastic.[3]

Pathology: Too superficial means too much wood activity compared to the amount of rest needed. Weak or hardly existing means exhaustion with inability to work. Superficial, hard and constricted means too much tension often with symptoms such as migraines.

DEEP *QI* WOOD

General picture: Deep *qi* wood comes quickly and firmly upwards as in spring; a flexible pulse.

Lu-11, *Shao Shang*, lesser *Shang*/metal; the deep *qi* wood of the lung is used to awaken *qi* or to revive consciousness. It affects growth in general, decision making and planning, especially when people are depressed. Lu-11 is a classical point to vitalize weakness of ancestral *qi* that goes together with tinnitus in the ear.[4]

The healthy pulse of the lung: Peaceful and as light as elm-seeds; feeble, floating and hasty in coming, scattered when going, or large, slow and like the touch of a feather.

Pathology: Too superficial, too big and hard means inflammation or another kind of congestion in the lung. Too weak means a weak lung *qi* in regard to respiratory system and consciousness.[5]

L.i.-3, *San Jian*, third space; the deep *qi* wood of the large intestine is beneficial in any case of physical growth retardation, in children (8–10 years of age) who remain small for no apparent reason, and in young women with amenorrhoea. It is also used to stimulate stagnant spiritual growth when people lack spiritual strength.

---

3   Elasticity is a water quality. It can be compared to a trampoline. If the trampoline is tensioned too weak, jumping is not supported; if it is tensioned too strong, people will be launched. Elasticity, the quality of the *qi* of the essence, can be diagnosed on the pulse by lightly pressing the pulse when you feel the beat.
4   The ear is equally the place of reunion of the ancestral energies.
5   See Chapter 27 under Seasonal point: Lu-11, *Shao Shang*, lesser *Shang*/metal.

The healthy pulse of the large intestine: Rather thick, comes up and disappears quickly, short, not much volume, a little superficial. Like stomach, but more superficial.

Pathology: Deviations in any one of the qualities of the large intestine pulse are a sign of improper functioning. For example, if the pulse disappears too slowly, it is a sign of heat. If there is too much volume, there is constipation (even if there is diarrhoea), meaning that the gut is too full.

DEEP *QI* FIRE

General picture: Deep *qi* fire moves the *qi* in all directions, especially upwards. It comes upwards quickly and goes away slowly, as in summer.

Sp-2, *Da Du*, great capital/organization; the deep *qi* fire of the spleen is needed for the digestive system, to be able to transform and to transport, for which damp is an indispensable element. Damp is the result of the encounter between water and fire to form the necessary conditions for transformation and transportation. It is a fragile balance. Too much or too little water or fire disturbs this balance of damp and creates a condition that causes stagnation.

Damp can be caused by external factors such as a humid climate, humidity in the house, wearing wet clothes and so on. Internal damp may develop when there is too little fire, for example due to poor (cold) food, overeating and a high-carbohydrate diet. In the initial yang phase of dampness, damp affects mostly the production of *qi* in general. In the more yin, chronic stage, damp affects the organs, channels and the skin. The use of the deep *qi* of the spleen should therefore often be accompanied by advice for a better diet. Damp and stagnation can cause heat, which must first be treated and removed before the deep *qi* fire of spleen can be used.

In addition the deep *qi* fire of spleen increases the spleen yang, which among other things supports concentration and positively influences mental sluggishness.

The healthy pulse of the spleen: A wave that softly flows to come together, then gently falls apart; broad, a little weak and soft. It is peaceful, soft and remaining apart, like a chicken treading the earth, slowly and spreading in four directions. This is a normal pulse for a spleen which has a balanced damp condition.

Pathology: The earthly fire of spleen goes upward and when it feels a little sharp like 'flames' it means pathology with too much heat and/or a lack of water. When it appears soft and dense or soft and loose, longer, little, taut, tense, or it pecks as a bird, the delicate balance of damp is disturbed and an internal disease is expected due to a lack of deep *qi* fire. Soft and deep means exhaustion during the day with a lack of concentration.

Ht-8, *Shao Fu*, lesser mansion; the deep *qi* of fire of the heart differs from the deep *qi* of fire of the spleen.

> When one's blood and *qi* are harmonious, his *qi* is flowing unhindered, the five viscera being shaped and the spirit stored in the heart causing thought and will, then he becomes a man.[6]

> The heart is the supreme commander, sovereign, or the monarch, master, of the human body, it dominates the spirit, ideology and thought of man.[7]

The heart and the *shen* are the sources behind all transformations and attune people to what is above everything and to the unity of life. In this way, it directs people to align individual choices with the shared universal source. The heart takes care of the emperor *and* his empire. Unlike the deep *qi* fire of the spleen, that involves organizing transformation and transportation throughout the body, the deep *qi* fire of the heart contributes to housing the *shen* on the one hand, and on the other hand it guides the blood to share the spirit and its nourishment throughout the body. The round, smooth image of the pulse of the heart is different from that of the spleen. It is a picture of wholeness and unity in which it can house the *shen* and at the same time be the vital source that maintains the body.

The healthy pulse of the heart: Steady flow, sliding as a string of pearls and smooth as jade stone.

Pathology: The heavenly fire of the heart feels like pearls and could be called 'slippery'. Any deviation from this normal pulse image means a form of pathology. It is recommended that treatment of the heart be done primarily through other channels such as the heart constrictor (see below).

---

6   *Ling Shu* Chapter 54.
7   *Huang Di Nei Jing Su Wen* Chapter 8.

DEEP *QI* METAL

General picture: The deep *qi* metal moves the *qi* towards the centre and can reveal itself in different ways. A little hard, even a bit flat, a little constricted or a little sharp like fire, but always directed to the centre.

Bl-67, *Zhi Yin*, arrival or extremity of yin; the deep *qi* metal of the bladder, which is felt superficially, differs from the deep *qi* metal of the kidneys, which is felt on the deep level. The bladder is the first layer through which the experiences, gained from the outside world and gathered by the deep *qi* earth of the small intestine, are filtered and offered to the inside. In contrast to the physical physiology where the non-useful fluids from the kidneys are presented to and excreted by the bladder, the deep *qi* metal of the bladder distinguishes and separates the useful from the useless and offers the useful to the kidneys, where it contributes to the power of the inner fire and continuation of life. The dry character of metal ensures that the healthy bladder pulse has a slightly dry and thin character, but not easy to push away. A really thin or fine pulse is an image of *xuè* insufficiency more than *qi* insufficiency; however, *xuè* insufficiency may lead to *qi* insufficiency. The deeper the thin pulse becomes, the more severely *xuè* is insufficient; the tighter, the more both *xuè* and yin insufficiency are present. The superficial, slightly hard, not easily pushable character of the bladder pulse is therefore an important reflection of a healthy deep *qi* metal of the bladder.

The healthy pulse of the bladder: A little superficial, a little hard, slightly thin.

Pathology: When life demands too much, the deep *qi* metal of the bladder gets out of balance first and shows itself in the bladder pulse as being too superficial, too hard, tense, tight or wiry. This is often accompanied by both acute and chronic back problems, for example a slipped disc, and when combined with heat it is an indication for cystitis.

Too sharp, flat, dry, hard, constricted and too deep are all signs of pathology of the deep *qi* metal. It should be noted that a deep *qi* metal pulse can be so constricted that it is difficult to locate. It is often diagnosed accidentally as a thin pulse, which should feel soft, weak and without strength, while this barely felt constricted pulse feels wiry or tight and thin, meaning obstruction or stagnation.

Ki-7, *Fu Liu*, returning current; the deep *qi* metal of the kidneys feels harder than the deep *qi* metal of the bladder due to more concentration and constriction.

In the autumn, *qi* and fluids concentrate in the deeper levels of the essence, preserving the life principle carried in water and fluids. The same takes place all year round through the deep *qi* metal of the kidneys to protect the power of the *jing*-essence. The deep *qi* metal of the kidneys ensures the absorption of water and solves problems with fluid balance by regulating pores and glands for sweating, creating the perfect conditions to enable inner fire and continuation of life.

The healthy pulse of the kidneys: Deep and rapid and somewhat hooky, hard on pressure. The term hooky in the classics is used to describe the gradual disappearing of a pulse, which is actually a property of a pulse in the summer. This, together with the increased speed of the pulse, describes the inner fiery character that is not expressed but rather concealed. The deep *qi* metal of the kidneys is located deep with some heat. This heat is not due to too much fire/heat but is a sign of the vitality that warms the body and ceases when we die.

Pathology: When the deep *qi* metal becomes too superficial and hard it means that there are congestions anywhere in the body. Deep and weak means exhaustion.

DEEP *QI* EARTH

General picture: The deep *qi* earth is a harmonizing pulse that feels soft as if putting your hand in a pot of loose earth with a certain resistance in the centre of the pulse.

Pathology of deep *qi* earth: Many pulse qualities are known as deviations of the deep *qi* earth. The rule of thumb, however, is that these pulses feel soft, spreading and/or yielding and may or may not have some resistance in the middle. There is insufficiency of deep *qi* earth when no centre of resistance can be felt. Too much resistance in the centre means overactivity and/or stagnation in the deep *qi* earth. Both situations create damp symptoms that can eventually also be accompanied by heat.

Liv-3, *Tai Chong*, great surge; as a seasonal point the liver is part of winter but mainly earth-related. It supports the transition of *qi* from winter to spring. The earth deep *qi* of liver has water properties. It supports free flow of *qi*, due to its property to build fluids in the liver. In women it is the point of heaven of the lower region according to the nine continents pulses.[8] About the artery located at this point it is said: 'If this artery beats, the patient will survive' and 'If a young girl of fourteen has this artery strongly beating, she can bear children.' This shows the intimate relationship of the earth deep *qi* of liver with water as the source of life and essence.

The healthy pulse of the liver: Gentle as a waving hand, as soft as the tip of a long bamboo, being lifted up – softly, weakly, a bit broad.

St-36, *Zu San Li*, leg three miles; as a seasonal point the stomach is part of spring but mainly earth-related. It supports the transition of *qi* from spring to summer. The earth deep *qi* of stomach has wood properties. It stimulates and vitalizes *qi* production, which in turn builds and helps the production of *ying qi* and *wei qi* – it balances the white blood cell count. It regulates the circulation of *qi* and *xuè* and is seen as a general tonification point for the body. In addition it can be used when there is a collapse of yang.

The healthy pulse of the stomach: Moderately superficial, slightly thick, short, less volume and superficial than large intestine, solid, firm but not hard.

However, this description of the pulse of the stomach is a general picture that changes qualities with the different seasons to guide health: In spring the pulse should be 'fine and delicate as the string of a lute' with moderate stomach *qi*; in summer the pulse is 'as the beat (resonating) of a fine hammer' with moderate stomach *qi*; in late summer the pulse should be 'soft and feeble' with moderate stomach *qi*; in autumn the pulse is 'small and rough' with moderate stomach *qi*; and in winter the pulse is 'small and like a stone' with moderate stomach *qi*. Over the years I have been able to observe that the pulse of the stomach resonates in the same way with the seasons. Nevertheless, despite the adaptation to the seasons, it must always have a certain earthy quality.

It should also be noted that the unique nature of the stomach and heart is emphasized by being the only channels that have an equal relationship of *wuxing qi* and deep *qi*.

S.i.-8, *Xiao Hai*, small sea; as a seasonal point the small intestine is part of summer but is mainly earth-related. It supports the transition of *qi* from summer to autumn. The earth deep *qi* of small intestine has fire properties.

The *qi* of the heart expresses itself in the world in different ways. The heart

---

8   *Huang Di Nei Jing Su Wen* Chapter 20.

constrictor is a filter and executive power for the heart; the *san jiao*, through its connection with the oneness, expresses the heart in connection with the multitude; the small intestine reveals the intentions of the heart in one-to-one relationships. The small intestine is connected on one side to the fire of summer and on the other it brings the experiences of the abundant flowering period into the reality and experience of the individual.

The earth deep *qi* of the small intestine is needed to find, physically and figuratively, balance and harmony in its function of separating the pure from the impure but also needs combining with fire to be able to digest food. The use of S.i.-8 is not without danger. When the (*wuxing*) earth *qi* of the spleen and stomach are too active – which is the case, for example, when people over-eat (but also when people place intellect and knowledge above intuition and intelligence) – the *qi* of the earth is easily transferred to the weaker fire via the reverse *sheng*-cycle. This may cause stagnation of the expressions of fire with symptoms such as insomnia, low back pain, itching, uterine diseases and so on.

The healthy pulse of the small intestine: Nicely formed, moderately superficial, not hard with a soft flow, less thin than *san jiao*.

Hc-7, *Da Ling*, great mound/hill; as a seasonal point the heart constrictor is part of autumn but mainly earth-related. It supports the transition of *qi* from autumn to winter. The earth deep *qi* of the heart constrictor has metal properties and has to do with defence and letting go; defence of the heart and the conditions of the natural continuation or ending of the cycle of life and the letting go of tension, fear, drives and so on but also letting go of any kind of motivation or urge for change. This *qi* has to do with finding the natural way, where expectations about the future and ideas about the past only get in the way.[9] This *qi* brings a person back to the present and to themselves. Too strong an urge to change is almost always found in too much constriction in the metal of the lung and large intestine, but even more so in the deep *qi* of the bladder and kidneys. When at the same time the heart *qi* is deficient, the deep *qi* of the heart constrictor, in particular Hc-7 (optionally with Liv-8, *Qu Quan*), relaxes and softens the metal pulses and creates calmness.

There is a special relationship between the heart constrictor and the heart. When the heart is underactive and weak, the heart constrictor becomes tight or wiry to protect it. In that case the heart should be treated to allow the heart constrictor to relax. When the heart constrictor pulse is too weak, the *qi* of

---

9   This has been discussed in Chapter 36.

the heart is unprotected. Sometimes that is compensated for by tight and wiry pulses in the first layer of defence, the *tai yang*: bladder and small intestine, where symptoms of disease can also be found. In that case the heart constrictor should be treated.

In the last decades I have seen a lot of young people where the heart *qi* is excellent and the heart constrictor *qi* seems to be too soft. These children are called indigo children,[10] new age children. They are children with a strong emotional life and the ability to navigate on intuition. They are independent and strong-willed, not easy to manage. Due to the uniqueness of their behaviour, they do not always meet the conditions set by parents and society. This often leads to diagnoses such as attention deficit hyperactivity disorder (ADHD) or the like. Treatment and guidance of the *qi* of the heart in these individuals is not to be found in the heart constrictor, but in the balance between the gallbladder and deep *qi* of the water so that more authentic ground is put under their feet, which calms their unlimited expression of fire.

The healthy pulse of the heart constrictor: Similar to the heart pulse but a little softer.

---

10   This term was coined by Nancy Anne Tappe and the concept was further developed by Lee Carroll and Jan Tober.

CHAPTER 39

LIKE *QI*

Constitutional acupuncture treats *qi* linked with the elements in the birth chart. These organs and channels are usually weaker and challenge the person to stay healthy. The practitioner promotes healthy individual development by strengthening the potentially weaker aspects to balance the innate *qi*, providing the patient with the tools for recovery. Constitutional acupuncture is dedicated to nourishing and guiding the individual destiny that aligns with the mandate of heaven, the individual nature, and the prevention and treatment of diseases.

LIKE *QI*

Like *qi* treatments are mainly used in preventive and nourishing treatments. Unlike *qi* is mainly used to correct the birth energy imbalances.

Table 39.1 Like *qi* of the earthly branches

Heaven	I *Zi* Gb	IV *Mao* L.i.	V *Chen* St	VIII *Wei* S.i.	IX *Shen* Bl	XII *Hai* Sj
Humanity	| Wood |	| Metal |	| Earth |	| Fire Prince |	| Water |	| Fire Min. |
Earth	Liv II *Chou*	Lu III *Yin*	Sp VI *Si*	Ht VII *Wu*	Ki X *You*	Hc XI *Xu*

CHALLENGES

This particular section is about finding the balance between the like *qi*-related organs and channels. When the challenges are properly understood and a natural balance is achieved, complaints and illnesses are prevented.

Earthly branch *Zi*, gallbladder, and earthly branch *Chou*, liver

I have noticed that challenges and lessons of life put people in situations that confronts them intensely with their destiny.[1] For example, people born with the earthly branch *Zi*, gallbladder, are challenged to align with the earthly branch *Chou*, liver. The challenge for these people is to maintain their own uniqueness in realizing plans and ideas, because the *qi* of the liver tends to prefer the drive to always seek renewal, move forward and focus on the future.

People born with the earthly branch *Chou*, liver, are challenged to align with the earthly branch *Zi*, gallbladder. The challenge for these people is to tune in and stay with an original thought or concept and resist the constant challenge of starting something new, because the *qi* of the gallbladder tends to always confirm the self by renewal.

Earthly branch *Yin*, lung, and earthly branch *Mao*, large intestine

The challenge for people born with the earthly branch *Yin* is to learn to exercise patience and focus on contentment and not just on innovation, because the tendency of the *qi* of the large intestine is to easily get excited about new developments.

The challenge for people born with the earthly branch *Mao* is to balance the dominance of their character and the space required for mutual interaction, because the *qi* of the lungs tends to affirm the self through social connection and thereby neglect reciprocity.

Earthly branch *Chen*, stomach, and earthly branch *Si*, spleen

The challenge for people born with the earthly branch *Chen* is to combine insight with execution rather than just thinking about it, because the *qi* of the spleen tends to focus on thinking only.

The challenge for people born with the earthly branch *Si* is to balance the value of insights about themselves and those of others, to find the way between stubbornness and indulgence, because the *qi* of the stomach tends to foster habits and safeguard pride.

Earthly branch *Wu*, heart, and earthly branch *Wei*, small intestine

The challenge for people born with the earthly branch *Wu* is finding a balance between stepping aside for the benefit of others, without losing authenticity and impairing themselves, because the *qi* of the small intestine tends to intellectualization and to undervaluing their own interests.

---

1   This is more true for the unlike *qi* than the like *qi*.

The challenge for people born with the earthly branch *Wei* is not to lose themselves in a relationship. A balance must be reached between the extent to which one must be there for the other and the degree of nourishment for one's own individuality, because the *qi* of the heart tends to find it difficult to balance self-love and compassion for others.

Earthly branch *Shen,* bladder, and earthly branch *You,* kidneys

The challenge for people born with the earthly branch *Shen* is to combine the inner life force with the tranquillity of taking a step back every now and then, because the *qi* of the kidneys tends to strengthen willpower, drive and pride to cover deep-seated fears.

The challenge for people born with the earthly branch *You* is to learn to rely on intuition, because adversity can make the *qi* of the bladder despondent, creating dogmatism that blocks reliance on intuition.

Earthly branch *Xu,* heart constrictor, and earthly branch *Hai, san jiao*

The challenge for people born with the earthly branch *Xu* is to keep inner peace in the event of adversity, to focus on the present rather than wanting to pre-serve the old, because the *qi* of *san jiao* tends towards prudence and an overly regulated lifestyle.

The challenge for people born with the earthly branch *Hai* is to let go of control and adapt to the rhythm of life and love, because the *qi* of the heart constrictor tends to compensate for personal pain; people tend to ignore and ward off the reality of pain by positive thoughts and behaviour.

CHAPTER 40

UNLIKE *QI* RELATIONSHIP BETWEEN *ZI* AND *WU*

The Vertical Axis of Renewal

When forces of the North and South converge
And tensions have been lifted
The sun rises in the East and shines.

Table 40.1 Unlike *qi* of the earthly branches

Heaven	I *Zi* Gb	II *Chou* Liv	III *Yin* Lu	IV *Mao* L.i.	V *Chen* St	VI *Si* Sp
Humanity	| Earth |	| Earth |	| Earth |	| Earth |	| Earth |	| Earth |
Earth	Ht VII *Wu*	S.i. VIII *Wei*	Bl IX *Shen*	Ki X *You*	Hc XI *Xu*	Sj XII *Hai*

CHALLENGES

People born with the earthly branch *Zi*, gallbladder, are challenged to align with the earthly branch *Wu*, heart. The challenge for these people is to be true to their own authenticity and uniqueness and to shape and express the 'self' in society. People born with the earthly branch *Wu*, heart, are challenged to align with the earthly branch *Zi*, gallbladder. The challenge for these people is to keep faith in their own strength and inner peace. This is particularly challenging when work and society require an inordinate amount of time and energy or when people face many setbacks or fears.

UNLIKE *QI* TREATMENT

The rule of thumb is to indirectly address the innate *qi* in the birth chart via related *qi* that balances the innate *qi*. This rule can also be applied when non-innate *qi* is affected. The treatment is carefully aligned with the *qi* design of the birth chart.

ZI, GALLBLADDER, AND DEEP *QI* WATER

Hexagram 24 *Fu*, Return, Revival, Renewal, Turning back.[1]

The trigrams *Chen*, Thunder, and *Kun*, Earth

The hexagram Return consists of the trigram Thunder at the bottom and the trigram Earth at the top. The bottom yang line represents renewed awakened consciousness, latent needs, ideas and desires that are ready to be realized by the five receptive yin lines. Unhindered growth of all that is hidden is made possible by the openness and receptivity of the trigram Earth.

The degree of fellowship, responsibility and compassion (the signature of the trigram Earth) evolves from the yang source of Thunder. When the initial growth of the source of life meets too much resistance, compassion is rooted only in the mind, but not in who we really are. Too much worrying, stubbornness, obsession and intellectualization may suffocate the newly born light, before it has really started well.

Deep *qi* water

Deep *qi* water matches the strong yang root of the first line of hexagram 24 Return.

> The highest good is like water. Water gives life to the ten thousand things and does not strive. It flows in places men reject and so is like the *Dao*. No fight; No blame.[2]

People with enough deep *qi* water of the gallbladder have the power to initiate renewal. They inspire, have new ideas and suggestions with unexpected mindsets. They can think out of the box and have the ability to revise and renew their own thinking models. They can do unexpected things and make changes that other people don't foresee. For those with deep *qi* water these changes

---

1   Hexagrams and trigrams are illustrated in Appendix II.
2   *Dao De Jing* Chapter 8.

are the only right and thoughtful options. To others they seem impulsive and unpredictable.

Too little deep *qi* water causes too little rooting. *Qi* rises too fast and too strong and can flow counter-current, leading to physical tension and stagnation. The rising *qi* may cause people to become too alert and irritable. They may even find it difficult to move with the normal cyclical movements of time, for example finding it difficult to wake up on time or to fall asleep easily, having problems with aging and so on. Any change in the status quo feels invasive and causes unrest and fear of the new. There is a tendency to keep control of everything and everyone. It manifests itself by tension and pain of the neck and shoulders with stiffness due to too little movement and goes hand in hand with restlessness and insomnia. These symptoms – not the underlying emotions, fears and insecurities – are usually the reason why they consult a therapist.

Spontaneity

Spontaneity is an unconscious impulsive urge that is manifested beyond the will. It can be compared to a river that emerges from a source. Spontaneity, the water of the river, flows within the boundaries of the dykes and banks, just as the limitation of a person's social communication skills determines the degree of flexibility of thoughts, prejudices, visions and opinions during a conversation.

Spontaneous actions are the sudden acceleration of the deep *qi* water of the gallbladder. The expression of this depends on the openness and flexibility of the trigram Earth, which determines the degree of identification with and compassion for others.

A point worth noting concerns the spontaneity of children, where too many impressions and overwhelming stimuli from an unsafe environment may cause strong emotional responses. There are roughly two types of behaviour in this instance: the yang way of shouting, crying, boundary-crossing behaviour, ego-centrism and impulsivity and the yin way of withdrawing, excessive vigilance, apathy, uncertainty and not crying. Children may have learned from an early age that control is a required quality because their spontaneity has been suppressed by being met with disapproval.

Stagnant *qi* of the Thunder and Earth are major causes of limited sponta-neity and creativity. These can cause diseases in the short and long term, for example digestive issues, complaints in the head due to counter-current *qi* of the gallbladder channel and sacroiliac joint issues. Treatment should start with releasing the tension of the trigrams Thunder (for example by using L.i.-9, *Shan Lian*) and Earth (for example by using points on the *ren mai* channel) and the deep *qi* of the gallbladder.

WU, HEART, AND DEEP *QI* FIRE

Hexagram 44 *Gou*, Encountering, Meeting together.

The dual world of yin and yang assumes that one yang line in hexagram 24 Return is linked to an opposite and complementary yin line: hexagram 44 *Gou*, Encountering.

Together they build the vertical axis of water and fire, distinguishable forces but not really separated. *Zi–Wu* is the axis of renewal that enables a cyclic movement of time, growth, flourishing, decay and death. *Qi* and *xuè* flow from *Zi* to reach their maximum in *Wu* and return to *Zi*.

The trigrams *Xun*, Wind, and *Qian*, Heaven

The structure of hexagram 44, Encountering, consists of the lower trigram Wind and the upper trigram Heaven. The bottom yin line of Encountering symbolizes the yin approaching in summer. Yin is still hidden and latent, but it suggests an important expected change.[3]

As the latent consciousness grows from the seed in the hexagram Return to bloom in summer, yin will indeed increase from this juncture of the hexagram Encountering. While the form perishes in autumn and winter, yin is in charge of the inner qualities of togetherness, relationships, contact, community, intuition, vulnerability and openness. The strength of these yin features originates from the initial yin line, the basis for the deep *qi* fire in hexagram 44, Encountering.

Wind dissolves rigidity. The bottom yin line of the hexagram/trigram represents the beginning of vitalization and the renewal of life through receptivity and approval. It ensures that the heart is brought into line with one's own authentic strength and, if possible, with the silence of one's own natural state. The yin aspect of deep *qi* fire is the threshold to the natural state of being, the acceptance of all that is happening. Yet reality is often different. To communicate with and relate to the demands of society, fire and the heart often follow the will of the mind, cognition, thought and emotion, rather than the will of heaven, the original nature, the inherent natural state characterized by spontaneity and originality without a to-do list.

The secret of the natural state lies in the power of letting go. It is not about letting go of thoughts and emotions, it is about letting go of the addiction to

---

3   The *Yijing*, the Book of Changes, starts with the hexagram *Qian*, Heaven, with six yang lines. At the time of the Xia and Shang dynasties, the pioneers of the *Yijing* are said to have started using yin-qualified hexagrams. It may be that yin then had a more positive connotation than the current well-known composition (where, for example, danger refers to water and yin). The later preference for yang could explain why the *Yijing* advises in hexagram 44 to stop the initial growth of yin below five yang lines. In this book I emphasize the positive properties of yin.

and the trap of thoughts and emotions. Yin is the unlimited space that perceives the limitedness of time, thoughts and emotions. It is the mind's addiction to knowledge and wanting to understand that limits the infinity of natural wisdom.

To connect with the natural state inside, the two upper yang lines of the trigram Wind can remove the obstacles of the addiction to thought and emotions, just as the wind clears the sky of clouds. Although the wind itself is uncontrollable, the sailboat's sail (yin) can catch the wind and navigate the boat well. In this way, with yin features such as openness, sensitivity and vulnerability, the heart and deep *qi* fire receive and cherish the flow of life, represented by the upper trigram Heaven that provides inner strength and inner stamina. It allows people to conduct self-examination and self-validation through introspection, even in difficult times.

The pitfall of yang
The power of yang is a serious pitfall for people born with the earthly branch *Wu* and/or for people who suffer from heart *qi* problems. When the yang lines of the trigram Heaven are understood as taking initiative and the desire for power and control, when people get lost in enjoying power, appearance and dominance, the tendency develops to focus on mere appearance and other yang behaviour. It easily causes diminished inner strength, insecurity and self-doubt, which is often offset by more dominance and external behaviour.

CLINICAL APPLICATIONS OF *ZI* AND *WU*
The excess of active yang of the summer hexagram Encountering, the heart and deep *qi* fire, is a pitfall for diagnosis. An insufficiency of the deep *qi* water of the gallbladder is easily missed due to the pulses of the heart and the related unlike *qi* gallbladder that appear strong and healthy. Strong symptoms of overactivity are indications to pay more attention to the absence or weakness of deep *qi* water.

The trouble of rising yang *qi* can be treated by Gb-41, *Zu Lin Qi*, to open *dai mai*, along with the deep *qi* water point on the gallbladder channel Gb-43, *Yang Ling Quan*. It corrects the flow of *qi* to descend again.

People born with the earthly branch *Zi*, gallbladder, who do not solve the demands and challenges of the unlike *qi* of the earthly branch *Wu*, heart, may have heart blood deficiency and heart yin deficiency. Heart blood deficiency gives palpitations in the evening, dizziness, insomnia, poor concentration and memory, anxiety and sometimes hypomania. Heart yin deficiency is caused by a long-term heart blood deficiency and is accompanied by the same symptoms but more severe and more likely to cause night sweats.

The use of the deep *qi* point on the heart channel Ht-8, *Shao Fu*, is possible only in severe heart yin deficiency with severe symptoms of loss of focus and depression.

For milder symptoms it is better to choose other points such as Cv-4, *Guan Yuan*, Cv-14, *Ju Que*, Cv-15, *Jiu Wei*, Bl-15, *Xin Shu*, Ht-5, *Tong Li,* with Ht-7, *Shen Men.*

CHAPTER 41

UNLIKE *QI* RELATIONSHIP BETWEEN *MAO* AND *YOU*

The Horizontal Level of Manifestation

CHALLENGES

People born with the earthly branch *Mao*, large intestine, are challenged to align with the earthly branch *You*, kidneys. The challenge for these people is to learn to trust their own inner strength and not get carried away by expectations that others impose on them.

For people born with the earthly branch *You*, the kidneys are challenged to align with the earthly branch *Mao*, large intestine. The challenge for these people is to develop courage to face their fear of the unknown (physical, emotional, mental and spiritual) and to learn to seek help from others.

MAO, LARGE INTESTINE, AND DEEP *QI* WOOD

Hexagram 34 *Da Zhuang*, Great strength.

When we consider the field of life and consciousness as the content of the circle of the earthly branches, the vertical axis in that circle (water–fire, *Zi–Wu*) initiates the developmental course of life and consciousness. On the yang side of the circle, from the earthly branch *Zi* to the earthly branch *Wu*, latent forces grow into manifested forms. On the yin side of the circle, from the earthly branch *Wu* to the earthly branch *Zi*, the life and consciousness of the manifested forms retreat through introversion and self-awareness.

The horizontal axis in the circle (wood and metal) represents manifestation in the physical realm. It divides the content of the circle of life and consciousness into above: yang, active, outer, awake, conscious; and under: yin, passive, inner, sleep, unconscious.

The origin and the degree of health of deep *qi* wood in the East depends on the correct alignment of the horizontal axis with the vertical axis and deep *qi* water and fire.

This concept of dependence has major implications for diagnosis and treatment. Water not only nourishes wood as known from the *wuxing*; in the concept of the deep *qi*, the vital *qi* of wood derives from the alignment and collaboration of water and fire. This implies that treatment should first focus on the balance and relationship of the deep *qi* water and fire when people suffer from deep *qi* wood problems.

The trigrams *Qian*, Heaven, and *Chen*, Thunder

The one yang bottom line in hexagram 24 Return has grown into three yang lines; the small latent stream of life has grown into a significant river. The three yang lines of the lower trigram Heaven represent the unified principle of life, which flows strong, calm and stable to create the 'ten thousand things'.

These yang lines depict the awakening light and life that becomes visible in the powerful rays of the rising sun in the East. Yang shows its strength and greatness, physically, but above all spiritually and morally.

The trigram Thunder of hexagram Return has been moved to the upper part of the hexagram Great Strength. The invisible collected light has finally become visible and shines over the 'ten thousand things'.

The fourth line of hexagram Great Strength is particularly important. This line represents the minister of the emperor.[1] The minister is involved in making decisions, finding the right ways, making choices and communicating with the outside world. He is steadfast and sincere. In the body, the fourth line of the hexagram represents the place of the middle burner, the area associated with desires for social cohesion and empathetic communication and human intelligence.

For people born with the earthly branch *Mao*, large intestine, the yang of the fourth line activates social activity, often so much that it exceeds their carrying capacity. They possess a lot of drive and energy, which easily masks an underlying tiredness. As a result, they cross their own boundaries unnoticed, especially since their motives behind servitude, loving attention, compassion and so on are positively appreciated. Exhaustion is usually discovered too late. These people are challenged to develop the objective observation of the unlike *qi* of the earthly branch *You*, kidneys, and to come to know their inner being

---

1   The fifth line represents the emperor.

through self-cultivation of the heavenly stem *Gui*. Taking up this challenge supports health more than the values derived from social affirmation.

> While writing this chapter I thought of a five-year-old girl, born with the earthly branch *Mao*. Her parents asked me for help in treating her chronic ear infections; she actually had a constant cold. The girl was known for her fine presence and tenderness.
>
> I remember that I initially mainly treated her symptoms, because she often suffered from high fever; at that time I believed this was the best approach. After a few treatments, she seemed to recover.
>
> I then got a call that she was sick again with high fever. When she came for an acute treatment the pulse picture in relation to the birth chart and further diagnosis led me to treat Ki-10, *Yin Gou*, yin valley; she appeared to have damp-heat in the lower burner manifested in cystitis, sore throat on the right and a lot of snot in the nose and pharynx. The outcome of that treatment taught me a lesson.
>
> She recovered in a few hours and, even more remarkably, her symptoms had disappeared and treatment was no longer needed. The next time she came for treatment her parents were laughing because she had disobeyed for the first time in her life. She finally stood up for herself.
>
> Because of her temperament – she kept pushing her limits, causing similar symptoms – I treated her more often, even when she was an adult.
>
> Of course, to decide on the treatment strategy, I research symptoms and focus treatment accordingly, but since that treatment I have focused more on the pulse picture in relation to the constitution rather than on symptoms, even in acute cases.

Collective sharing

The bottom two lines of a hexagram reflect the seeds of unconscious feelings and collective inherited background. The two middle lines represent the conscious area in which the unconscious seeds have germinated and evolved into manifested forms. The top two lines show the mental-spiritual qualities of the individual independent person.

The two yang lines of the third and fourth positions of hexagram 34 Great Strength express the power by which the unconscious and collective field, shared by people, is transmitted and consciously realized at the level of humanity.

The influence of the unconscious collective background and the spiritual legacy of parents and ancestors influence people in general, but especially children born with the earthly branch *Mao*, hexagram Great Strength and the deep *qi* wood. Family suffering is easily passed on to these children and affects their behaviour. Complaints in the area of the deep *qi* wood that may arise as a result are abdominal pains, sudden high fevers and irritable bowel syndrome (IBS).

Usually, diseases that originate from the collective shared field disappear while growing up, partly because children learn to shut themselves off from this collective field. This developmental stage can be accompanied by nightmares and insomnia. Fortunately, complaints due to collective sharing are relatively easy to treat in children via the deep *qi* wood of the large intestine.

As people get older, the influence of the collective field can (again) recur and people may suffer from fears and pains. And, although the resulting diseases are mainly expressed physically, the cause often lies in childhood trauma. Healing personal trauma from the past contributes to the well-being of everyone embedded in the collective field. The key to this healing can be found in hexagram Great Strength and the deep *qi* wood of the large intestine within the balance of deep *qi* water and fire.[2]

L.i.-3, *San Jian,* third interval

The deep *qi* point on the large intestine channel L.i.-3 is indicated for stiff joints and heaviness in the body, facial pains, shoulder complaints, dry eyes, sensitivity to strong emotions and overload of the mind. These symptoms can all be signs of unconscious resistance to getting in touch with personal and collective trauma.

Patience, gentleness and love, compassion and empathy are the tools that soften the seemingly rough paths to personal and collective grief and fear and give people the courage to view these inwardly. The deep *qi* point L.i.-3 balances the wood–metal horizontal axis of manifestation.

Deep *qi* treatments of soul problems caused by imperfections in the *po* and *hun* are only meaningful when the individual natural balance of the vertical axis of water and fire has been achieved, which, as you will understand, requires a more extensive treatment, though L.i.-3 can pave the way for that trajectory.

YOU, KIDNEYS, AND DEEP *QI* METAL

Hexagram 20 *Guan*, Watching, Contemplation.

The two top yang lines come from heaven, the two bottom yin lines are the latent, unconscious parts of human consciousness in which the universal light

---

2   It is advisable to treat this process together with a counsellor.

is mirrored. The two central yin lines depict the manifested receiving conscious-ness of the self.

The trigrams *Kun,* Earth, and *Xun,* Wind

The Earth at the bottom of this hexagram represents, among other things, the subjective self, which is open to receive and respond to the impressions of the object world. A healthy self is calm and tension-free, even when observing unrest and tension.

Calm and tension-free behaviour, guided by the characteristics of the trigram Earth, is the true nature of meditation: alertness, watching and calm diagnos-tic observation of body, mind and spirit.[3] The features of the trigram Earth, together with those of the deep *qi* metal of the kidneys, open the pathway to that authentic footing.

However, usually, due to the impulses of the external world, the ego's will intervenes. The personal will deviates from calmness, openness and authen-ticity. The ego seeks self-affirmation and escapes the complicated feelings that might come when discovering the authentic self. It looks for the understandable, limited and measurable. It is driven by desires and passions of the heart-mind that change the blood (*xuè*), intent (*yi*) and will (*zhi*) and with these the deep *qi* metal of the kidneys.

Wind at the bottom of hexagram Encountering (earthly branch *Wu*, heart) has moved to the top of hexagram 20 Watching. Latent and subjective motives are now manifested and objectified. They gently touch the world enabling the qualities of earth to perceive, observe and nourish.

The top trigram Wind enables the spiritual universal spark to express itself authentically in all forms. However, there is the resistance from the will of the ego driven by instincts, emotions and thought. The ego redirects and makes impressions and experiences personal. The hexagram is an example of the power of yin observing and perceiving life in a receptive and responsive way, so that the ego does not intervene or (re)act (again).

The two central yin lines at the level of humanity illustrate internal calmness and gathered inner strength. They receive the influence of the two top yang lines, the manifested virtues of heaven and impressions of nature, and the two bottom yin lines, the manifested reflection of heaven in the unconscious. In this way, yin represents the inner established universal values generated by

---

3   What is discussed about the trigram Earth also applies to the hexagrams 23 *Bo* and 2 *Kun*, respec-tively related to the earthly branches *Xu*, heart constrictor, and *Hai, san jiao.*

the inner universal spark of each individual authenticity that expresses itself uniquely and freely in the self.

Observation

This hexagram could be an example of the ideal diagnostic conduct of a practitioner and for any person interested in spiritual growth. Observation, attention and meditative watching mean that the object or point of attention is viewed with the qualities of Earth; with full attention, openness, without prejudice or involvement. It sounds rude to call people objects, but I don't mean anything disdainful. With the distinction subject–object, I mean that the object is something perceived by subjective consciousness. In fact, a person who examines their own self has also become an object for the same self ...

Impressions can be observed objectively and subjectively. Objective observation focuses on and evaluates one's own behaviour in response to impulses from others and the self. Subjective observation focuses only on inner motives.

Both ways of self-examination lead to more insight. The calmer the (un)conscious mind – the four yin lines – the purer the impressions which are received, and the purer the view regarding facts and reality.

When deep *qi* metal is excessive, it can subdue the free flow and strength of the deep *qi* wood. When too weak, it loses the ability to strengthen and nourish the shape and can easily be influenced by powerful or confusing thoughts or the intense emotions of wood. The *qi* is sent out and up.

Both excessive and insufficient deep *qi* metal can lead to similar complaints and symptoms: prostate pain, prostatitis, prostate cancer, stricture of the ureter, cystitis, kidney stones, cramps in the back and leg muscles, eye diseases, osteopetrosis, osteoporosis, pelvic floor problems with prolapse and instability of the pelvis and hips.

In these cases, the balance between the deep *qi* metal and wood must be addressed, bearing in mind that when such problems are caused by underactivity of the deep *qi* wood, the deeper cause may lie in the relationship between the deep *qi* water and fire.

The deep *qi* metal pulse

The deep *qi* metal in pulse diagnosis has been described as a movement of *qi* toward the centre. It may reveal as hard, even a little flat, or a bit constricted or a little sharp like fire, but always directed towards the centre. This movement should never come at the expense of relaxation and space for the *qi* of the middle.

The surface must be light and empty, with no force emanating from there. In the depth, the pulse shows its inner strength without further tension. It is a delicate balance because the demands of the ego often cause tension in both the superficial (Wind) and the deep part (Earth). Healing can only take place when the will calms down and sufficient attention is paid to objective and subjective observation of the self.

Ki-7, *Fu Liu*, returning current

Chapter 34 has already discussed a few aspects of Ki-7. The power of the deep *qi* point on the kidney channel is the return to the source of yang: to return to the conditions of regenerating life and to give impetus to the development of authenticity and the cultivation of inner virtues.

CHAPTER 42

UNLIKE *QI* RELATIONSHIPS BETWEEN *SI* AND *HAI*, *YIN* AND *SHEN*

Heaven–Earth and the Axis of Humanity

There is another intersecting link besides the link between the vertical creative axis *Zi–Wu* and the horizontal axis of manifestation *Mao–You*. The axis *Si–Hai*, fire–water (hexagrams Heaven-Initiative and Earth-Responding), takes on its true meaning in manifestation of humanity, human consciousness and the reality of everyday life reflected in the *Yin–Shen* axis (hexagrams Advance and Standstill). The description, meaning and significance of the last two hexagrams stem from the convergence of the forces of heaven and earth.

CHALLENGES

People born with the earthly branch *Si*, spleen, are challenged to align with the earthly branch *Hai*, *san jiao*. The challenge for these people is to create a balance between originality, community spirit and care.

For people born with the earthly branch *Hai*, *san jiao*, it is the challenge to align with the earthly branch *Si*, spleen; to develop the courage to choose for themselves and to be able to execute unpleasant, difficult choices.

People born with the earthly branch *Yin*, lung, are challenged to align with the earthly branch *Shen*, bladder. The challenges for these people are to occasionally do nothing, to exercise patience and to master the art of letting go.

People born with the earthly branch *Shen*, bladder, are challenged to align with the earthly branch *Yin*, lung. The challenge for these people is to learn that staying true to principles and retreating into seclusion does not come at the expense of vitality and reciprocity. The creative power of life lies in togetherness and alignment.

SI, SPLEEN, AND THE DEEP *QI* FIRE
Hexagram 1 *Qian*, Heaven, Creative, Initiative.

The hexagram Heaven, the earthly branch *Si* and the deep *qi* fire of the spleen are characterized by active functional vitalities: creative, initiative, completion and preserving what is created. It is up to humans to learn to live according to their nature (heaven) and to express their true being and consciousness in everyday life by nourishing everything and everyone they feel connected to.

Twice the trigram *Qian*, Heaven
The trigram Heaven was discussed in previous chapters; Heaven stands for firmness and strength. Its dynamism emphasizes correct and superior action, thus providing the impetus for initiative to bring about change at the right time. The trigram Heaven contains the four emanations – *yuan, heng, li, zhen* – preparing the conditions to govern the four directions and bring about changes.

The original unchangeable realm of 'non-duality' (Heaven) expresses itself in the changeable world through action, initiatives and transformations in the 'four directions' and is available when and where it is needed. Heaven is the supreme power of life from which all form arises; it is the source of freedom of the true human being, and can be heard as the inner voice of truth.

Every person has access to the truth of the inner voice. It is supported by experiences and dreams, not accessible by the mind or will. This also means that what is learned, including the subjects in this book, must not be accepted as truth or compared to learned knowledge, but always freely compared to the always present inner voice of truth. After all, the truth is unique to every person, no one has a monopoly on absolute truth. Any suggestion in this direction should be mistrusted.

The secret of the hexagram Heaven, the earthly branch *Si* and the deep *qi* of the spleen lies precisely in the invisible and hidden; the voice of everyone's inner nature, which is a reflection of the way of heaven.

Unfortunately, this fundamental principle of life is nowadays often undermined and destroyed by intellectual thinking and excessive zest for life. These ways of life can harm health; excessive intellectual thinking may lead to stagnation and heat in the spleen that damages the heart *qi* via the reverse *sheng*-cycle relationship from spleen to heart, and the heat of excessive zest for life might damage the *qi* of the spleen and pancreas, that can also adversely affect heart *qi*.

When the nature of change (the unchanging element of change) is understood, people no longer focus solely on the ever-moving outside world. They most likely feel the need to turn inward and pay attention to the eternal source: the silent, the limitless and the unpolarized. The eternal source of life is undefined yet complete in itself, hidden in the ever-changing self and in all that exists. Understanding the quality of the hidden nature of change offers alignment with the heart-*shen* and provides insight, overview, transparency and a broader perspective on the changing reality. Understanding begins with stepping back, creating an overview, along with the sense of mutual connection and commitment.

The pendulum clock is a nice metaphor for understanding the deep *qi* fire and the way it creates overview from a distance. The changeable world is the reciprocal movement of the pendulum. From the stationary suspension point of the pendulum, variability in movement and direction is easier to perceive and comprehend than when the observer is part of the movement of the pendulum.

Understanding through the deep *qi* fire and the heart-*shen* contributes to self-knowledge and self-awareness and to having constant and stable relationships between the ego and its environment: everything that falls under non-ego. Our profession can make a distinctive contribution to the recovery of the relationship between the pureness and feelings of the heart-*shen* by aligning the understanding of deep *qi* fire of the spleen with the heart-*shen*, by connecting understanding and feeling.

Sp-2, *Da Du*, great capital/organization

The outcome of treatment is strongly determined by the psycho-emotional state of the person treated. When the ego mainly focuses on outer appearance, the deep *qi* point on the spleen channel stimulates the zest for life; when the ego mainly focuses on the mental realm, Sp-2 stimulates intellect; when the ego mainly focuses on self-cultivation, it strengthens feelings of the heart-*shen*.

In addition Sp-2 activates the mind to act in cases of lack of concentration or lethargy.

SAN JIAO AND THE DEEP *QI* WATER
Hexagram 2 *Kun*, Earth, Receptive, Responding.

What has been seeded by *Qian* is brought forth by *Kun*.

Twice the trigram *Kun*, Earth

The features of the hexagram Earth are characterized as yin, gentle, submissive and following, yet yin remains firm and inert when it is set in motion. Although it appears beneficial to achieve goals through gentleness and perseverance, in the development of diseases these properties might lead to persistent chronic complaints; too late or too little initiative can cause *qi* to stagnate.

The spiritual aspects of the hexagram Earth and the earthly branch *Hai*, *san jiao*, are characterized by non-conceptual consciousness, openness and the connection with the Now. The personal path of the deep *qi* water of *san jiao* is somewhere on the path between the ego that seeks a position and affirms its right to exist, and the ego that is aware of greater wholeness and focuses on adjustment, involvement and acceptance instead of action and purposefulness.

In practice, involvement means that people need to learn to let go of expectations (often initiated by upbringing) and to connect with the Now; to relate with what currently IS present and to let go of the rest. Unfortunately, due to the enormous possibilities of the Now, people face fears. The seeking ego simply cannot let go of control and understanding. Allowing limitlessness in making choices can be awfully complicated, though the accompanied love of the omnipresent creative impulses of existence of the Now may be the reward of bliss. Love contributes to peace and wholeness as it transcends and eliminates duality. It is the unchanging constant that makes uncertainties, changes and contradictions bearable.

As the cause of the ever-present inevitable transformative power of change is hidden in the hexagram Heaven, so Love is hidden in the hexagram Earth and appears by experiencing the Now.

Much of this book was written during the Covid-19 crisis. Even before the crisis started, I noticed with pulse diagnosis that the deep *qi* water of the *san jiao*[1] was changing from a deeper to a more superficial position and from a thinner and slightly watery pulse into a wider and softer pulse. In a very large proportion of patients the *san jiao* pulse was too shallow, too wide and too soft. This commonly found pulse announced that something was about to happen collectively and

---

1   The *san jiao* activates *yuan qi*, regulates the movements of waterways and *qi* in general and is involved in generating warmth of the spleen and kidneys and transformation of *qi*, food and fluids. The *yuan qi* is a pre-heavenly essence that connects people to everything in the past. It is a dynamic force, the basis of inherited vitality, that makes it possible to facilitate individual transformation. The *san jiao* regulates, generates and transforms through adaptation and acceptance, just as water adapts to and limits itself in the specified solid forms in which it resides. As the river flows within its banks, the deep *qi* water allows the *san jiao* to connect to all parts of the body. In this sense, the deep *qi* of the *san jiao* has the same relationship with spontaneity as the deep *qi* of the gallbladder.

that (collective) aspects of the *yuan qi* opened up to be revealed. Inherited and epigenetic factors became available to the individual consciousness and helped people to develop and mature. However, associated fears have also led people to project and transfer their emotions onto others.

During this crisis, many people were (un)consciously confronted with intense personal life questions and people's experiences and insights have probably changed them forever. Earth and the deep *qi* water of *san jiao* focus on the deepest essentials and activate these for the purpose of maintenance of revealed life. When the nature of the unchanging element of change is known, people no longer focus solely on the ever-moving outside world, but may turn inward and pay attention to the eternal source; that is: the silent being, the boundless, unpolarized, undefined yet complete self within itself.

Sj-2, *Ye Men*, fluid door

The deep *qi* point on the *san jiao* channel balances the heart and kidneys, calms the heart and attachment to past experiences, reduces focus on expectations and brings people into the moment.

YIN, LUNG, AND THE DEEP *QI* WOOD

Hexagram 11 *Tai*, Advance, Peace.

The trigrams *Qian*, Heaven, and *Kun*, Earth

The three yang lines represent Heaven, the creative principle of life, the strong, united, calm and stable source behind the 'ten thousand things'. The bottom yang line in hexagram 24 Return has grown into three yang lines in hexagram 11 Advance.

Although the hexagram corresponds to the initiating creative principle of the emanation *yuan*/wood, that is rooted in the emanation *zhen*/water, hexagram 11 Advance and the associated deep *qi* wood of the lung mainly arises out of the meeting and merging of heaven and earth, fire and water that evoke movement, change and *qi*.

Heaven has three major lights: the sun, moon and stars; earth has three seeds of *qi*: water, fire and wind;[2] and humans have three treasures: *jing*, *qi* and *shen*.

Equal to these trinities, the three different deep *qi* water, fire and wood are inseparable and dependent on each other. The planets, moon and, in humans,

---

2   Wind is breath, *qi* and movement: the universal rationale, the essence of the power behind all growth and change.

the heart-*shen* receive and reflect the light and breath of the universe. The human spirit and mind (the heart-*shen*) are co-responsible for the health of the cosmic living network in which we all participate, including the network of organs and channels, which is the microscopic equivalent of the macrocosmic features of the sun, moon, planets and Earth. This omnipresent task of responsibility for the health of this network is felt by people born with the earthly branch *Yin*, lung, and is expressed by the deep *qi* wood.

Heaven and earth

> Heaven and earth are moving together
> An image of advance
> In correspondence with this,
> The ruler gives full play to his ability and wisdom
> To complete the Tao of heaven and earth
> And assists their suitable arrangement,
> To influence people[3]

The trigram Heaven at the bottom position of hexagram 11 ascends and meets the trigram Earth on the top position that descends. This expresses their nature of attraction and leads to movement and change.

The trigram Earth allows unhindered expression of the yang of heaven. It requires openness, receptivity, fellowship, responsibility and compassion to express the magnificence of the formless inspiration. As discussed with hexagram Return (24), the manifestation and realization of ideas and inspiration can be blocked due to the incorrect function of Earth. The degree of realization depends on *conscious* choices and motives in contrast to hexagram Return of the earthly branch *Zi*, gallbladder, which is in an unconscious state.

The latent stimuli of life principles in the deep *qi* water have changed into conscious stimuli in deep *qi* wood. People born with deep *qi* water (*Zi*, gallbladder) take on the challenge of learning to sit back until the latent stimuli will reveal themselves. People born with deep *qi* wood (*Yin*, lung) face the challenge of having faith in inner latent forces and unconscious motives that want to reveal themselves as movement and change. The condition for this accomplishment is a proper balance between deep *qi* water with fire!

In practice this means that in cases of insufficiency of the lung *qi* and reduced strength of *wei qi*, the lung *qi* should be treated indirectly by restoring the

---

3   *The Complete I Ching* by Taoist Master Alfred Huang (1998, 'Commentary on the Symbol').

balance between deep *qi* water and fire, in order to optimize the deep *qi* wood to improve the function of lung *qi* and increase the strength of the *wei qi*. One of the eligible points for achieving this balance is Ki-16, *Huang Shu*.

> An example: Emphysema can be caused by an excessive activity of the deep *qi* wood of the lung *qi* or when wood invades metal. The expansion of wood is too dominant and hinders the normal contraction (metal) of the lungs. The walls of the alveoli are damaged and as a result they collect fluids which diminishes their normal function.
>
> The excessive deep *qi* wood is often not caused by an imbalance of lung *qi* only and therefore it makes little sense to treat the lung *qi* only. The cause of the disease is often found in the *qi* of the axis water–fire, *san jiao*–spleen, perpendicular to the horizontal axis wood–metal, lung–bladder. For instance, malfunction of *san jiao*, which can be the result of an imbalance between the deep *qi* water of *san jiao* and the deep *qi* fire of spleen, causes disturbances in *jing qi* and kidney *qi*.
>
> This does not mean that in cases of emphysema the deep *qi* wood of the lung should not be treated, but it should be accompanied and preceded by balancing the deep *qi* water and fire, thereby positively influencing the function of the deep *qi* wood of the lung *qi*.

Lu-11, *Shao Shang,* lesser *Shang*/metal

The deep *qi* point on the lung channel is known for its ability to treat sore throats and wind-heat. It is also a point for reviving consciousness. The latter function refers to the deep *qi* wood of the lung that activates and awakens *qi*. Therefore, one should generally be careful to sedate or disperse Lu-11, as this downgrades consciousness and awareness.

SHEN, BLADDER, AND THE DEEP *QI* METAL

Hexagram 12 *Pi*, Hindrance, Standstill.

Hexagram 12, Hindrance or Standstill, is oriented in the West, the direction of sunset and decay. The West is the symbol of sleep, the dying process and death.

Sleep and standstill, as well as the unconscious, facilitate processes by which the essences of experiences can be processed in stillness, encouraging 'the self' to develop. In that sense these phenomena are the gates of spirituality. The only force that can hinder this development is the power of the ego itself.

People born with this hexagram and deep *qi* metal live somewhere on the path between an ego that is flexible, adaptable and gentle and an indifferent and petrified ego that deems life meaningless. The harder the ego has become, the more problems can occur, such as rigid blood vessels and stiff muscles and nervous system. It once again explains why a good sense of humour, which is an aspect of spirituality and opposite to indifference and hardening, is so important to make *qi* flow.

The trigrams *Kun*, Earth, and *Qian*, Heaven

Like the hexagram Advance and deep *qi* wood, hexagram Standstill and deep *qi* metal are the result of a process that takes place between heaven and earth.

The trigram Heaven on the top position of the hexagram Standstill ascends and separates from the descending trigram Earth at the bottom position. The separation of the universal forces results in standstill and obstruction.

Usually, standstill comes unexpectedly and unintentionally. Due to illness or other events, people sometimes suddenly have to stop working and are forced to change their life path. Often this is interpreted as unfortunate, and often it is, but not always! The secret of healing and enrichment can be found precisely in standstill; it is a powerful gateway to change.

Confirming the unbearable situation, recognizing and observing (deep *qi* metal of the kidneys) the obstacles can lead to the necessary relaxation in due time. Either way, the primary focus of treatment is relaxation and changing the pursuit of improvement. People may then find some peace and inner silence and learn to use the inner antennae for natural change. Strangely enough, the focus is often only on having positive thoughts and action – and this may certainly be necessary in many situations – but the reality of the unbearable nature of the situation can create space for sadness and pain that hindered change.

In the sense of being receptive to and restoring the natural flow of life (in wholeness and healing), the deep *qi* metal of the bladder is involved in this process of humanization.

This hexagram is usually associated with grief and misfortune and people are therefore advised not to move, especially not to intervene and above all to wait patiently.

In my opinion, it pays to take a closer look at this opinion. Standstill has potential; it is not the same as patiently waiting for better times.

Standstill is characterized by withdrawing from action and distancing your-self from the known, and from being in the spotlight. Standstill may change the feeling that 'the self' needs confirmation; it is the transition from the experiences in the outside world to the consciousness of the inner spiritual world. This does not mean that there is immediate peace, quite the opposite. Incorporating emotions and thoughts into the inner being and being able to endure the ordeal of not giving in to the instinctive forces to turn inner tensions into power, social adaptation and aggression is hard labour!

The ego goes through a special transformation during standstill. Giving up external affirmation, external power, knowledge and dignity and giving up the importance of 'itself' is part of inner maturation and, with the help of others and circumstances, the personality can become an 'instrument', a transit point for Love.

The merging of heaven and earth in the hexagram Advance and the deep *qi* wood opens the gates of vitality, breath and growth; the separation of heaven and earth unlocks the gates of change to create the new. The special feeling with such experiences is the deep connection with something bigger than the self.

People born with the earthly branch *Shen*, bladder, and anyone confronted with it, can feel the burden of suffering. The art of healing is to surrender to the situation, to release any kind of pressure, even to release the pressure of letting go itself, but above all to learn to relax into the situation as it is, so that eventually, usually after a long time of sweating, hard labour, pain and swearing, the realization comes that it is as it is. The pursuit of change dissolves. This is the beginning of healing of the self.

Dependency, attachment versus emancipation

We are lonely in the deepest sense of the word. In the state of being alone, we might experience that we are part of a larger whole and feel connected to it. Some call this experience of wholeness the collective consciousness, others universal nature, others the higher self or heaven. The words and meanings don't really matter, the inner process they evoke does.

We are born alone and die alone, and since in youth no one usually teaches us to deal with loneliness, which is ideally the experience of connection with the universal, loneliness can easily lead to dependency and attachment. As people grow older and the inner finds more peace and quiet, there might be a greater longing for being alone, which is not experienced as loneliness but as nourishing and connectedness.

During childhood we need the protection and enclosure of our parents. While growing up, we slowly learn to stand on our own two feet, but the feelings of loneliness, which certainly comes along in this learning process, are unpleasant and in response we look for security in the form of connections, but also dependency and attachment to others, work, habits, religions, knowledge, things and so on.

Usually, loneliness has a negative connotation, as something that we should avoid. That is too bad because the positive aspect of loneliness is innovation and creativity, the power to invent something out of nothing. It is a state in which dependency and attachment to the well-known, the old, the conditioned and so on can be released, creating space for renewal.

The cautious manifestation of renewal takes place in the earthly branch *Zi*, gallbladder, hexagram 24 *Fu*, Return. The birth of the new can be discovered in the state of standstill of hexagram *Pi* and the deep *qi* metal of the bladder. People are able to free themselves, emancipate and identify with all parts of the self, even with loneliness (!), by letting go of the old and transforming dependence and attachment into interdependence with autonomy and freedom.

Bl-67, *Zhi Yin*, arrival or extremity of yin

The deep *qi* metal point is indicated to guide people who suffer. It can dynamically turn a person's chaotic, suffering *qi* into acceptance and a new perspective on a purpose in general.[4]

---

4 Sedation or tonification; it depends on the quality of the pulse.

CHAPTER 43

UNLIKE *QI* RELATIONSHIPS BETWEEN *CHOU, CHEN, WEI* AND *XU*

The Field of Transformation

Table 43.1 The inner structure of the hexagrams of the field of transformation

Earthly Branches					Unlike *Qi*		
Chou	Liver	Approaching	䷒	䷗	Retreat	*Wei*	Small intestine
Chen	Stomach	Resolution	䷪	䷖	Splitting apart	*Xu*	Heart constrictor
Wei	Small intestine	Retreat	䷠	䷒	Approaching	*Chou*	Liver
Xu	Heart constrictor	Splitting apart	䷖	䷪	Resolution	*Chen*	Stomach

The four trigrams used are the Lake,[1] Mountain,[2] Heaven[3] and Earth.[4]

The various deep *qi* earth of the earthly branches *Chou, Chen, Wei* and *Xu*, related to the liver, stomach, small intestine and heart constrictor respectively, are determined by the inner structure of the following hexagrams: 19 Approaching, 43 Resolution, 33 Retreat, 23 Splitting apart. The four trigrams used in these hexagrams are *Dui*, Lake, *Ken*, Mountain, *Qian*, Heaven, and *Kun*, Earth.

- **Unlike *qi*:** All yang and yin lines of the hexagram associated with the

---

1 *Dui* ☱
2 *Ken* ☶
3 *Qian* ☰
4 *Kun* ☷

earthly branch are changed to their counterparts in the unlike *qi* of the earthly branch.

- **Unfolding *qi***: The three bottom lines of a hexagram reflect the subjective, latent, unconscious motivation for development. The three top lines of a hexagram reflect the objective situation into which the latent motivations develop.

The lower trigram Lake of hexagram Approaching appears in hexagram Resolution as the upper trigram. The lower trigram Mountain of hexagram Retreat is the upper trigram of hexagram Splitting apart.

The deep *qi* earth of liver and small intestine associated with the hexagrams Approaching and Retreat have the lower located trigrams Lake and Mountain: the quality that is more internal and potentially present.

The upper located trigrams Lake and Mountain in the hexagrams Resolution and Splitting apart manifest the unfolding deep *qi* earth of the liver and small intestine into the stomach and heart constrictor. The process of unfolding *qi* from internal and potential towards manifestation and expression is made possible successively by the features of the trigrams Earth and Heaven.

PRACTICAL APPLICATION OF UNFOLDING *QI*

Insufficient deep *qi* earth of the stomach might be caused by insufficient deep *qi* earth of the liver. The trigram Lake in the hexagram Approaching refers to rooting at the level of the feet and of the lower burner. Both regions have the potential for growth and expansion of opportunities. The yang lines of the hexagram and trigram represent the support of growth of the potential that will unfold in due time.

Physically, this initial unfolding manifests itself in the deep *qi* earth of the liver: the reservoir that manages the power of defence, that allows the liver to move and warm *wei qi*, that nourishes *ying qi*, ascends, decides, makes plans, guarantees free flow of *qi* and so on. Spiritually it governs the ability to respond correctly – that is, responsibly: not giving in to desires, personal intentions and conditional behaviour, but listening to and being open to the unfolding of the rhythm of life and acting with upright *qi*. Through the unfolding qualities of the deep *qi* earth of the liver, expressed in the upper trigram of hexagram 43 and the deep *qi* earth of the stomach, these qualities allow the stomach to firmly refuse or accept food in the broadest sense of the word.

For instance, a restless, too active and alert deep *qi* earth of the heart constrictor might be a (unconscious) defence mechanism to protect inner uncertainty. A calming treatment of the heart constrictor weakens the defence and increases uncertainty and exacerbates the situation. The inability to turn inward, relax and find peace and stillness stems from the insufficiently unfolded deep *qi* earth of the small intestine. The Mountain, lower trigram in the hexagram Retreat, portrays the correct condition for individuation, providing grounding and stability through silence and tranquillity.

Disturbances of deep *qi* earth of the liver and small intestine can manifest in disturbances of the deep *qi* earth of the stomach and heart constrictor: abdominal pains, heartburn, Crohn's disease, fainting, urethritis, madness, heat disorders, pain in the area of the scapulae and so on.

Disturbances in unfolding *qi* also occur in other deep *qi*; for instance, a disturbance in the lower hexagram Thunder with the deep *qi* water of the gallbladder can be manifested in the upper trigram Thunder with the deep *qi* wood of the large intestine. For example, complaints to the feet and ankles that arise from malfunction of the deep *qi* water of the gallbladder can cause muscle complaints in the lower back and lead to constipation.

However, the disturbances of unfolding *qi* in the deep *qi* earth-related channels are more common than with other deep *qi*. This might be caused by climate change and bad eating habits.

CHALLENGES

People born with the earthly branch *Chou*, liver, are challenged to align with the earthly branch *Wei*, small intestine. The challenge for these people is to find balance in supporting inner growth and growth of their surrounding group.

People born with the earthly branch *Chen*, stomach, are challenged to align with the earthly branch *Xu*, heart constrictor, and to unfold the properties of the earthly branch *Chou*. The challenge for these people is to combine a certain degree of egocentrism with loyalty and compassion for others and to master acceptance and to be free from habits.

People born with the earthly branch *Wei*, small intestine, are challenged to align with the earthly branch *Chou*, liver. The challenge for these people is not to lose sight of their own interests in representing the interests of others.

People born with the earthly branch *Xu*, heart constrictor, are challenged to align with the earthly branch *Chen*, stomach, and to unfold the properties of the earthly branch *Wei*. The challenge for these people, especially in times of adversity and difficulty, is to feel inner confidence and faith and to share presence and commitment.

CHOU, LIVER, AND THE DEEP *QI* EARTH
Hexagram 19 *Lin*, Approaching.

Table 43.2 Liver axis

☰	Heaven	Upper Dan Tien	DM-20	*Bai Hui*
☵	Water	Middle Dan Tien	Liv-14	*Qi Men*
☲	Fire	Middle Dan Tien	Liv-13	*Zhang Men*
☷	Earth	Lower Dan Tien	Liv-3	*Tai Chong*

The *qi* of heaven is received by the water of the earth. The water and fire of the earth transform the *qi* of heaven for the creation and manifestation of human life. The vertical life-giving creative axis heaven–earth–human is answered by humans via the liver axis; the quality of the root of the deep *qi* earth of the liver determines the quality of the human response to the heaven.

Liver channel and liver axis
The liver channel starts at Liv-1, *Da Dun*, at the medial side of the nail of the big toe. It runs over the foot to Liv-4, *Zhong Fen*, goes to Liv-5, *Li Gou*, via Sp-6, *San Jin Jiao*, runs over the medial side of the leg to the medial side of the knee at Liv-8, *Qu Quan*, ascends to Liv-11, *Yin Lian*, in the groin. Via Sp-12, *Chong Men*, and Sp-13, *Fu She*, to collect and support the yin in general, the channel goes further to Liv-12, *Ji Mai*, in the groin. From Liv-12 the channel flows around the genitals, meets Cv-2, *Qu Gu*, Cv-3, *Zhong Ji*, Cv-4, *Guan Yuan*. From the abdomen it ascends through the stomach area, some authors say Cv-12, to Liv-13, *Zhang Men*. On the left side of the body it rises directly to Liv-14, *Qi Men*; on the right side it first connects to the liver and wraps around the gallbladder to meet Liv-14. From Liv-14 as well as from the liver the flow ascends through the thorax and throat to the eyes.

My teachers had different opinions about the continuation of the channel from Liv-14; one trajectory described is more superficial along the sternum to connect with the stomach, lung and heart to ascend to the eyes. Another trajectory described is more internal: It passes through the diaphragm and touches the flanks of the thorax to rise up via the throat to the forehead and the area of the eyes. I assume both trajectories are correct.

From the eyes, a branch descends to the inside of the cheeks and encircles the mouth. One branch rises up from the area of the eyes to meet the *du mai* at Gv-20, *Bai Hui*.

My *qigong* teachers mentioned another branch, called the liver axis. It starts from Cv-2 and goes internally to the lower burner, where it meets *Bao Zhong*.[5] One of my teachers just mentioned the word *Bao*.[6] From the lower burner the liver axis ascends vertically and pierces the diaphragm to pass through the heart, the lungs, throat and brain to Gv-20. From Gv-20, it descends via the ventral side of the spine toward the pelvic area to complete the cycle at Cv-2. The liver axis is first of all accessible via Cv-2, the acupuncture point that carries and supports life in general and strengthens perseverance and self-confidence, Cv-3, the acupuncture point that empowers the depths of a person's being, and Cv-4, the acupuncture point that roots *qi* in the basic principle (*yuan qi*).

Liv-3, *Tai Chong* (Liv-8[7]), Liv-13, Liv-14 and Gv-20 are used to activate the flow of *qi* in the liver axis in relation to the acquired quality of the human response to heaven.

Liv-3, *Tai Chong*, supreme rushing, the deep *qi* earth point of the liver channel

Liv-3 is perhaps the most widely used acupuncture point in Chinese medicine. The mobilizing and moving actions on the *qi* are founded in the meeting of the liver channel with the lower burner at Cv-2, Cv-3 and Cv-4. The lower burner regulates and generates a base of purity from which the *qi* in general is enabled to move. Due to the deep *qi* earth and the connections to the lower burner, Liv-3 provides a solid foundation through which people can physically and spiritually individualize, yet stay connected to their ancestors.

Liv-3 unites with the network of the basic principle: The original source of *qi* divides into two kidneys after which the triple warmer, *san jiao*, spreads the *qi* across the body to, for example, the back *shu* points. A proper free flow of *qi* in the lower burner is a prerequisite for Liv-3 to generate free flow of *qi* throughout the body. There is also another precondition.

The two bottom lines of trigram Lake in the hexagram Approaching refer to the basic rooting, as discussed in the text on unfolding *qi*. The unfolding of deep *qi* earth can stagnate in the middle burner due to obsessive or too thoughtful behaviour, worrying, excessive damp or mucus or little exercise. It would be good to focus the treatment first on the cause of possible stagnations, before Liv-3 ensures good rooting and free flow of *qi*.

---

5   In women, *Bao Zhong* is considered the uterus, in men the chamber of sperm, possibly the prostate.
6   *Bao* is another word for the lower *dan tien* area.
7   Liv-8 is mentioned, but has a lesser effect than Liv-3.

Liv-13, *Zhang Men,* veil or camphorwood door, gate of order, door of shelter

Liv-13 on the right and left side have different features. Liv-13 on the right side relates to the trigram *Kan,* water, on the left side to the trigram *Li,* fire.

Liv-13 on the right produces, distributes, maintains and manages the principles of yin. It is used in issues of form principles, *xuè,* the physical, the material, due to stagnation of yin-flow of *qi.* For example, it is used for problems with breastfeeding, abdominal distension, vomiting, indigestion, lumbar pain that feels like a fracture, difficulty urinating, internal cold.

Liv-13 on the left is called the palace of life. It transforms and moves *qi,* managing the life principles at the level of humanity, the principles of yang and vitality. It moves and inspires the form, which in turn stimulates organs to produce *qi* and *xuè.*

Liv-13 is indicated when inactivity and stagnation prevail. People can feel blocked while they still feel like doing something. This feeling is usually accompanied by considerable uncertainty and chronic doubt. It manifests itself physically in pain in the rib cage and at the top of the lumbar spine when people lie down (Liv-13 left), or in the elderly as shortness of breath and a swollen abdomen (Liv-13 right).

The yin line in the third position of the hexagram Approaching allows the two bottom yang lines to bring about change. It stands for the calmness of the surface of the water of the lake. The calmer the surface, the better the deep *qi* earth of the liver is gathered.

The lower burner

The third line of any hexagram corresponds in the body to the lower burner area. The state of calmness of the lower burner is crucial in keeping the deep *qi* earth of the liver, the two yang lines, gathered. Unrest, weakness or stagnation in the area of the lower burner, the thighs, waist and groin, in general but especially in people born with the earthly branch *Chou,* liver, suggests problems in gathering the deep *qi* earth of the liver in the basic principle (*yuan qi*).

Unrest with weakness may lead to yang bursting out, resulting in various types of skin diseases, for example. In its extreme form it can cause severe disruption of the *qi,* resulting in cancers such as prostate cancer, ovarian cancer, leukaemia, and bone and bone marrow cancer.

Stagnation may lead to introvertedness and the unpleasant feeling that life just doesn't flow and is hindered.

The lower burner region is very much influenced by *dai mai,* the channel that is crucial for the balance between gathering and spending *qi.* In some traditions

Liv-13 is considered a point of *dai mai* and is treated when people develop block-ages of *qi* in the lower burner. This especially occurs when people are unable to accept powerlessness, quite common among people who feel trapped in their busy schedules or in complicated family problems. Gb-27, *Wu Shu*, fifth pivot, may be helpful here; it is a central axis point that helps yang to descend and yin to ascend and spreads the *qi*. Distended abdomen, menstrual spasms, joint problems, pain in deep levels of muscles, prolapse of the uterus can be treated on the condition that people find a better balance in gathering and spending *qi*. Treatment of Gb-27 supports this process.

Liv-13 clears stagnation by passing the stagnated yin into the network of the gallbladder and liver channel by needling Liv-13 towards the gallbladder (channel) or towards *dai mai*. This is a necessary treatment to obtain access to the liver axis.

Liv-14, *Qi Men*, gate of cycle, gate of hope, door of epoch

The names of Liv-14 suggest an end and a beginning. At least three functions of Liv-14 meet this suggestion. The final point of the liver channel bridges the *qi* through the last gate of the cycle into the first channel, the lung. Liv-14 controls the end of yin and the transformation towards yang: the end of the night and the beginning of the day, the end of winter and the beginning of spring. *Qi* finishes its cycle to begin another new cycle.

Second, Liv-13, the other gate, is called the camphorwood door that refers to death and suggests that the spirit of the dead has been released and passed on to the next exit, Liv-14, where the *hun* can permanently leave the body.

The third option at Liv-14 is the gate of hope. Hope can be a solution to an uncertain expectation but that is not what is meant here. The hope of Liv-14 is beyond doubt. It is real and waiting for the chance when authentic collected deep *qi* earth of the liver flows freely to the head, eyes and Gv-20, when openness and responsibility secure the *zheng qi* to reunite with heaven.

When motives, beliefs and instincts calm down, inner strength is gathered in a natural, authentic way depicted in the two lower yang lines of hexagram Approaching. The open, receptive yin of the other levels invites *qi* to come into quiet contact with the head, eyes, mouth and Gv-20. The eyes shine brightly and the mouth speaks with virtue. The permanent spark of the basic principle comes into contact with the eternal in Gv-20.

A subtle spiritual development can begin, returning the markings in Gv-20 to Cv-2 and the lower burner via an internal channel on the ventral side of the spine where it enriches and purifies the yin-supporting structure of the whole being. Then the spirit shows itself through wisdom. From Cv-2, the enriched deep *qi* earth of the liver ascends again along the liver axis to express its light. The human being has become a light bearer.

The guidance of the natural path of development of the deep *qi* earth of the liver axis begins in Liv-3 and evolves during life through a free functioning lower burner. Liv-13 opens the yin, physical material existence, to the yang, spiritual consciousness. It continues its path through the gate of hope in Liv-14, to connect with the subtle realm of heaven in Gv-20.

Liv-14 is used in cases of stagnant blood and liver *qi*, yin obstructions in the thorax and epigastric region with yang fullness above or as a point of the *yin wei mai* to relieve menopausal symptoms.[8] Treatment of these types of complaints may have a better outcome if the previous preconditions are first taken into account. Any further spiritual development is purely individual and unfolds in its own time.

CHEN, STOMACH, AND THE DEEP *QI* EARTH
Hexagram 43 *Guai*, Resolution, Eliminating, Breakthrough.

The trigrams *Qian*, Heaven, and *Dui*, Lake
Commentators on the Book of Changes describe the receptive yin line at the top of hexagram Resolution as exhaustion of yin which is about to turn to yang. The fullness and strength of the five other yang lines, led by the supreme fifth line,[9] easily eliminates the yielding properties of yin.

However, the peaceful quality of the upper yin line is the strength of the trigram Lake. It rests, reflects and receives humbly, accepts and has no objections. Its satisfaction comes from silence that keeps the vitality and strength of yang inside.

Stomach deep *qi* earth and heart-*shen*
The stomach channel runs along the eyes, nose, mouth and ears, after which it collects the impressions in Gv-24, *Shen Ting*, spirit courtyard, the palace of the original spirit. Touching all the senses in the head makes the stomach channel an important gate and protector of the heart-*shen*. The deep *qi* earth of the stomach perceives and accepts to digest and transform the acquired impressions

---

8   Ki-9 governs the period of birth to puberty, Sp-15 from puberty to menopause, Liv-14 from menopause till death.
9   The fifth line represents the emperor, the ruler and organizer.

and offers these to the heart-*shen*.[10] Everything perceived is 'swallowed' as food and presented to the brain, mind and heart by the deep *qi* earth of the stomach.

The receiving qualities of stomach and spiritual qualities of the heart-*shen* are reflected in the locations and functions of the first nine points of the stomach channel ending in St-9, *Ren Ying*, man's welcome, also called *Wu Hui*, five celestial meetings.[11] St-9 is a window of the sky point, a point through which earth communicates with heaven. Heaven is not only the idea of a subtle realm outside, but is also embodied in the subtle realm of the heart-*shen*. This quality is represented by the five yang lines of the hexagram Resolution.

St-9 enables people to welcome and receive the love of life. It can be used when people have turned inward and cut themselves off from the world and/or feel unloved, suspicious and paranoid. It is only indicated when people are ready to change without setting too many conditions. St-9 balances the *qi* between the head and the thorax and is used, for example, in *yang ming* headaches, congested thorax and hindered breathing. It descends counter-current *qi* and takes too much yang from the area of the thorax to the head.

The deep *qi* earth of the stomach meets the unfolding *qi* of the deep *qi* earth of the liver and balances the inner and outer world in line with the individual basic principle (*yuan qi*).

The creative forces of the three yang lines of the lower trigram Heaven easily influence the will of the ego to fulfil desires. It interferes with the character of receptivity and acceptance of the upper yin line. People born with the earthly branch *Chen*, stomach, easily become addicted to sensations of pleasure, excitement, sports and goal setting.

The personal desire for well-being prevails over susceptibility and adjustments. Possible fears and uncertainties are preferably not regarded but sublimated in overexcitement. The will and desires guide the ego. This combination of forces can be the cause for people to be perceived as overactive and/or stubborn.

The pulse shows a full stagnated deep *qi* earth pulse with a strong and solid core; the ego's desires are leading and there is not enough room for creative initiating communication that is fruitful and satisfying for the heart-*shen*.

Stagnation due to lack of stillness and receptivity of the upper yin line can lead to various heat symptoms in the stomach, *xuè* or heart-*shen*. This manifests itself in cold or canker sores, rheumatoid arthritis, concentration disorders, hay fever, hyperventilation, panic attacks and so on. In addition to treatment people

---

10 All senses report to the heart-*shen*.
11 Five can reflect the breath of life, the five senses, the five heavens, the five seasons, the five organs. In addition it is the number of change.

may be advised to only do things that bring inner satisfaction and happiness. Following one's bliss is healthier than external appreciation and affirmation.

A docile, unwilling ego can also cause stagnation in the deep *qi* earth with the same symptoms as a desiring ego. But in that case the deep *qi* earth pulse is different. It is stagnant, but has a yielding core instead of a strong and solid core. It is recommended to treat the deep *qi* earth point St-36, preferably with moxa.[12]

The ego can be too compliant and docile due to loss of vitality of the will of the inner heaven: the heart-*shen*. One of the symptoms of this insufficient heart-*shen* condition is that people want to stay at home. Their condition resembles hibernation.

WEI, SMALL INTESTINE, AND THE DEEP *QI* EARTH
Hexagram 33 *Dun*, Retreat.

The trigrams *Ken*, Mountain, and *Qian*, Heaven

Hexagram Retreat shows the Mountain under Heaven. The mountain symbolizes silence and its expanse radiates holiness. The features of Mountain accept limitations and are aware that heaven is always within reach to receive and collect its *qi*. The withdrawal of *qi* can be accepted as in accordance with the will of heaven and natural development.

The front *mu* point of the small intestine, Cv-4, *Guan Yuan*, the gate of *yuan qi*, has another name: *Kun Lun*, a nine peak sacred mountain range with a mountain lake in its centre. This water symbolizes a heavenly pond in which the collected *qi* is the origin of all water circulation. It is the residence of the Mother of the West, the direction of sunset. The stillness of the mountains represents the withdrawal of visible and well-known integrated actions. Stillness is the needed precondition to enter the world of sleep, 'death' and non-action: the spiritual world of the ever-shining inner lights.

The Kun Lun Mountains are known as the mountains of immortality. They refer to people who walk the central path in accordance with heaven and earth and form the space in which silence and peace reign. This opens the path of individuation and the process of becoming who you are at heart.

Heaven on top of Mountain shows retreat. It is a way to maintain strength, to be obedient to the natural development of time and seasons and accept that growth development is accompanied by decline; that birth includes death and

---

12   For people not born with the earthly branch *Chen*, stomach.

action is accompanied by rest. The ego knows when to act and when to keep quiet.

> If one loves others and they do not respond in the same way, one should turn inward and examine one's own love. If one treats others politely and they do not return politeness, one should turn inward and examine one's own politeness. When one does not realize what one desires, one must turn inward and examine oneself in every point.[13]

The text encourages people to explore the latent forces of the unconscious – the three lower lines in the hexagram. Although many points on the small intestine channel mainly treat channel problems, their functions also refer to internalization and self-examination and evoke stillness.

For instance, S.i.-19, *Ting Gong*, listening palace, the exit point of the small intestine channel, treats many ear disorders and brings yang to the centreline, collects *qi* and calms the mind, as does the deep *qi* earth point of the small intestine, S.i.-8, *Xiao Hai*, small sea. It calms the fullness of *du mai*, calms the mind, stimulates water (with S.i.-7, *Zhi Zheng*, upright branch, branch to correct) and brings grounding and stability.

XU, HEART CONSTRICTOR, AND THE DEEP *QI* EARTH
Hexagram 23 *Bo*, Splitting apart, Decline, Erosion, Falling away.

The trigrams *Kun*, Earth, and *Ken*, Mountain
The Earth carries the Mountain. The Mountain rests on the safe wide base of the Earth.

Unfortunately, if the properties of the lower trigram Earth are not somewhat mastered, stillness of the mind and heart hardly unfolds. The central theme of the trigram Earth in this location is to step back, be patient, careful and cautious. It is not appropriate and meaningful to continue to achieve goals simply because it is desired. Loyalty to alignment with the natural development of decay liberates people from their compelling will.

The main difference to hexagram 20 *Guan*, Watching, is the fifth line that has changed from yang to yin. The five yin lines together, despite being stable, responsive and yielding, can still push the solid yang line over the edge. Yet the sixth line represents the central theme of the hexagram; it carries the seed for

---

13   Huang (1998), Hexagram 39: Mencius resonating with Confucius.

the next cycle that begins with hexagram 24, Returning, and the deep *qi* water of the earthly branch *Zi*, gallbladder. The proper unfolding of the upper trigram Mountain is crucial for a new life cycle and for the aligned inner human response to the pure and natural *qi* of heaven. This change requires patience in tuning in and waiting for the right time.

The Book of Changes states that yin functions in this hexagram can only be completed if the only present yang line changes into yin. However, when that hexagram changes too quickly, people lose the opportunity to learn the special power of this yang line; the top yang line of the hexagram is the peak of the upper trigram Mountain, which depicts keeping still, silence and completion.

Mountain is the gateway to completion and shows the continuation of a process that seems to have ended but manifests itself in a new way. Such a gate must be reliable, stationary and silent so that the essential movement of renewal can pass through. In the body the Mountain is represented by the uterus. Only when the growth of a foetus comes to an end does the uterus open to generate the next stage of life.

In addition Mountain represents the grip of the hands. Holding on to something unnecessarily or unnaturally long or tight and clinging to something that you know is passing are expressions of the dominance of the yang will and hinder the unfolding and manifesting qualities of the deep *qi* earth of the heart constrictor into the deep *qi* earth of the small intestine. I mean that being 'hard on yourself' or 'finishing something because you have to' often comes from setting expectations and goals. As a result, the deep *qi* earth of the heart constrictor stagnates and as a result the heart constrictor cannot listen to the messages of the heart-*shen*, ultimately causing an imbalance in the deep *qi* earth of the small intestine.

Stillness

The heart constrictor envelops the heart. It protects the heart and expresses the qualities of the heart in the world. It acts like an aura by which it defines the scope of the consciousness of the heart. When the emperor/heart is strong and pure, the *qi* of the minister/heart constrictor follows the 'commands' of the heart by keeping its own impulses calm. In that way it protects the body through an aura of purity and health.

When the heart is weak, the heart constrictor becomes restless and is influenced and controlled by its own and other people's emotions and passions. The minister no longer listens to his emperor but leans toward the unrest of the people in the country. This principle also applies to the heart constrictor and the heart affecting the human soul and the body. The heart constrictor's internal branch to the abdomen communicates with the body (country) through the connection with the three burners.

The internal channel starts in the chest around Cv-17, *Dan Zhong*, chest centre, and descends to the abdomen to make contact with the middle burner at Cv-12, *Zhong Wan*, middle stomach, and the lower burner at Cv-7, *Yin Jiao*, yin crossing. These are the three front *mu* points of the three burners that allow the heart constrictor to align with the *qi* of all organs.

The deep *qi* earth of heart constrictor is based on observation and aligned with yin properties such as vulnerability and sensitivity. This yin state of the deep *qi* earth of the heart constrictor may seem inactive, but it is a state of awareness: waking presence and mindfulness that listens to the sound in the stillness of the being. This state is the secret behind the initiative of yang, creation and renewal.

Stillness is a state of being, not achieved by willpower, but by self-knowledge allowing the activity of the self to become quiet. When the deep *qi* earth of the heart constrictor becomes as quiet as a mountain, it can hear the sounds of the heart and the authentic self.[14]

The one yang line on top of five yin lines depicts a house with a roof (the yang line) that holds the walls together (the yin lines). If the roof is strong, flexible and sufficiently adaptable the house will stand. If it is stiff, or otherwise inflexible, the house will collapse easily and leave its heart unprotected.

Completion

The inner voice that calls from the depth of the heart is the voice that silently experiences completion. This is not the same completion as described in the discussion about the emanation *heng* at the beginning of the book, but it refers to completion before manifestation as we know it, before completion was time bound. Nevertheless, this completion does affect manifestation and time.

The inner voice that emerges from completion is the seed for the new, the inner living vibration of love that nourishes and renews the intimate connections with the self, others and the collective consciousness.

When each one of us fulfils and heals the bliss of consciousness of the heart, all personal puzzle pieces are placed in the collective wholeness. In this sense each person contributes to the healing of the whole. The deep *qi* earth of the heart constrictor is the silent doorkeeper of completion, which is usually found only in death. However, many spiritual schools explore this door to completion. The accompanying lessons turn out to be a lifelong learning experience.

---

14   This is in line with the inner attitude of someone who makes a (pulse) diagnosis.

The network of deep *qi* earth

Problems with the deep *qi* earth of the heart constrictor can be approached through the deep *qi* earth of the stomach (unlike *qi*). It should be borne in mind that the deep *qi* earth of the stomach may arise from the improperly unfolded deep *qi* earth of the liver. In addition deep *qi* earth issues of the heart constrictor may arise from stagnated deep *qi* earth of the small intestine.

It is worth mentioning that all deep *qi* earth problems should always be compared to the condition of the heart *qi*, which includes the mandate of heaven, the central theme, which is reflected in the deep *qi* earth.

Many heart constrictor points affect the health of the stomach, the heart and to a lesser extent the small intestine and liver.

Hc-3, *Qu Ze*, clears heat in the stomach and harmonizes the intestines.

Hc-5, *Jian Shi*, descends rebellious *qi* in the chest and stomach and promotes proper function of the stomach.

Hc-6, *Nei Guan*, tonifies and regulates the stomach when the stomach and spleen are not in harmony.

Hc-7, *Da Ling*, eases the chest, relieves tension in the stomach and harmonizes the intestines.

Hc-1, *Tian Chi*, is the meeting point of *jué yin* and influences the liver. All heart constrictor points have an influence on the balance between liver and heart constrictor, both part of *jué yin*.

Hc-7, *Da Ling,* great mound

Hc-7 strongly affects the heart, especially used in cases of rising heat. It is indicated for the treatment of restless yang behaviour, which occurs when people listen more to impulses from the environment rather than their own thoughts and feelings. Hc-7 soothes the excess yang deep *qi* earth and opens its yin qualities. During the treatment it is therefore advisable to remain silent and to facilitate relaxation.

CHAPTER 44

THREE DYNAMIC FIELDS

In addition to the four earthly branches that have just been discussed, there are two other combinations of four earthly branches that together create a dynamic field. The three fields as a group can be placed in the created concept of heaven–humanity–earth. Heaven can be seen as the initiating stimulus from nature coming directly from the Great One or Oneness. The earth rules over all materially created manifestations and humanity acts in between these two realms.

Heaven:	Zi-Mao-Wu-You	gallbladder – large intestine – heart – kidneys
Humanity:	Yin-Si-Shen-Hai	lung – spleen – bladder – *san jiao*
Earth:	Chou-Chen-Wei-Xu	liver – stomach – small intestine – heart constrictor

Creating balance in dynamic fields often takes precedence over other treatments.

HEAVEN
Zi and *Wu* establish the creative vertical axis within the dynamic field of heaven and people born with either the earthly branch *Zi* or *Wu* are challenged to express their authenticity in everyday life. The created horizontal axis between *Mao* and *You* is the level in which the authenticity of *Zi–Wu* manifests and expresses itself.

For people born with *Zi* or *Wu*, the search for authenticity and the mission to express it can become quite difficult when the horizontal *Mao–You* axis is imbalanced and large intestine and/or kidney *qi* problems are present.

People born with the earthly branch *Mao* or *You* must feel that daily life is safe and organized, which means that the horizontal *Mao–You* axis is in balance, which can then create alignment with their authenticity. In times of stress, inward focus on authenticity, righteousness and independence by treating the vertical *Zi–Wu* axis can help people born with either the earthly branch *Mao* or *You* to regain balance.

The square of heaven particularly focuses on issues of the *shen* and *jing* in relation to the *hun* and *po*.

HUMANITY

People born with the earthly branches *Yin*, *Shen*, *Si* or *Hai* are challenged to balance practicality with spirituality – what's the point, what do you do with it? Spirituality must be practical and applicable in life and cannot only be an end in itself.

People born within the dynamic field of the square of humanity must find a practical balance between the objective calmness and clarity of heaven and the stability and care of earth. It means that there should be awareness and consideration for themselves as well as for everyone they are in contact with.

A calm, clear mind and a balanced emotional life are prerequisites for heavenly inspiration, but being too quiet and introvert can lead to disconnection. A little challenge is needed to inspire people born with the earthly branch *Yin* or *Shen*. In times of stress and overstimulation, treating the vertical *Si–Hai* axis can bring back calmness and balance to the *Yin–Shen* axis.

Spiritual inspiration is a calling for people born with the earthly branch *Si* or *Hai* but it has to manifest and be made visible and tangible in everyday life. The power of inspiration becomes reality and takes form at the level of *Yin–Shen*. This requires individuality and independence, combined with compassion and thorough self-knowledge, to which the *Yin–Shen* axis makes a great contribution.

EARTH

In people born with one of the earth-related earthly branches, *Chou*, *Chen*, *Wei* or *Xu*, there is a desire to be nourishing and caring. In a tolerant and non-intrusive way, these people seek change in the self and others.

If the change happens too suddenly, too fast or is too intense, it will seriously affect the ego and lead to tension within the ego. Change is one of the most important features of life, but the biggest challenge is to find balance and stability within change.

People born with the earthly branch *Chou* or *Wei* seek individual growth. Feelings of loneliness can be hidden behind social overcompensation, too much identification with role models and overwhelming symbiotic (co-dependent) relationships.

The solution can be found in the *Chen–Xu* axis, where the dynamic between egocentrism and altruism prevails. Here, people must learn to develop one without abandoning the other.

People born with either earthly branch *Chen* or *Xu* are challenged to balance individual growth of the *Chou–Wei* axis with developing sympathy and empathy.

A female patient was born with a dominant earthly branch *Chen*, stomach; dominant because *Chen* is the earthly branch of the year, month and day of the date of birth. It is very likely that the challenges of staying healthy, to find the right balance between weaknesses and strengths, are found in the innate weaker qualities of the unlike *qi*, the earthly branch *Xu*, heart constrictor. Treatment of the heart constrictor *qi* might only give a temporary result, since the axis *Chou–Wei*, liver–small intestine, is the level to which the *Chen–Xu* axis attunes.[1] Although symptoms and diseases may be less present in the *Chou–Wei* axis than in the heart constrictor, in order for treatment to take hold, the treatment of the *Chou–Wei* axis should precede the treatment of the heart constrictor.

The heart constrictor channel affects the mental-emotional state. The patient has lower back pain, is nervous, has panic attacks and is always afraid to be late. She is extremely self-centred, defensive and insecure.

Diagnosis clearly shows an insufficient deep *qi* earth of the heart constrictor with symptoms of rising *qi* and superficially a too yang quality in the heart constrictor pulse. The choice of acupuncture naturally goes to the direction of the heart constrictor, for example Hc-7, *Da Ling*, to calm the mind, soothe the excess yang and open the yin qualities. However, if the diagnosis shows that the liver *qi* or small intestine *qi* is affected in any way, it is better to start the treatment with the liver and/or small intestine before treating Hc-7. In this specific case I treated Liv-3, *Tai Chong*, with Hc-7. The order in which the points were needled is important to achieve the desired result.

---

1   The vertical pair in each square manifests through the horizontal and the horizontal pair attunes with the vertical pair.

⇒ CHAPTER 45 ⇐

THE FOUR POSSIBILITIES[1]

The interactions between the great movement and heavenly stem as discussed in Chapter 22 must take into account the deep *qi* of the related organ, leading to four possibilities instead of two.

AN EXAMPLE OF THE FOUR POSSIBILITIES
'*Bing*, S.i. in water'

The small intestine belongs to the fire phase in the five phases theory and has deep *qi* earth.

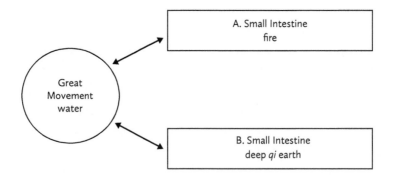

Option A: Great movement water and fire phase
The great movement water can influence the fire aspect of the small intestine. Interestingly, practice shows that other fire-related organs and channels can also be affected via the fire aspect of the small intestine. This is probably because we

---

1   This chapter concludes Chapter 22 in which we discussed the mutual influences of the qualities of the great movements and the heavenly stems.

are dealing with the great movement. The fact is that in practice we see that the great movement water can affect the small intestine, the heart, the *san jiao*, the heart constrictor and the spleen, because the spleen's deep *qi* is also fire. When fire becomes too watery it may cause the heart to become too cold. It can result in insufficiency of fire of the heart leading to, for example, cold hands, pale face, palpitations.

Conversely, the water of the great movement may receive too much fire from the small intestine. It can affect all *qi* that belong to water: the bladder and kidney, the gallbladder and *san jiao*, the latter two channels having deep *qi* water. Too much fire in the bladder and kidneys can lead to a wilful character, headaches, dark coloured urine and exhaustion due to excessive willpower. It can cause urinary tract infections when damp affects the heat in the bladder and kidneys.

Option B: Great movement water and deep *qi* earth

Not only the fire aspect but also the deep *qi* earth aspect of the small intestine can be affected by the great movement and vice versa.

The water of the great movement affected by too much earth can cause problems in the bladder, the kidney, the gallbladder and the *san jiao*. Too much damp in the kidneys can disturb the flow of fluids leading to, for example, puffiness in the skin, water retention in the abdomen with abdominal pains, easy weight gain.

Earth affected by too much water can cause coldness in all earth-related organs and channels: the stomach, the spleen, the liver, the small intestine and the heart constrictor. Too much water gives coldness in the spleen sub-duing the fire needed for transformation and transportation. It may lead to spleen yang insufficiency with symptoms such as cold hands and feet, a desire for hot food and drink, abdominal pain after eating cold food, diarrhoea with undigested food.

The potential imbalances discussed are just tendencies that may further be affected by predisposition due to heredity, behaviour and dietary preferences. But if one or more of the four possibilities occur in the pulse, it nearly always manifests in symptoms. However, caution is advised because the pulse adapts to the seasons and should not have the same image throughout the year. For example, the wood-related channels need a little more water in the summer to soothe the rising *qi*, but in autumn too much water is actually damaging. This shows that accurate examination of the seasonal differences in the pulse is indispensable.

Table 45.1 Four possibilities

Four Possibilities	GM → HS/phase	GM → Deep *qi*	HS/phase → GM	Deep *qi* → GM
1. *Jia* Gb in earth	Wood – E↑	Water – E↑	Earth – Wo↑	Earth – Wa↑*
2. *Yi* Liv in metal	Wood – M↑*	Earth – M↑	Metal – Wo↑	Metal – E↑
3. *Bing* S.i. in water	Fire – Wa↑	Earth – Wa↑*	Water – F↑	Water – E↑
4. *Ding* Ht in wood	Fire – Wo↑	Fire – Wo↑	Wood – F↑*	Wood – F↑*
5. *Wu* St in fire	Earth – F↑*	Earth – F↑*	Fire – E↑	Fire – E↑
6. *Ji* Sp in earth	Earth – E↑*	Fire – E↑	Earth – E↑*	Earth – F↑*
7. *Geng* L.i. in metal	Metal – M↑*	Wood – M↑*	Metal – M↑*	Metal – Wo↑
8. *Xin* Lu in water	Metal – Wa↑*	Wood – Wa↑*	Water – M↑	Water – Wo↑
9. *Ren* Bl in wood	Water – Wo↑	Metal – Wo↑	Wood – Wa↑*	Wood – M↑*
10. *Gui* Ki in fire	Water – F↑*	Metal – F↑	Fire – Wa↑	Fire – M↑*

*The interactions that are seen most in clinic are indicated with ***

Constitutional acupuncture not only looks at where such tendencies manifest, but further as to which constitutional imbalance might be the cause. 'Spleen too watery' for example can occur in '*Bing*, S.i. in water', but also in '*Jia*, Gb in earth' and '*Gui*, Ki in fire'.[2]

Constitutional treatment is only given if the diagnosis is confirmed through (pulse) diagnosis and corresponds to the innate imbalance that is apparent from the birth chart. Only when someone is born with '*Bing*, S.i. in water', '*Jia*, Gb in earth' or '*Gui*, Ki in fire' is a constitutional treatment considered.

This raises the question: What is a constitutional treatment?

---

2 The water aspect of kidney influences the great movement fire that causes coldness of deep *qi* fire of the spleen.

UNLIKE *QI* OR NOT UNLIKE *QI*, THAT IS THE QUESTION

In Chapter 38 we discussed a treatment I had observed with J.D. van Buren in which he treated Sp-2, *Da Du*, in a patient born with '*Bing*, S.i. in water'. Didn't he mention in his teachings that the unlike *qi*, in this case '*Xin*, Lu in water', was the best option for treatment? What was the reason that he didn't choose the unlike *qi*? Would that not balance the great movement and reinstate the balance between the great movement and heavenly stem? Or does the deep *qi* imply other rules? These were the questions I struggled with for a long time.

I still remember that, with this patient, the lung *qi* was insufficient and thus open to treatment. After having diagnosed the pulse, if asked, I would have suggested treating the lung. Months after this event, I discussed my doubts and struggle over his chosen point. His answer was short, delicate and thoughtful: 'The spleen is the mother of the lung, so the lung *qi* recovered as well.'

That answer turned my world upside down. Slowly I learned that my rationale, a result of my Western education in cause and effect thinking – that the cause is an imbalance in the great movement, therefore the solution is the unlike *qi* – does not fit into the Chinese philosophical way of analogous thinking. Using the unlike *qi* certainly wouldn't have been wrong, but it wouldn't have done justice to what was needed at the time. The renewed balance in the spleen *qi* was what this patient needed at that moment and it reinstated the great movement imbalance indirectly as well.

This treatment was a turning point in my training. I learned not just to blindly follow fixed rules from the teachings but to have a free mind in which the same results can be achieved without violating existing theories.

Coming back to the original question asked, what is constitutional treatment? The answer is any treatment that takes into account the constitution depicted in a birth chart made according to the philosophy of heavenly stems and earthly branches. The specific treatment with Sp-2 was therefore a constitutional treatment.

A CASE STUDY THAT TAUGHT ME A LOT

The patient was born in 1954.

'*Jia*, Gb in earth'. Like *qi*: liver; unlike *qi*: spleen

Wu, Ht, deep *qi* fire. Like *qi*: small intestine; unlike *qi*: gallbladder

Other weaknesses

Tendency for weakness in the great movement water.

The gallbladder as unlike *qi* further weakens the tendency to water weakness.

Four possibilities

- Wood too earthy – gallbladder, liver, large intestine, lung
- Water too earthy – bladder, kidney, gallbladder, *san jiao*
- Earth too woody – stomach, spleen, liver, small intestine, heart constrictor
- Earth too watery – stomach, spleen, liver, small intestine, heart constrictor

Diagnosis: Emphysema

Emphysema is a lung condition that causes shortness of breath. The alveoli in the lungs are damaged. Over time the surface area of the lungs is reduced, resulting in a reduced amount of oxygen reaching the blood. When exhaling, the damaged alveoli don't work properly and old air becomes trapped, leaving no room for fresh, oxygen-rich air to enter.

In Chinese medicine this is a condition where wood invades metal/lung (reverse *ke*-cycle), which causes improper contraction of the lungs due to a lack of lung *qi*. There is too much expansion and people have trouble exhaling. Often patients with emphysema have chronic bronchitis with damp-phlegm conditions.

One day this patient called me to ask if I could treat him and his acute symptoms. The medicines prescribed by the GP did not help and someone had advised him to see me.

When he entered the clinic room, he looked very unhealthy. His face was pale white and he had a dark, almost blue, colour under his eyes and a greenish-blueish colour around his lips. The tip of his nose and cheekbones were bright red.

The clear visible complexion points in the direction of deep *qi*.

- The clear pale white: metal, bladder and kidney deep *qi*
- The clear dark, almost blue, colour under his eyes: water, gallbladder and *san jiao* deep *qi*

- Clear redness of the tip of the nose and cheekbones: fire, heart and spleen deep *qi*

The area and vague greenish-bluish complexion around the lips are a sign of extreme coldness or of a liver issue (vague means five phases-related).

Shock

These are signs of an emotional shock, and when I asked what had happened, he could hardly speak because he started crying. One of his children had recently had an accident and was hospitalized. He had barely slept for a few days.

An emotional shock damages the *qi* of the spleen and the heart. The fear for the condition of his child and the lack of sleep may have exhausted his *jing* and kidney *qi*.

These assumptions were confirmed by pulse diagnosis. It was a very fiery pulse, emphatically found in the spleen *qi* and heart *qi*. The *san jiao, jing* and kidney *qi* were insufficient, thin, spreading and deep. The liver *qi* was stagnant with heat. The lung *qi* felt superficial, big and hard – these are signs of too much wood in the lung which was, however, not visible in the complexion; there were no clear green-blue (*qing*) colours.

My initial treatment strategy was to treat the spleen and heart *qi* to treat the shock, together with the *jing* and the kidney to treat the failure of grasping the lung *qi* that led to breathing difficulties.

The great movement earth was active, leading to a tendency for the great movement water to become insufficient. It strengthened my motivation to treat the water aspects with kidney *qi*. In addition the lung might need to be treated for shortness of breath. Still, I was unsure about my choices and I suddenly remembered that J.D. van Buren had taught me that insufficient water is often better treated with gallbladder and *san jiao* than with bladder and kidneys. In this case, gallbladder is unlike *qi* of the earthly branch *Wu*, heart, and mental-emotional health issues, especially when they are acute, can be better treated via earthly branches than through great movements and heavenly stems. The field of the great movements and heavenly stems is more essential and inner-personal, while the field of earthly branches is more psycho-emotional and interpersonal.

I decided to feel the pulse again to see if I had missed something. The gallbladder pulse felt too deep and slightly constricted, indicating that there was too little water deep *qi*. The constriction also indicated that this patient was doing his utmost to 'gather' water.

These observations, in combination with the excess fire, made me decide to change my original plan and to first treat the deep *qi* of the gallbladder as unlike *qi* of the innate earthly branch *Wu*, heart, and unlike *qi* of the harmed spleen. I also planned to treat *jing* and kidney *qi* to root the lung *qi*, and the stagnated liver *qi* to treat the congestion in the thorax. Moreover, a released liver *qi* supports the lung *qi* in the Chinese hourly clock.

The points I wanted to use were Sj-4, *Yang Qi*, pool of yang, Gb-40, *Qiu Xu*, hill ruins, and Liv-5, *Li Gou*, calf drain or woodworm canal. This combination regulates the liver and gallbladder *qi*, clears stagnation of the liver *qi* and generates free flow of *qi*. It separates the liver and gallbladder pulse. This combination is especially good for treating fear and nervousness due to emotional turbulence. Sj-4 with Liv-5 secures the *jing* and allows people to be in contact with their own wisdom and calmness.

However, since the gallbladder was his innate *qi*, I couldn't use Gb-40, despite it being unlike *qi* of the earthly branch. I therefore looked to the unlike *qi* (spleen) to treat the ill gallbladder.

I chose Sp-18, *Tian Xi*, heavenly stream, to treat the ill gallbladder, to open and treat the congestion in the thorax and to promote the downward flow of *qi*. Liv-5 clears liver stagnation, is good for fear and nervousness and together with Liv-10 it clears heat and encourages sleep.

Treatment: Sj-4, Liv-5, Liv-10, Sp-18

During the treatment the pulse and complexion normalized and the shortness of breath disappeared. To my surprise, the pulses of the lung, *jing* and kidney recovered very quickly, even better than I had anticipated. At the time I thought that the function of the lungs improved mainly due to the improved function of the *jing* and kidney *qi* to grasp the lung *qi*. However, after further investigation of the pulse, I understood that the restored vertical axis of the deep *qi* water of the gallbladder and *san jiao* with the deep *qi* fire of the heart had normalized the deep *qi* wood function of the lung on the horizontal axis.

CHAPTER 46

DYNAMICS OF INVERTED HEXAGRAMS

Opposite hexagrams, where yin lines are changed into yang lines and vice versa, reflect the unlike (deep) *qi* relationships between the earthly branches. Unlike *qi* relationships in general challenge human physical, psycho-emotional and spiritual behaviour.

For example, to stay healthy, a person born with the earthly branch *Xu*, hexagram 23 *Bo*, Retreat, heart constrictor, is challenged to keep the unlike deep *qi* of the earthly branch *Chen*, hexagram 43 *Guai*, Resolution, stomach, dynamic. It means that they must learn to consciously say yes or no to what is presented. Due to loyalty – the hallmark of their earthly branch *Xu*, heart constrictor – these people tend to say yes too easily. As a result, exhaustion and overload lie in wait. The energetics of the unlike *qi* of the earthly branch *Chen*, stomach, challenge people to first distinguish the pleasant and unpleasant. From there, they can decide about yes or no.

The meaning of the relationships of the earthly branches related via inverted hexagrams is different from that of opposite hexagrams. The inverted hexagrams display each other's mirror image, through which they provide insight into the complementary forces that are present in the self. They usually manifest themselves later in life and demand attention as inner critical voices.

In an esoteric sense, the external world of shapes is seen as a reflection – and therefore a reversal – of the spiritual world. In hexagrams 23 *Bo*, Retreat, and 24 *Fu*, Return, this reversal occurs when yang moves from the top to the bottom line and appears as an inner voice, the hidden revelation of light and love. Something similar happens to the only yin line in hexagrams 43 *Guai*, Resolution, and 44 *Gou*, Encountering. The five yang lines remove the yielding power of the yin at the top of hexagram 43 *Guai*, which reappears in hexagram 44 *Gou* as the bottom line: Inner receptivity and sensitivity become the sources of vitality.

People born with the earthly branch *Xu*, heart constrictor, with hexagram 23 *Bo* are challenged in unlike *qi* earthly branch *Chen*, stomach, with hexagram 43 *Guai*. However, they increasingly may feel, over the course of their life, the need for authenticity and the need to listen to the impulses of the inner voice to renew themselves to a more authentic expression of themselves. This is motivated by the inverted hexagram 24 *Fu*, Return, gallbladder. The inner, often still unconscious, voice makes itself heard more and asks the ego to attune thinking and feeling to inner values. People want to synchronize with themselves and manifest themselves more authentically.

Over the years I have observed that disturbances in the earthly branches often do not occur *directly* in the unlike *qi* of the innate earthly branch. Instead they are frequently announced in the deep *qi* of the earthly branches associated with the inverted hexagrams of both the innate branch and its unlike *qi*.

For example, with stomach channel issues in people born with the earthly branch *Xu*, hexagram 23 *Bo*, heart constrictor, the impulses and deep *qi* of the inverted hexagrams of both *Xu* and its unlike *qi Chen*, stomach, must be diagnosed and addressed first when diseases appear that are caused by an imbalance within that unlike *qi* relationship (between earthly branch *Xu*, hexagram 23 *Bo*, heart constrictor, with the earthly branch *Chen*, hexagram 43 *Guai*). So in this case only when the relationship of the deep *qi* of the inverted hexagrams – the earthly branch *Zi*, gallbladder, hexagram 24 *Fu*, and earthly branch *Wu*, heart, hexagram 44 *Gou* – is restored does an unlike *qi* treatment on the stomach channel (earthly branch *Chen*)[1] itself have a long-lasting effect.

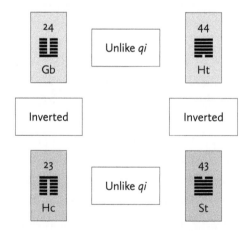

Figure 46.1 Inverted and unlike qi group 1

---

[1]   Often the treatment of the inverted hexagrams has already restored the original unlike *qi* relationship and such treatment is no longer necessary.

OTHER EXAMPLES

In someone born with the earthly branch *Zi*, gallbladder, disorders first arise in the balance of heart constrictor and stomach, before they arise at the level of the unlike *qi*, in this case the heart.

In someone born with the earthly branch *Mao*, problems with the balance between the liver and small intestine may arise before the unlike *qi* of the kidney is affected.

In the field of humanity, disorders related to the hexagrams and related earthly branches that belong to the Heaven–Earth axis – spleen and *san jiao* – often first arise at the level of the humanity axis – lung and bladder – and vice versa, because the inverted hexagrams either show the same picture or are equal to the opposite hexagram. Heaven–Earth is first treated at the level of humanity and vice versa.

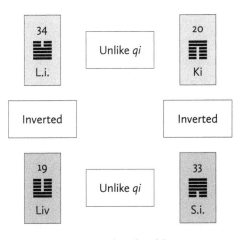

Figure 46.2 Inverted and unlike qi group 2

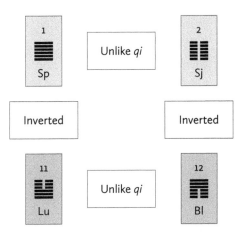

Figure 46.3 Inverted and unlike qi group 3

CHAPTER 47

HIDDEN STEMS

When I studied at the ICOM Institute, the subject of hidden stems was not taught and it is only in the last twenty years that I have been working with it.

When I was first introduced to constitutional acupuncture it was still normal practice to directly address the insufficient channels related to the innate earthly branch. The practice of stems and branches has developed further since then and it became increasingly clear that it is better not to treat the innate *qi* directly. The results are positive in the short term; however, in the long term, direct treatment of the innate *qi* could negatively affect the essential *qi*. It was then decided that treatment of a channel/earthly branch involved in the same field of tension as the innate earthly branch should be preferred over direct treatment. Initially, these channels were mainly the like *qi* and unlike *qi* relationships.

During my work as an acupuncturist and teacher I regularly came across insufficient channels related to the innate earthly branch. Since the results of like and unlike *qi* were not always satisfactory, I started looking for a method to treat the insufficient innate earthly branch more directly. Pulse diagnosis guided me. New mindsets often have their origins in mental processes but, in this case, practice showed me the answer to my question, and it was up to me to perceive, understand and describe the thinking model behind the answer.

The hidden stem philosophy offered me the solution I had been seeking, and I started working with it more systematically around the year 2000 and obtained satisfactory results.

Table 47.1 Hidden stems

I Zi	II Chou	III Yin	IV Mao	V Chen	VI Si
10 Gui	6 Ji	1 Jia	2 Yi	5 Wu	3 Bing
	8 Xin	3 Bing		10 Gui	7 Geng
(9 Ren)	10 Gui	5 Wu	(1 Jia)	2 Yi	5 Wu

VII *Wu*	VIII *Wei*	IX *Shen*	X *You*	XI *Xu*	XII *Hai*
4 *Ding*	**6 *Ji***	**7 *Geng***	**8 *Xin***	**5 *Wu***	**9 *Ren***
6 *Ji*	2 *Yi*	9 *Ren*		4 *Ding*	1 *Jia*
(3 *Bing*)	4 *Ding*	5 *Wu*	(7 *Geng*)	8 *Xin*	(5 *Wu*)

The hidden stems are known in the *bazi* system,[1] a Chinese astrological system that determines a person's fate or destiny via the heavenly stems and earthly branches of the year, month, day and hour, the so-called four pillars of destiny. These four pillars are also used in constitutional acupuncture.

The hidden stems are called hidden because they are the heavenly stems hidden behind the earthly branches.

Each earthly branch contains one or more hidden stem that represent the hidden potential of the earthly branch. In *bazi* the hidden stems reveal hidden characters, possibilities, feelings, talents and so on.

In the theory of constitutional acupuncture the heavenly stems and earthly branches are mutually dependent on each other. The heavenly stems express themselves through the earthly branches and the vitality of the earthly branches depends on the heavenly hidden stems.

In an insufficient channel/earthly branch, the related heavenly hidden stem is not able to express and manifest itself through that earthly branch. The converse is true: when the heavenly stem is underactive/insufficient, the vitality of the earthly branch weakens.

I found that I achieved the best results when I worked with the bold heavenly stems in the table. The points used are the stem points. There are two ways to use this in practice:

---

1   The schedule of the earthly branches and hidden stems comes from *bazi*, meaning 'eight characters'. *Bazi* is a very old form of astrology in which four heavenly stems and four earthly branches are determined (the year of birth, month, day and hour). With this information, the destiny, fate and character of a person can be divined. People who are very adept at *bazi* may find things like the number of children born to a marriage or the dates of accidents that have occurred or will take place. The bold printed hidden stems in Table 47.1 are called regular, those below, successively middle and residual. At the residual level, the Korean scheme contains a number of extra hidden stems compared to the usual schemes. These hidden stems in brackets come from Tae Hunn Lee, a valued colleague and close friend, who received this through his family in Korea. The patient's pulse image often points to the hidden stem of the regular field, rarely to one of the other fields. Usually, it concerns underactivity of the quality of the *qi* of the great movement within the channel. For example, the liver *qi* with too little metal (gathered) and too much wood (dispersed, scattered), or the bladder *qi* that has too little wood and stays deep and watery, or the spleen *qi* that has too little earth with dryness or fire-yang.

1 TREAT THE HIDDEN STEM OF THE INSUFFICIENT INNATE CHANNEL/EARTHLY BRANCH WITH THE STEM POINT

For example, for someone born with the earthly branch *Yin*, the vitality depends on the strength and quality of the hidden stem *Jia*, and vice versa. When *Yin*, lung, is insufficient, it may be caused by an underactive hidden stem *Jia*. *Jia* is first treated with Gb-34, *Yang Ling Quan*, only if (pulse) diagnosis confirms and allows this treatment.

This example does not apply to people born in 1974 (year *Jia-Yin*), because the hidden stem is the innate heavenly stem of the date of birth. It is better to choose the unlike *qi* of *Jia* or one of the other hidden stems (*Bing* or *Wu*). Practice has taught me that pulse diagnosis shows the way.

2 TREAT THE HIDDEN STEM OF THE INSUFFICIENT CHANNEL/EARTHLY BRANCH WITH THE STEM POINT

Regardless of the constitution, anyone can at times be confronted with weakness in a channel/earthly branch.

For example, when people are confronted with letting go, such as when losing a job, a relationship ends, a loved one dies or something else of that kind, the bladder *qi*, the earthly branch *Shen,* is insufficient. In a large number of cases the hidden stem *Geng*, large intestine, is underactive. The bladder *qi* is insufficient in its metal quality.

At first glance this is often not noticeable because a shortage of metal leads to more wood and a pulse that appears clearer and more superficial will cover its insufficiency. By treating the stem point L.i.-1, *Shang Yang*, both the large intestine and the vitality of metal in the bladder *qi* are restored.

In general, constitutional acupuncture chooses to work with few needles to clearly convey the message behind the treatment principle. This is certainly a requirement when the hidden stems are addressed.

CHAPTER 48

THE DYNAMIC EGO[1]

Our being is in a symbiotic state with the mother when we are in the womb. After birth, the safe space usually given by the parents can provide the ego with the necessary security from which it can slowly detach, separate and empower itself. The ego develops from a dependent individualistic being into an autonomous social being by gradually finding its own place and identity[2] in the world with which it must learn to deal. It learns to adapt, to defend, to know its weaknesses and strengths, to distinguish itself and so forth.

The development of the ego goes through the same stages as the development of humanity. From an original focus on survival and symbiosis with nature, human beings developed from a tribal group identity that had to defend itself against other groups into the reasonably autonomous beings of the twenty-first century. Yet many people, groups and countries are still in the phase of finding their own identity through power conflicts. It seems usually to be the only way in which egos, groups and countries give themselves the right to exist. But it can also be different.

The development of humans and humanity continues as ego orientation develops from self-centredness into a we-oriented society in which there is positive interconnection. We-orientation leads to mutual respect, where the commonality of people is seen as the higher good. In Chinese philosophy that would be heaven: the subtle power which inspires the group and the subtle power in the human themselves that we call true self[3] or authenticity.

The subject of this chapter is particularly close to my heart. It deserves to be elaborated on more extensively in a book that discusses purely and only this

---

1   The centre of human consciousness from which a person is in relation to both society and the true self.
2   The awareness and ability to evaluate the self and ego in its actions. Identity develops into a social being: Who am I?, What can I do?, What do I want?
3   The central point of the total personality, the true nature. It is distinct and distinguishable from self-image and identity.

topic. Yet it also belongs in this book because the development of humans and humanity proceeds according to the twelvefold division of their constitution. This is why I will try and discuss its essence in a short summary.

In this chapter I would particularly like to share a vision of human development that is in relationship with the cycle of the twelve earthly branches. The goal is to provide tools that help people understand each other better. This chapter grew out of what I learned from my teachers and patients. Both opened up to me and invited me into their life history. I am extremely grateful for that and hope that what they have taught me can be a positive contribution for you, the reader, and your patients.

THE EGO HAS ITS UNIVERSE

The earthly branches *Hai, Zi, Chou* and *Yin* (*san jiao*, gallbladder, liver and lung) are dominant in babies and small children. These earthly branches participate in processing the sensory information required to build the ego. During this period, feelings of well-being are dominant and the instinct for self-preservation is developed. In young children the objective external and subjective internal world are inextricably intertwined and are hardly distinguishable from each other. During the first years of life the distinction between these two worlds gradually becomes clearer, but babies do not yet distinguish the objective from the subjective. The mother's or father's hands and their own hands are part of the same amorphous whole. The sound of their own laughter is not experienced differently from the sound of the radio. Children feel an uncomfortable atmosphere between parents as if they themselves were uncomfortable and can respond to it with, for example, reactive or even hyperactive behaviour. This happens without the child knowing or thinking about it. Babies and children slowly learn in time to discern what enters through their senses and what is their own.

The specific function of these earthly branches in building the ego, in making it strong and important, continues when childhood is over. The other earthly branches nuance the qualities of the ego. For some, however, that first phase continues to dominate all of life.

The verb that expresses this stage is 'to have'. Behaving accordingly should be dominant throughout this phase. The subjective ego or 'I am' principle needs to have desires during the first period of life to confirm its existence. When 'having' continues to be dominant as an adult, it may cause diseases such as high blood pressure and chronic back pain. Long-term and excessive desires to possess significantly affect the gallbladder, liver and lung channels, and to a lesser extent the *san jiao*.

Characteristic of the first four earthly branches and channels is the influence of the external world on the subjective, inner world of the ego. The receptiveness of the ego and its responses to stimuli is necessary for the development of instincts for self-preservation and adaptation, but also for physical growth, learning and well-being. These earthly branches and channels play a major role in the treatment of children born with a disability due to brain damage and are essential for the treatment of people who have problems with their social position and interactions.

The earthly branch *Hai, san jiao*

The earthly branch *Hai, san jiao,* is essential for all other earthly branches and channels. The *san jiao* is the activator and messenger of *yuan qi*,[4] without which life does not unfold. *San jiao* activates the *yuan qi* and guides it to all organs, channels, *qi* and *xuè*.

The *san jiao* represents the whole area of existence in which we live. It is the ultimate expression of love and commonality rooted in the One.[5]

The *san jiao* is deeply involved in every expression of the ego. The ego of babies and small children identifies and is one with the environment. Therefore 'to have' at this age has a different meaning from when the ego has learned to distinguish itself from the environment. A baby who puts something in its mouth experiences 'desiring and wanting to have' from an inherent place of unity. This unconscious involvement changes when the ego becomes stronger; gaining ego power goes hand in hand with the instinct to distinguish.

Later in life, we may learn to consciously engage in a world of duality and continuous distinction. The quality of the *san jiao* is our guiding principle in that world.

The earthly branch *Zi,* gallbladder

The earthly branch *Zi*, gallbladder, is in charge of seeds, the concentrated primal force of life. It manages first impulses and impressions, unhindered by acquired visions, ideas and concepts. The uninhibited instincts and responses to stimuli that arise from upbringing, education and the direct environment are extremely important for the development of children and their brains.

The developed adult brain takes control of what is felt or thought and quickly

---

4 *Yuan qi* is the root of all living, the *san jiao* the governor of all *qi*. The *yuan qi* is stored in the kidneys. Some sources state that the *yuan qi* is stored in kidney yang only, others mention *Ming Men* or the space between the kidneys. The *Nan Jing* uses the term *dong qi* or moving *qi*. The similarity between these locations is that *yuan qi* is hidden deep and *san jiao* is its messenger.
5 See the discussion of the earthly branch *Xu* in this chapter.

labels first impressions before they get the chance to actually land. The step of paying attention to the effects that impressions have on the being is often skipped. If impressions are not obstructed by preconceived thought models and biased feelings and thoughts, they are given the opportunity to land and penetrate deeply into someone's being. In the short time before impressions enter the cognitive and emotional mind, inner alignment, understanding and intuitive knowledge come about. That moment is the domain of *Zi*, gallbladder.

The earthly branch *Chou*, liver

The earthly branch *Chou*, liver, is involved in patiently supporting growth. *Chou*, liver, supports learning to find a place, the feeling of being someone who belongs in the world. This developmental phase of the ego is the basis for asking questions. It is the 'why phase' when children of about 2–3 years old come up with questions like 'Why is that a cow?', 'Why is the sky blue?', 'Why do I have to sleep?' This phase remains present but becomes less dominant in later life: 'Where and when do I feel comfortable or uncomfortable?', 'Why do I want to leave?', 'Why do I stay in this relationship?' These kinds of questions are typical of the earthly branch *Chou*, liver.

First impressions are managed by the earthly branch *Zi*, gallbladder, whereas dominance, flexibility, rigidity, shyness, the way people inhabit their space and position in the world – also the clinic room! – are managed by the earthly branch *Chou*, liver.

The earthly branch *Yin*, lung

Communication is controlled by the earthly branch *Yin*, lung. This earthly branch provides the first conscious contact with the external world. During childhood, the 'why phase' develops further due to the conscious experience of the surrounding world. The amount of information received causes an irresistible desire to organize the (overwhelming) world. It passes when the world takes on meaning and its structure and systematizing is better understood. A child finds its place in the world through the earthly branch *Chou*. Through the earthly branch *Yin* it learns to relate to the environment, to create and maintain relationships, to connect through commonality.

The nature of communication and interaction provides a lot of information about the condition of the lung *qi*. Questions like 'How are you?' can be asked out of habit or arise out of real interest. Questions might be defensive, interactive, resentful, empathetic and so on. The way people express themselves in communication shows the nature of the flexibility, openness, strength and expression of the lung *qi*.

THE EGO BECOMES INDEPENDENT

The next four earthly branches and channels establish a field in which object and subject – world and ego – have independent and opposite positions. It is the phase in which children get to know their own autonomy. They feel a boundless curiosity to discover the world.

In general most adults become more independent over time, even if the initial phase was difficult. Inner strength and confidence of the ego grows, because it is partly freed from the influence of the world on which it was initially so dependent. The ego finds its own safe place within a (new) family, friends and work, which are safe havens to share feelings. This safety shows itself through a relaxed and comfortable posture and behaviour.

When the ego feels unsafe, dependent and insecure, people may stretch the body and look overconfident to enforce appreciation and confirmation or, conversely, bow their head and tend to depression, inertia and heaviness. Weakness of the ego shows itself in weakened muscle strength, connective tissue and general posture. This might be caused by severe emotional neglect in childhood. It strongly depends on the resilience of the person involved, exactly how and when that challenging period can be processed and overcome. Finding a quiet solid core in the ego does not just come naturally! Underlying patterns of anxiety are deeply ingrained in the ego, so treatments, given once a month, can take several months or even years before such patterns are resolved. Changes in the ego encounter a lot of internal resistance and only happen slowly. The help of a psychologist is recommended.

Balancing the first four earthly branches in line with the birth chart strengthens the foundation on which people can slowly build their confidence.

The next group of earthly branches, *Mao*, *Chen*, *Si* and *Wu* (large intestine, stomach, spleen and heart), is very different from the first. The second group assesses and investigates the impressions of the outside world and what is accepted after careful and critical evaluation is then broken down into manageable chunks so that the inside can process it.

The ego becomes more personal once a child has learned to say 'I am', at first unconsciously but, as people get older, they consciously learn to organize the outside world through analysis, critical questions, distinguishing, differentiating and the merging impressions and experiences. As a result, the attitude of the ego gradually changes from 'desire and having' to 'wanting to become'. The ego learns to work with its environment from the image of two opposing forces. Through this, the ego finds its own individuality. Children learn to perceive and create the world from a more independent position. The ego inhales the world and exhales itself out into the world.

The earthly branch *Mao,* large intestine

Through the earthly branch *Mao*, large intestine, one gets to know the order of the world and its influences. The meaning and content of communication becomes clearer. The condition of the large intestine is visible in the way people present themselves in clinic. How long does it take before patients give substantive information? How much insight does the patient have into the origin and content of the complaints and symptoms and how is it communicated with you? When was the essence of the problem discussed?

The clarity of the shared content and the strength, weakness or perseverance of communication are diagnostic tools for the condition of the *qi* of the large intestine. The actual content of the communication has no bearing on the nature of the *qi* and therefore the practitioner can only properly assess the *qi* of the large intestine if ideas and potential judgements about the content such as good and bad, correct and incorrect and so on are not transferred.

The earthly branch *Chen,* stomach

The condition of the earthly branch *Chen*, stomach, determines the power and authority of the slowly evolving independent centre of the ego universe.

People with weak stomach *qi* tend to fully transfer the responsibility for recovery to the practitioner: 'Here's my problem, please treat me and heal me.' The weak *qi* may be hidden and compensated for by a big mouth, tough behaviour and an arrogant attitude. The condition is serious if that occurs in someone with *Chen* as birth *qi*. Then recovery is likely to take a long time and may never be complete.

When the stomach *qi* is strong and healthy, people are able to effectively conduct the process of life, which ideally involves processes of self-development and self-examination in order to gain an overview of the role of the ego in family, work and friends. 'What are the reasons that I do the work that I do?' and 'I like to take care of others, but where inside me does that impulse actually come from?' are typical questions of earthly branch *Chen*, stomach. People whose stomach *qi* is in overdrive tend to overcontrol the process of life and dominate others; this easily causes heartburn.

Patients having a healthy stomach *qi* take responsibility for their health and desire to contribute to the healing process. They often ask questions about their behaviour and diet. The implementation of the advice given is managed by the *qi* of the spleen, whereas the ability to reflect and the willingness to take personal responsibility are part of stomach *qi*.

A healthy stomach *qi* means that the mutual vitality of relationships is well nourished and maintained. Generally, with healthy stomach *qi*, there is balance between the needs of the ego and the demands of the surrounding world, although this might only appear to be so on the outside because people born with the earthly branch *Chen* can often have an intense inner emotional life that is not easily shared with others.

The earthly branch *Si,* spleen

Birth is a brutal disturbance of the symbiotic arrangement in the womb. By listening to inner instinctual needs, desires and the necessity for survival are evoked in the newborn being. Desires are first fulfilled by parents and caregivers. The baby wants to eat, sleep, drink or be reassured when it feels uncomfortable. But, in time, humans have to learn to support themselves and this process is initially founded on the same principle of desire.

In the earthly branches discussed so far, desires led to the manifestation of an ego-consciousness that managed to positively establish itself securely more and more in society. The spleen is the manifestation of the desire to root the ego in one's own being and existence. To do this, the ego uses its environment. Impressions, food and drink are transformed and transported in such a way that the ego and the being can digest them and use the positive elements for the preservation, growth and development of the wholeness of the body. The earthly branch *Si*, spleen, manages the care of health and the balance of the inner being. The execution of the process to live a healthy life in accordance with the self and the environment is carried out by the spleen. It must act within the possibilities that exist: what diet is followed, what interest there is, the mental and emotional state, how life is organized and so on. A healthy spleen *qi* can cope well with all conditions encountered. The effects of a weak spleen *qi*, such as malnutrition, that is common today, are often only subtly visible to the eye, but quickly noticeable upon pulse diagnosis.

The earthly branch *Wu,* heart

The cycle of the earthly branches is built around the *Zi–Wu* axis, gallbladder and heart. The first part of the cycle we have discussed so far awakens and supports the ego in its growth and expression.

The second part of the cycle, which begins with the earthly branch *Wu*, may be initiated by a reduced focus on I-ness and increased sense of we-ness, togetherness. The ego changes from a separate to an integrated individuality.

The development of humans and humanity reaches its turning point in the earthly branch *Wu*. It is the crossroads at which the human being chooses either to continue to follow its own needs and desires to enforce happiness and health, or to experience happiness and health through engagement with compassion for others.

Integration through the heart-*shen* is the trademark of togetherness. The heart-*shen* regulates emotions, perceives sensory stimuli and organizes the body, mind and consciousness. Integration is a precondition for real presence, connection and mutual cooperation between the ego, the true self and its environment. Heart-*shen* integration safeguards the connection between people, enabling the sharing of moral values, the connection of thoughts, the unifying of emotions and behaviour, the health of the body ... the list is endless. Without integration an individual becomes chaotic, stagnant, isolated and sick. In short, you could say that integration transforms people into fellow human beings. Learning, listening and receiving are the first steps towards integration, where the ego considers the true content and reciprocity of a relationship more important than ego self-affirmation. Promoting integration creates wholeness and togetherness between egos rather than competition, status and separation. It is important to note that issues of disintegration need to be looked at in the light of all four of these earthly branches (*Mao, Chen, Si* and *Wu*).

THE EGO IS EMANCIPATED, LIBERATED, SELF-CONTAINED AND INSPIRED BY A LIVING DYNAMIC

The discussion of the following earthly branches and channels is the record of my own path and quest. The study of Chinese medicine and philosophies, meditation, self-cultivation and experiencing the beauty of nature and music and other wonders of life turned my passions into compassion. This is the main reason to write this book and share what I have received.

Characteristic of the second group of four earthly branches and channels is the interaction between the external and internal world from independent positions, where the two influence each other. The last group of four earthly branches describes the development of the ego towards we-ness rather than I-ness.

A creative togetherness between the inner and outer world occurs when the ego emancipates itself and can freely move and realize itself as part of a unity. The outside world then changes from external to an integrated wholeness with the ego, which then becomes part of the rhythm of everything and everyone: the realization that we are all one. The verb associated with this stage is 'to be'.

The awareness of 'to be' opens the connection to the shared dynamic life source in the depth of the self. This path directs inward to self-knowledge, life experience and empathetic understanding. In addition to the fact that heaven is an abstraction of the supreme oneness that expresses itself in nature and beings, it is the life-giving source, the spark of life that illuminates the true Self.

I would like to start the discussion of the earthly branches *Wei*, *Shen*, *You* and *Xu* (small intestine, bladder, kidney and heart constrictor) with a meditation rather than transferring knowledge. Meditation begins with and is silence. So ... let's be silent together for ten minutes.

If you are not used to meditation and even if you are, most likely there was no silence but a chicken coop of thoughts and feelings and maybe unrest in the body.

This unrest, if present, originates from the *qi* and *xuè* of the earthly branches *Wei* and *Shen*, small intestine and bladder, the *tai yang* division. It is the most superficial layer of the six divisions and the first line of defence, *wei qi*.

Wei qi enters the body at the time of *Zi*, gallbladder, and exits at the time of the earthly branch *Yin*, lung, at 3 a.m. It then rises to the head where it pours into the *tai yang* division upon awakening, flowing from S.i.-19, *Ting Gong*, listening palace, to S.i.-1, *Shao Ze*, little marsh, and from Bl-1, *Jing Ming*, bright eyes, to Ht-9, *Shao Chong*, lesser surge, to contact and activate the heart-*shen*.

Wei qi awakens and keeps people alert but, as you may have noticed, also causes restlessness when there is a sudden quietness. Being silent more often trains the *wei qi* to be calmer.

Wei qi is not guided by willpower. If the will was in charge of our defence, *wei qi* would likely be always too late to intervene when external pathogenic factors present themselves. Instead the *wei qi* works autonomously and unconsciously. The tricky part of any involuntary, autonomous, unconscious system, however, is that it involves the involuntary emergence of movement, feelings, thoughts and moods, which, when we are silent, automatically take the lead. In addition, the *tai yang* division contains more *xuè* than *qi*, making these channels more sensitive to thoughts and emotions experienced throughout the day.

At night, when the *hun* and *shen* reside in the liver and heart, these thoughts and emotions are digested and purified, but when they are too strong or when the *hun* and *shen* do not rest, restlessness and insomnia arise and the blood remains 'infected' with 'impure' (unprocessed) thoughts and emotions.

It is therefore important to become acquainted with a place within from which careful observation of the involuntary can be observed without the mind being taken along unintentionally.

The earthly branch *Wei*, small intestine

The earthly branch *Wei*, small intestine, is linked to the heart. At first sight this is a peculiar combination, because these organs apparently have nothing to do with each other. The heart-*shen* constitutes the basis of all spiritual actions and considerations and is involved in consciousness, thinking, intuition, memory, emotions and the alternation of waking and sleeping. The small intestine in apparent contrast is mainly involved in digestion. This organ ensures that food is broken down into liquid parts. After food has passed the small intestine and the particles have come into contact with the blood vessels surrounding the small intestine, the food is no longer an object and something from the outside world, but something that now belongs to the subject, the internal world. At the physiological *qi* level, the small intestine is responsible for separating the pure from the impure. It is an organ that seems to separate and distinguish without hesitation and with clear vision and decisiveness. On a mental level, these critical dynamics of the small intestine behave in exactly the same way; our thoughts almost never stand still. There is constant judging and placing of impressions in the invisible drawers of good and bad, useful and useless, agree and disagree, acknowledge and dispute and so on.

With a healthy earthly branch *Wei*, the small intestine makes its decisions in agreement with the orientation of heart-*shen*. It commits to and integrates the pure with mutual alignment.

The heart-*shen* automatically connects to the radiance and vibration of everything and everyone it perceives. The mutual resonance between the heart-*shen* and that which it perceives determines the alignment and thus the flow of *qi*. The mental material mind, also part of both the heart-*shen* and the small intestine, makes choices through thinking and comprehension.

Returning now to our meditation: The restlessness of thoughts, emotions and body during meditation are, as it were, viewed from a distance. It is as if the ego watches someone else's ego. That is actually very strange, because the one ego looking at the other restless ego is the same ego. This is a trick of the mind: It is trapped by the judging abilities of earthly branch *Wei* and bypasses the attunement of the small intestine with the spiritual aspects of the heart-*shen*, which is the alignment with the collective vibration.

The assessment of judging pure and impure, good and bad is actually the pitfall of the earthly branch *Wei*. Ideally instead, the physiological aspects of the small intestine are reflected in the psychological character: non-judgemental and purely acting, not by choices based on time-related thoughts, but by in the moment alignment with the heart-*shen* and by being a mutual part of the process.

Illness due to an imbalance in the last four earthly branches manifests itself when the interaction between the external form and behaviour is no longer aligned with the inner being and the relationship is strongly disturbed. It often stems from too much motivation and drive to prove or achieve something. People try their best to deal with and master the stresses of life, but exhaustion means they don't know where to find the energy to recover. Overly restrained and self-protective behaviour are other possible manifestations of this imbalance.

Treatments in these cases should always start with the earthly branch *Wei*, small intestine, which creates the conditions for insight, attunement and coordination. *Wei* is the natural link from outer appearance and vanity to inner life through simplification and inner strength.

The earthly branch *Shen,* bladder

It is not immediately obvious, but due to its yang character and connection with *wei qi*, the earthly branch *Shen*, bladder, serves renewal. It mobilizes yang to go to yin, to the root of existence in the depth of one's being. It inspires life in oneself for which the earthly branch *Wei* created the conditions. In particular the connection of Bl-1 with the divergent channels[6] of heart and small intestine (fire), spleen and stomach (earth) and bladder and kidneys (water) and the connection with the *luo* channels of heart (fire), stomach (earth) and bladder (water) offer the possibility of assimilation of *qi* and *xuè* within the vertical axis fire–earth–water or heaven–earth–humanity. It is the inner lifeblood, the *qi* that represents the expression of the human response to the Universal Spark of life.

LETTING GO

I have treated so many people who could no longer cope with the pressures and demands of society – apparently you attract what you have to learn yourself. The required change to a different way of life is accompanied by the release of adjustments to the demands of society. Only then can the being come into contact with authenticity and heal the connection between self and ego. Letting go seems so difficult, until you realize that letting go is actually letting go of suffering. The suffering of the ego polishes and shapes the self.

The (often sudden) choice to let go and turn to another direction of life is made in the depth of one's being. Afterwards, I have heard patients say that, though the misery of suffering had been annoying and frustrating, they would

---

6　Historically, the idea of divergent channels seems to be older than the eight extra channels, although they meet in their relation to the source of all *qi* that is hidden deep and described as constitutional.

not have missed this opportunity. In the future, they will listen to themselves faster and better because they now feel more attuned to themselves.

Bl-67 activates this process of renewal. It can change someone, new life goals can be set, but it is all about the right timing...

No doubt it is clear that many patients don't experience these psychological problems consciously. People come to the clinic with trigeminal neuralgia (stomach), a herniated disc with pins and needles in the legs (gallbladder and bladder) or other diseases such as infertility or chronic bowel disease, but not so often with problems of the ego, difficulties with making friends or feeling stagnated in a midlife crisis. Yet, psychological health problems often cause physical problems that can be a result of stubbornly clinging to what should actually be released, the theme of the earthly branch *Shen*, bladder.

The earthly branch *You*, kidneys

We have arrived at the source of life, the essence of existence and the ultimate expression of we-ness.

We are all conceived from the genetic material of our parents, who were conceived from the genetic material of their parents and so on. It means that we stand on the shoulders of all who have been before, which is the actual meaning of the pre-natal, deeply hidden hereditary *qi* in everyone's being, *jing qi* and *yuan qi*.

The *jing qi* is divided into two parts: The pre-natal *jing qi* comes from the *jing qi* of both parents. It stores the memory of the true self and the mandate of heaven. This *jing qi* is the most physical, dense aspect of the body and provides the material for creating a new life. The post-natal *jing qi* stores the memory of a person's own life experiences, nourishes the body, controls growth, is involved in reproduction and further development throughout life. The post-natal *jing qi* is derived from the digestive and respiratory system.

The *yuan qi* precedes everything that is and is also passed on to children. It is the dynamic source of life, the basis of hereditary vitality, always available during life and facilitates all transformations in the body. The survival and evolution of humans and humanity is determined by the quality of the *yuan qi*.

The *san jiao* is the activator of the *yuan qi* and the messenger that transfers *yuan qi* to all different parts of the body. It is the power of unity that is spread in all parts of the being, a perfect metaphor of a collective unity shared in diversity.

This cohesion is the beauty but also the pitfall of the earthly branch *You*, kidneys. Sometimes people can only develop self-knowledge through cohesion with society and going out and therefore do not pay so much attention to authenticity. That is not to say that going out cannot be authentic, self-knowledge is indeed founded in relationships. The root of an emancipated, liberated, self-contained ego lies in the dynamics of the *yuan qi* and the memory of the true self found in the pre-natal *jing qi*, the inspiration of the living dynamic source. It is comparable with the many different branches of a large tree experiencing commonality in the root system that nourishes them all. The true wisdom of humanity lies in the togetherness of what we share.

And so back to our meditation; if we are able to turn the attitude of having and becoming into being, to stop pursuing goals, to live without predetermined blueprints, even of meditation, a consciousness can arise that brings natural order to the abundance of our impressions.

A teacher once told me: 'Meditation is about the silence that is found by silence in the mind, but is not experienced as silence, because then there is no more silence.'

Life is the revelation of love that resides in the depths of the dynamic ancestral *qi* as a potential and is realized and expressed by the heart-*shen*. The origin and carrier of the warmth and vibrancy of the heart-*shen* lies in the original fire of the *yuan qi* and pre-natal *jing qi*. This can be a blessing and a reassurance, because everything that is observed, learned, rejected, everything that is felt, done, spoken and thought, is in accordance with the transgenerational inner values of humanity and implies a testimony to the wholeness of existence.

The source from which we are nourished has its roots in the communality of heaven, which is visible for human beings not only as the sky or nature, but in the authenticity of our being.

The earthly branch *Xu*, heart constrictor

Henri Borel, writer, journalist, interpreter of the Chinese language and sinologist, lived from 1869 to 1933. About his work *Wu Wei* (1911), which is included in his larger work *Wisdom and Beauty from China* (1919), he said: 'It is my favourite work to the extent that I wouldn't care if all my other publications were burned, provided *Wu Wei* was preserved.' I completely agree with him. This book is a jewel of my library and would definitely be one of the books I would like to take to a desert island.

When my writing arrived at the earthly branch *Xu*, heart constrictor, I knew I needed to describe the beauty and wonder of Love and I hesitated. While theoretical aspects of *Xu* in relation to the evolution of the ego and Love are known to me, the subject continues to remain a source of inspiration. The process of practical implementation of Love in everyday life has inexhaustible resources and possibilities. The veils are thinning, making me a servant and apprentice of the reality of Love. In my hesitation, I picked up the book and read the following beautiful short story again. It is dear to me. I ask you to accept these words of Henri Borel as a gift of Love.

'Love is no other than the rhythm of Tao. I have told you: You are come out of Tao and to Tao you will return. Whilst you are young – with your soul still enveloped in darkness – in the shock of the first impulse within you, you know not yet whither you are trending. You see the woman before you. You believe her to be that towards which the rhythm is driving you. But even when the woman is yours, and you have thrilled at the touch of her, you feel the rhythm yet within you, unappeased, and know that you must forward, ever further, if you would bring it to a standstill. Then it is that in the soul of the man and of the woman there arises a great sadness and a look at one another, questioning whither they are now bound. Gently they clasp one another by the hand and move on through life, swayed by the same impulse, towards the same goal. Call this love if you will. What is a name? I call it Tao. And the souls of those who love are like two white clouds floating softly side by side, that vanish, wafted by the same wind, into the infinite blue of the heavens.'

'But that is not the love that I mean!' I cried. 'Love is not the desire to see the loved one absorbed into Tao; love is the longing to be always with her; to deep yearning for the blending of two souls in the one; the hot desire to soar, in one breath with her, into felicity! And this always with the loved one alone – not with others, not with Nature. And where I absorbed into Tao, all his happiness would be forever lost! Oh let me stay here, in this goodly world, with my faithful companion! Here it is so bright and homely, and Tao is still so gloomy and inscrutable for me.'

'The hot desire dies out,' he answered calmly. 'The body of your loved one will wither and pass away within the cold earth. The leaves of the trees fade in autumn, and the withered flowers droop sadly to the ground. How can you love that so much which does not last? However, you know, in truth, as yet, neither how you love nor what it is that you love. The beauty of a woman is but a vague reflection of the formless beauty of Tao. The emotion it awakens, the longing to lose yourself in her beauty, that ecstasy of feeling which would lend wings for the flight of your soul with the beloved – beyond horizon-bounds, into regions of bliss – believe me, it is no other than the rhythm of Tao; only you know it not. You resemble still the river which knows as yet only its shimmering banks; which has no knowledge of the power that draws it forward; but which will one day inevitably flow out into the great ocean.

A poet looks upon a woman, and, swayed by the "rhythm", he perceives the beauty of the beloved in all things – in the trees, the mountains, the horizon; for the beauty of a woman is the same as that of Nature. It is the form of Tao, the great and formless, and what your soul desires in the excitement of beholding – this strange, unspeakable feeling – is nothing, but your oneness with this beauty, and with the source of this beauty – Tao. And the like is experienced by your wife. Ye are for each other angels, who lead one another to Tao unconsciously.

When you are absorbed into Tao, then only will you be complete, eternally united with the soul of your beloved, with the souls of all men, your brothers, and with the soul of Nature. And the few moments of blessedness fleetingly enjoyed by all lovers upon earth are as nothing in comparison with that endless bliss: the blending of the souls of all who love in an eternity of perfect purity.'

The *Ho t'u*

The *Ho t'u*, the Yellow River map,[1] is a mystical arrangement and symbol that hides the expressions of heaven and the four emanations in the form of numbers and directions. The beauty of symbols lies in their multi-interpretable meaning, which may lead to a better understanding of how the nameless expresses itself in the named, such as the four emanations, the *wuxing*, the heavenly stems, the seasons, the trigrams and hexagrams and the earthly branches. This map has kept me busy for over forty years and continues to do so. Unfortunately the topic is too extensive to discuss in detail here, but I would like to make a few comments to invite the interested reader to further study this topic.

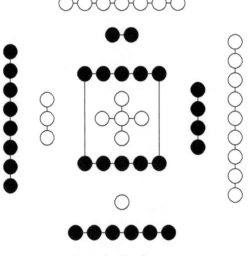

Figure I.1 Ho t'u map
Heaven, yang, odd numbers, white.
Earth, yin, even numbers, black.

---

1   There is a story that the legendary emperor Fu Xi received the *Ho t'u* via a mythical dragon horse from the Yellow River. The first trigrams that are the basis of the *Yijing* would have arisen from the *Ho t'u*.

At the heart of the map is a yang point with four other yang points in the North, South, East and West that surround the centre point and are connected to it. They might symbolize the four emanations that emanate from the heavenly origin. These five life forces animate and transform all that exists. The centre point is the earthly reflection of the heavenly oneness in humans. It represents the central heart that enters life of all that exists. After all, it's always about what people intend from their hearts.

Just as waves in the water expand in a circle from a point where a stone is thrown into the water, the central consciousness expands. To the North, on the larger circle of a denser plane of existence, is another yang point. It is the original potential force into which everything has withdrawn into a seed. It is the original manifested source, the power of authenticity that is within everyone.

At the same time the numbers two and three are created in the South and East. Along with duality in the South, yin and yang, up and down, within and without, the three emerges. Three is the intermediate consciousness that connects the dual powers of number two. The potential and probabilities of the 10,000 things of the North are being realized through the central intermediate factor in the East. It is *qi* that manifests and brings forth a new world that houses consciousness precisely because of the limitation of dualities. The rising sun symbolizes the vitality of the movements and possibilities of *qi*, with which the idea of time is perceived.

The yin number four in the West receives time in its space and divides it into segments such as the four seasons, the four quarters of the day and hours, and so on.

A denser plane of existence is accomplished by the interaction between the initial numbers[2] and the central life-giving forces of the number five. The one in the North gives rise to the yin number six which houses the six *qi* by which all living forms are animated and organized. It enables the twelve channels[3] that interact between the flow of *qi* from heaven and the receiving qualities of the earth. The latent power of duality, hidden in the yin number two in the South, is accomplished by the yang number seven, which represents the completeness of the manifestation. The North and South are the two extreme forms of revelation. The withdrawn life in the North is in full bloom in the South. Their partnership is observable in the sky as the North Pole Star and the Big Dipper's seven stars.[4] The North Pole Star is the place of the heavenly emperor, the Big

---

2 The numbers one through five are called initial numbers, the numbers six through ten are called the accomplished numbers.
3 It is the hidden start of the flow of the twelve earthly branches and twelve main channels.
4 The North Pole Star (Polaris, Alpha Ursae Minoris) can be found by extending the distance of the last two stars, Dubhe and Merak (α Ursae Majoris and β Ursae Majoris), of the Big Dipper (Ursa Major) six times until a reasonably bright star is found.

Dipper, his chariot. The handle of the Big Dipper is a pointer of a clock that points to the compass point of the current season. It points East in spring, South in summer and so on. It shows the completeness of the possibilities of life and expresses the vitality of all the possibilities hidden in the North.

The culmination of the manifestation of forms opens the way inward, back to the origin of life. The expected turnaround, the centripetal movement, accentuates the number seven associated with the seven senses and seven emotions.

The yang number three in the East is accomplished in the yin number eight which stands for differentiation and integration. Eight divides and organizes the different divisions to collaborate.

The boundaries indicated by the number three are further ordered by the number eight. We see this for example in the eight compass points, the eight trigrams, the eight extra channels, the eight winds.

The yin number four in the West is accomplished in the yang number nine. The space of the number four is divided into three sections heaven–earth–human, each section of which is also divided into three parts. Nine shows the achieved wholeness of human development. This condition implies standstill and termination. So, nine is the number of major changes that become possible after reaching an end, a goal, a life and so forth.

The yin number ten is placed in the centre of the diagram. It accomplishes the number five and thus encompasses all other realizations of numbers and represents all distinguishable qualities of heaven on earth. The five emanations reveal themselves in five forces above and five forces below. This image corresponds to the five heavens in the sky and the ten great movements and ten heavenly stems, five of which are yang and five yin. They describe the movements and developments on earth.

Trigrams and Hexagrams

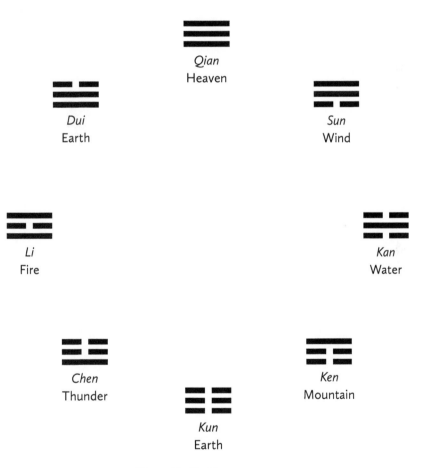

Figure II.1 Fu Xi arrangement

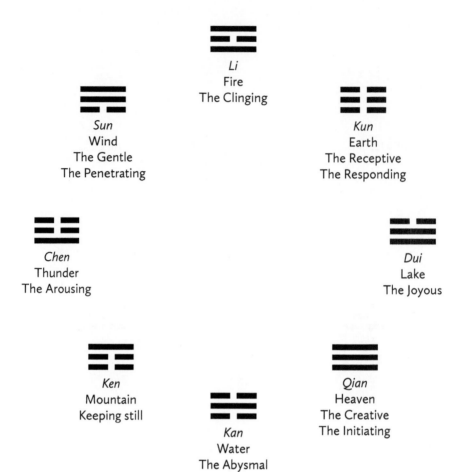

Figure II.2 King Wen arrangement

Table 11.1 Trigrams, *Fu Xi* arrangement and heavenly stems

| Trigrams | Trigrams and Heavenly Stems | | Heavenly Stems |
	Arrangement of *Fu Xi*		
▤ *Qian* Heaven	• The creative, initiative powers • Power of light • Yang, positive, Heaven • Formless • *Qian* relates to success and to spirituality • Strong in its enclosed unity	甲 *Jia* Gb Yang of wood	• First manifestation of the vital spark of life on Earth • Life meets form • Heavenly, intuitive inspiration • Idea, first impulse
▤ *Kun* Earth	• The receiving and the responding • Dark, yin, negative, Earth • Principle of matter and form • Strong in its enclosed unity	乙 *Yi* Liv Yin of wood	• Transformation and growth of form guided and supported by the vital spark • Growth and protection • Guidance of heavenly *qi* • Inner knowledge

▤
Ken
Mountain
	• In its positive aspect *Ken* relates to silence, meditation
	  and prayer
	• Calmness in body and mind necessary for concentration
	• In its negative aspect *Ken* nourishes egoism and
	  egocentricity
		丙
		Bing
		S.i.
		
		Yang of
		fire
			• Limitation of vitality through form gives a sense of
			  separation; start of duality, digestion and understanding
			• Thought and insight into heavenly source of life
			• Understanding the heavenly *qi*. Insight

▤
Dui
Lake
	• A mirror in which Heaven can reflect itself
	• *Dui* spreads spiritual energy on Earth
	• *Dui* represents the giving powers of energy and
	  intelligence from *Qian*
	• The holding of a religious belief
		丁
		Ding
		Ht
		
		Yin of
		fire
			• Awareness and consciousness through relationship to
			  others and the self are possible now
			• Ability to go deep and find meaning and reach out to life
			  with love and compassion
			• Desire to connect to the light that supports us all
			• Benevolence
			• New life becoming fully grown, limitless inspiration

cont.

Trigrams and Heavenly Stems

Trigrams	Arrangement of *Fu Xi*		Heavenly Stems
䷁ *Kan* Water	• Coldness • *Kan* represents matter and the body's powers • *Kan*, Water, is seen as the manifestation of 'lower' aspects • Form on Earth	戊 *Wu* St Yang of earth	• Oneness of Heaven on Earth, life-giving source that creates and supports life and all forms postnatally • Centre within that reflects the qualities of *Qian*, Heaven • Stable, firm and harmonious • Formation and limitation; transformation of the heavenly *qi* = unlimited love
䷝ *Li* Fire	• Heat • *Li*, Fire, is seen as the manifestation of 'higher' aspects • Spirit on Earth • Life	己 *Ji* Sp Yin of earth	• Individual form is completely vitalized and inspired by the spark of life • With acceptance and integrity, awareness of distinction between ego and its environment, individual and universal self is possible • Process of individualization and individuation, emancipation and self-realization starts here • Reliability • Completion of the form; centralization
䷲ *Chen* Thunder	• *Chen* accelerates *qi* • *Chen* represents the birth of the 10,000 beings • *Chen* expresses itself in all growing things • *Chen* strives towards the light with its roots in the Earth	庚 *Geng* L.i. Yang of metal	• Power to protect internal and external life; to gather fluids and what is essential for continuation and nourishment of the source of life and to let go of what is not • Instinctive abilities, clarity, focus and introspection guided by compassion and righteousness aid the process of purification, inner development and cultivation of the self • Making the world a better place by clarity, strength, 'fight', righteousness and cutting off

Trigram	Attributes	Stem / Element	Qualities
☴ *Sun* Wind	• *Sun* represents air (breath) • *Sun* vitalizes breath of the spirit, the renewal of life. The link between the spirit and the body (Heaven and Earth) • Receptiveness for the quality of feelings that open themselves to all living forms on Earth	辛 *Xin* Lu Yin of metal	• Strength to protect and order the source of life and synchronize all life processes accordingly • To generate inner transformation that will illumine the *shen* • Withdrawal and silence • Acceptance of what there is • Being awake in silence
☰ *Qian* Heaven	• The creative, initiative powers • Power of light • Yang, positive, Heaven • Formless • *Qian* relates to success and to spirituality • Strong in its enclosed unity	壬 *Ren* BI Yang of water	• Internalization and attunement, being sensitive to the unfolding and expression of life from the hidden source of authenticity and accepting and surrendering to its course • Inner strength and stability to meet the challenges of life and integrate experiences • Openness, vulnerability, acceptance and silence • Time to receive the heavenly *qi* for personal creation. Life is hidden deep inside
☷ *Kun* Earth	• The receiving and the responding • Dark, yin, negative, Earth • Principle of matter and form • Strong in its enclosed unity	癸 *Gui* Ki Yin of water	• By attuning to the vital spark within, the inner source of heavenly *qi*, one can sacrifice personal gain and will. This can lead to a true connection and devotion to life and humanity • Being in harmony and balance • Responsible on all levels of the being after transformation and receiving all information • Expression of heavenly *qi* in humans and humanity

Table 11.2 Trigrams, King *Wen* arrangement

Trigram	Attributes	Expression	Cycle of Life	Development of Consciousness	Body Area and Function
☳ *Chen* Thunder The Arousing L.i.	• Beginning of the King *Wen* arrangement • The East, direction of sunrise • Wood and early spring • 6:00 • Eldest son • Burst of growth • Activity and movement • *Chen* relates to swiftness	• Things that are new • Emotions and excitement • Expansion • Setting in motion • The release from tension after its build-up and growing from it (attachment, growth and letting go)	• At birth, we are full of excitement and new beginnings	• Subject: we start to recognize the self	• Feet • Mobility
☴ *Sun* Wind The Gentle/ The Penetrating Lu	• The Southeast • Wood and late spring • 9:00 • Eldest daughter • *Sun* relates to flexibility and adaptability	• *Sun* makes things flow into their natural form • *Sun* relates to a gentle, warm wind that opens the blossoms and establishes firm growth • *Sun* describes the nourishment of form and the perception of form • The lungs give rise to *qi*, which in turn gives rise to form	• Coming into your own; ripening and maturing	• Object: we start to recognize the non-self, the objective, the world	• Thighs • Receptivity

Li Fire The Clinging Sp	• The South • Fire and summer • 12:00 • Middle daughter • Fire, light • Intelligence, intuition, devotion, clarity	• The high sun of summer: everything has grown into its form and the light of the long days makes everything visible • Fire needs something to attach and cling to in order to be able to express itself • The quality of the *shen* is only visible through substance	• We can see and be seen • Visuality: the mechanism by which the eyes make something visible; the process of becoming visible	• Self-consciousness • We start to act on intuition (the power of fire)	• Eyes • Visibility
Kun Earth The Receptive/ The Responding Liv/Ki *Ren Mai*	• The Southwest • Earth and late summer • 15:00 • Mother • Inactive, yielding, passive, receptive and responsive • Female • Receiving the powers of light and heat and responding by nourishing all • *Kun* is responsive and does things by the simplest route	• *Kun* relates to *xuè* • *Kun* relates to the forming of seeds. Seeds symbolize the most concentrated potential and nourishment of (plant) forms	• We take responsibility for what we have gathered to be able to contribute to Life • Devotion to Life • Fellowship • Service	• We-consciousness • Awareness and understanding of unity and compassion • Human contribution to Heaven	• Abdomen • Digestion

cont.

Trigram	Attributes	Expression	Cycle of Life	Development of Consciousness	Body Area and Function
☱ *Dui* Lake The Joyous Ht/Hc	• The West • Metal and early autumn • 18:00 • Youngest daughter • *Dui* symbolizes strength within and gentleness without • Joy of the harvest • *Dui* means to receive the harvest with humility • Satisfaction	• A time of peace, joy, silence and contemplation • A time to review gains and what has been reaped	• Joy is an important quality of life • Contentment • Serenity • Inner smile	• We realize that happiness and joy lie within	• Mouth and tongue • Nourishment
☰ *Qian* Heaven The Creative The Initiating Gb/Bl *Du Mai*	• The Northwest • Metal and late autumn • 21:00 • Father • Active, strong, firm, creative • Male • *Qian* initiates • *Qian* produces the invisible seeds of all development	• In autumn, all material existence seems to die and nothing but the seeds of Life remain • Struggle to let go, finding the potential in the hindrance • Process of regeneration and birth	• A time of struggle and endeavour • One has to learn to let go, only taking in what is really needed for the continuation of Life and for the self • If a person is stuck and in despair, there is an opportunity to find the invisible seed of creativity which can open a new door	• We experience introspection, self-questioning and self-validation • Self-awareness is important for the development of consciousness	• Head • Awareness

䷜ **Kan** Water The Abysmal St	• The North, direction of the source of Life • Water and winter • 0:00 • Middle son • The will to survive • Yang is deep inside the yin (protected by the cold of winter) • Within the darkness is the light of yang	• Relationship with springs of water, flowing streams as well as hidden, deep-seated emotions • *Kan* represents effort and exertion • Fight for survival at the deepest level	• The time when we start to contact the subconscious • A time that asks for perseverance, endurance, effort and determination • These times cannot be avoided, denied or lived without	• We come into contact with our innermost being (the vertical axis) • *Li*, fire, intuition versus *Kan*, water, the subconscious/shadow side	• Ears • Space
䷚ **Ken** Mountain Keeping still S.i./Sj	• Hidden beginning of King *Wen* cycle • The Northeast • Earth and late winter • Eldest son • Late in winter, before the beginning of spring, there is a clear and bright stillness; cold and unmoving to end the year's cycle • *Ken* holds the potential for movement • The porch through which energy moves out (in springtime)	• The hidden meeting of yin and yang before manifestation • Opening of gates or doors • Time for silence and standing still, allowing space for movement	• Silence and peace • Acceptance and completion	• *Ken* allows transition and change	• Hands and fingers • Trust and forgiveness

Table II.3 Hexagrams and earthly branches

	24. Fu **Return/Renewal** Change spontaneously, at the appropriate time	子 *Zi* Gb	• *Zi* receives the seed to regenerate and renew life • The *qi* is still hidden and in harmony with Heaven: not conscious yet • Time to be assertive, decisive, determined and compassionate with good judgement • Virtue: Self-assertion
	19. Lin **Approaching** Acting in the right way	丑 *Chou* Liv	• *Chou* represents a centre from which it supports the growth of the seed: It is aware of the possibilities for growth and change while remaining firmly rooted • A bridge of encounter between the nourishing *qi* of Earth below and the vitalizing *qi* of Heaven above • Virtue: Flexible power
	11. Tai **Advance/Peace** In harmony with the laws of nature Act according to the central path	寅 *Yin* Lu	• Meeting the world: Any kind of encounter and communication is an expression of the *qi* of the earthly branch *Yin* • Life is being awakened and follows the rhythm of Heaven based on a firm structure, freedom and vitality • Virtue: Peace
	34. Da Zhuang **Great Strength** Inner strength	卯 *Mao* L.i.	• *Mao* pushes the *qi* forward and upwards • *Mao* represents the strength that comes from knowing your essence within through emotions and feelings and from there to experience the world without • Letting go and moving forward • Virtue: Courage
	43. Guai **Eliminating** Rely on courage and resourcefulness No force but tolerance	宸 *Chen* St	• Life is ever-moving and ever-changing; we have a past from whence we came and a future we move towards • *Chen* represents the stillpoint, the centre that is aware of it all, giving us the opportunity to come into contact with the source of Life, vitality and change that lies within • Virtue: Stability

▬▬▬▬▬▬	*1. Qian* **Initiating** Understanding the nature of change The Dao of heaven – the Dao of human. Maintaining balance	巳 *Si* Sp	• After connecting with the source of Life and vitality within, we can recognize and re-connect with source of life without • We can organize and align our internal life with the order and virtue of Heaven • Form has reached its peak and it's important to turn our awareness inwards: meditation through self-contemplation • Virtue: Positivity
▬▬▬▬▬	*44. Gou* **Encountering** Act without tolerance but no fight Careful	午 *Wu* Ht	• We can connect with and serve Life, humanity and the world with true compassion and love • Life begins to turn inwards and the journey to understand the self begins • Virtue: Love
▬▬▬▬	*33. Dun* **Retreat** Walking the central path Central and obedient	未 *Wei* S.i.	• *Wei* connects to the depth of our being to understand our essence and the essence of our experiences • *Wei* represents a centre in the depth of our being in which everything comes together to unite, fertilize and transform • Awareness of the present moment • Formation of new seeds and true nourishment is possible through *Wei* • Virtue: Perseverance
▬▬▬	*12. Pi* **Hindrance** Restrain, no attachment Acceptance	申 *Shen* Bl	• *Shen* represents silence, peace and hidden strength necessary for the new Life to appear in spring • *Shen* represents the heavenly, intuitive inspiration in humans and our responsibility of responding from a sense of unity and compassion • Inner awareness to realize the light that shines deep within and throughout all that exists • Virtue: Humour
▬▬	*20. Guan* **Watching** Careful attention, alertness Watching one's self and reactions of others	酉 *You* Ki	• The realization that we all contribute to the light of life, humanity and the universe gives humans the responsibility to preserve the essence and the seed of life within • Through contemplation and allowing to be, new potential and creativity/yang concentrates hidden deeply within the yin, ready to express itself when the time is right • Virtue: Responsibility

cont.

	23. Bo **Falling away** Act in accordance with the situation Keeping still	戌 *Xu* Hc	• *Xu* acts as intermediate between the self and the world and has difficult choices to make, and whichever choices we make, there are those we don't make: We have to choose wisely as our choices affect everything else • *Xu* represents the centre that unites with love and makes true inner transformations and new directions possible through unconditional loyalty to the continuation of Life and self and by letting go of behavioural patterns, attachments, identifications and desires • Virtue: Freedom
	2. Kun **Responding** Submission and responding Flexibility, devotion, humility, gentleness Straight and square, upright	亥 *Hai* Sj	• *Hai* represents the merging and unification of Heaven and Earth, yin and yang. A space that both generates and accepts change and thus allows Life to take its course • *Hai* represents unity and harmony: The light of Heaven shines and infuses everything and the Earth receives and responds in the appropriate way • *Hai* allows for conception and physical and spiritual awakening • Virtue: Humility

References

Bertschinger, R. (1991). *The Golden Needle and Other Odes of Traditional Acupuncture.* New York: Churchill Livingstone.

Bing, W., Wu, N. L. and Wu, A. Q. (1997). *Yellow Emperor's Canon Internal Medicine.* China Science and Technology Press.

Borel, H. (1911). *Wu Wei: A Phantasy Based on the Philosophy of Lao-Tse.* Authorized version by M.E. Reynolds. London: Theosophical Publishing House.

Borel, H. (1919). *Wijsheid en schoonheid uit China.* Amsterdam: Van Kampen.

Borel, H. (1931). *De Chineesche filosofie, toegelicht voor niet-sinologen: III Meng TSZ (Mencius).* Amsterdam: Van Kampen.

Campbell, J. and Moyers, B. (2011). *The Power of Myth.* New York: Anchor.

Ellis, A., Wiseman, N. and Boss, K. (1989). *Grasping the Wind.* Boulder, CO: Paradigm.

Fisch, G. (1973). The triple-burner and its significance in energy pathogenics. *The American Journal of Chinese Medicine 1*, 1, pp. 99–104. Available at https://doi.org/10.1142/S0192415X73000097.

Giesen, P. (2019). Analyse Geluk onder jongeren. *De Volkskrant*, 28 December.

Huang, T. M. A. (1998). *The Complete I Ching: The Definitive Translation by Taoist Master Alfred Huang.* Rochester, VT: Inner Traditions.

Jung, C. G. (1968). *Alchemical Studies*, Collected Works vol. 13. Princeton, NJ: Princeton University Press.

Kluwer, P. S. (1995). *Daodejing (Tau teh tsjing).* Deventer: Ankh Hermes, Uitgeverij.

Larre, C. and de La Vallée, É. R. (2004). *The Heart: In Ling Shu Chapter 8.* London: Monkey Press.

Lee, C. B. (1982). *System of a New Philosophy by the Dualistic Monism.* Seoul: Korea Academic Institute of A new philosophy.

Lu, H. C. (1990). *A Complete Translation of Yellow Emperor's Classics of Internal Medicine (Nei-jing and Nan-jing).* Vancouver: Academy of Oriental Heritage.

Matsumoto, K. and Birch, S. (1986). *Extraordinary Vessels.* Boulder, CO: Paradigm.

Merton, T. (1965). *The Way of Chuang Tzu.* Boulder, CO: Shambhala Publications.

Ming, L. (2016). *Observing. Wuwei: The Heart of the Daodejing.* Translation and Commentary by Liu Ming. California: Da Yuan Circle.

Ortiz, A., et al. (2021). Chronic kidney disease is a key risk factor for severe COVID-19: a call to action by the ERA-EDTA. *Nephrol Dial Transplant 36, 1*, pp. 87–94.

Shou-Zhong, Y. trans. (1997). *The Pulse Classic: Translation of the Mai Jing by Wang Shuhe.* Boulder, CO: Blue Poppy Press.

Twain, M. (1972). *Mark Twain's Fables of Man*, vol. 7. Ed. J. S. Tuckey. Los Angeles: University of California Press.

Unschuld, P. U. (1986). *Nan-ching the Classic of Difficult Issues*, vol. 18. Los Angeles: University of California Press.

van der Leeuw, K. (2008). *Mencius: Inleiding, vertaling en commentaar.* Budel: Uitgeverij DAMON.

Wu, J. C. H. (1989). *Lao Tzu/Tao Teh Ching.* Boulder, CO: Shambhala Publications.

Wu, J. N. (1991). *Yi Jing.* Honolulu: Taoist Center/University of Hawaii Press.

Wu, J. N. (1993). *Ling Shu: or the Spiritual Pivot.* Honolulu: University of Hawaii Press.